Pediatric Maxillofacial Surgery

Guest Editors

BRUCE B. HORSWELL, MD, DDS, MS
MICHAEL S. JASKOLKA, MD, DDS

ORAL AND MAXILLOFACIAL SURGERY CLINICS OF NORTH AMERICA

www.oralmaxsurgery.theclinics.com

Consulting Editor
RICHARD H. HAUG, DDS

August 2012 • Volume 24 • Number 3

SAUNDERS an imprint of ELSEVIER, Inc.

W.B. SAUNDERS COMPANY
A Division of Elsevier Inc.

1600 John F. Kennedy Blvd. • Suite 1800 • Philadelphia, PA 19103-2899

www.oralmaxsurgery.theclinics.com

ORAL AND MAXILLOFACIAL SURGERY CLINICS OF NORTH AMERICA Volume 24, Number 3
August 2012 ISSN 1042-3699, ISBN-13: 978-1-4557-4962-1

Editor: John Vassallo; j.vassallo@elsevier.com
Developmental Editor: Teia Stone

Oral and Maxillofacial Surgery Clinics of North America (ISSN 1042-3699) is published quarterly by Elsevier Inc., 360 Park Avenue South, New York, NY 10010-1710. Months of issue are February, May, August, and November. Business and Editorial Offices: 1600 John F. Kennedy Blvd., Suite 1800, Philadelphia, PA 19103-2899. Periodicals postage paid at New York, NY and additional mailing offices. Subscription prices are $355.00 per year for US individuals, $522.00 per year for US institutions, $159.00 per year for US students and residents, $414.00 per year for Canadian individuals, $621.00 per year for Canadian institutions, $476.00 per year for international individuals, $621.00 per year for international institutions and $216.00 per year for Canadian and foreign students/residents. To receive student/resident rate, orders must be accompanied by name or affiliated institution, date of term, and the *signature* of program/residency coordinator on institution letterhead. Orders will be billed at individual rate until proof of status is received. Foreign air speed delivery is included in all *Clinics* subscription prices. All prices are subject to change without notice. **POSTMASTER:** Send address changes to *Oral and Maxillofacial Surgery Clinics of North America,* Elsevier Periodicals Customer Service, 11830 Westline Industrial Drive, St. Louis, MO 63146. Tel: 1-800-654-2452 (U.S. and Canada); 314-447-8871 (outside U.S. and Canada). Fax: 314-447-8029. E-mail: journalscustomerservice-usa@elsevier.com (for print support); journalsonlinesupport-usa@elsevier.com (for online support).

Reprints. For copies of 100 or more, of articles in this publication, please contact the Commercial Reprints Department, Elsevier Inc., 360 Park Avenue South, New York, NY 10010-1710. Tel.: 212-633-3812; Fax: 212-462-1935; Email: reprints@elsevier.com.

Oral and Maxillofacial Surgery Clinics of North America is covered in *MEDLINE/PubMed (Index Medicus), Science Citation Index Expanded (SciSearch®), Journal Citation Reports/Science Edition,* and *Current Contents®/Clinical Medicine.*

Printed and bound by CPI Group (UK) Ltd, Croydon, CR0 4YY

Transferred to Digital Print 2012

Contributors

CONSULTING EDITOR

RICHARD H. HAUG, DDS
Carolinas Center for Oral Health,
Charlotte, North Carolina

GUEST EDITORS

BRUCE B. HORSWELL, MD, DDS, MS, FACS
Director, First Appalachian Craniofacial
Deformity Specialists, Charleston Area Medical
Center-Women and Children's Hospital;
Clinical Assistant Professor, Department of
Surgery, West Virginia University-Charleston
Division, Charleston, West Virginia

MICHAEL S. JASKOLKA, MD, DDS
First Appalachian Craniofacial Deformity
Specialists, Charleston Area Medical
Center-Women and Children's Hospital;
Department of Surgery, West Virginia
University-Charleston Division, Charleston,
West Virginia; Adjunct Clinical Instructor,
Department of Oral and Maxillofacial Surgery,
University of North Carolina, Chapel Hill,
North Carolina

AUTHORS

SHELLY ABRAMOWICZ, DMD, MPH
Instructor, Department of Oral and
Maxillofacial Surgery, Harvard School of Dental
Medicine; Attending Surgeon, Department of
Plastic and Oral Surgery, Children's Hospital
Boston, Boston, Massachusetts

MICHAEL S. BEASLEY, MD
Private Practice of Otolaryngology, Eye and
Ear Clinic Physicians, Charleston, West Virginia

JOLI C. CHOU, DMD, MD, FRCD(C)
Assistant Professor, Department of Oral and
Maxillofacial Surgery and Pharmacology,
University of Pennsylvania School of Dental
Medicine, Philadelphia, Pennsylvania

BERNARD J. COSTELLO, DMD, MD, FACS
Chief, Division of Craniofacial and Cleft
Surgery; Professor and Program Director,
Department of Oral and Maxillofacial Surgery,
University of Pittsburgh School of Dental
Medicine; Chief, Pediatric Oral and
Maxillofacial Surgery, Children's Hospital of
Pittsburgh, Pittsburgh, Pennsylvania

AMELIA F. DRAKE, MD
Newton D. Fischer Distinguished Professor
of Otolaryngology/Head and Neck Surgery,
Department of Otolaryngology/Head and
Neck Surgery, University of North Carolina,
Chapel Hill, North Carolina

MICHAEL R. GOINS, MD
Assistant Clinical Professor of Otolaryngology,
West Virginia University-Charleston Division;
Ear, Nose and Throat Associates of
Charleston, Charleston, West Virginia

BRENT A. GOLDEN, DDS, MD
Assistant Professor, Department of Oral and
Maxillofacial Surgery; Adjunct Professor,
Department of Pediatrics, University of
North Carolina at Chapel Hill, Chapel Hill,
North Carolina

NICHOLAS J.V. HOGG, MD, DDS
Private Practice, London, Ontario, Canada

LARRY H. HOLLIER Jr, MD
Professor and Residency Program Director,
Division of Plastic Surgery, Baylor College of
Medicine, Houston, Texas

BRUCE B. HORSWELL, MD, DDS, MS, FACS
Director, First Appalachian Craniofacial
Deformity Specialists, Charleston Area Medical
Center-Women and Children's Hospital;
Clinical Assistant Professor, Department of
Surgery, West Virginia University-Charleston
Division, Charleston, West Virginia

SHARON ISTFAN, MD, FAAP
Assistant Professor of Pediatrics, Department
of Pediatrics, West Virginia University-
Charleston Division; Co-Medical Director,
Child Advocacy Center, Children's Medicine
Center, Charleston, West Virginia; Adjunct
Clinical Instructor, Department of Oral and
Maxillofacial Surgery, University of North
Carolina, Chapel Hill, North Carolina

MICHAEL S. JASKOLKA, MD, DDS
First Appalachian Craniofacial Deformity
Specialists, Charleston Area Medical
Center-Women and Children's Hospital;
Department of Surgery, West Virginia
University-Charleston Division, Charleston,
West Virginia; Adjunct Clinical Instructor,
Department of Oral and Maxillofacial Surgery,
University of North Carolina, Chapel Hill,
North Carolina

GEORGE M. KUSHNER, DMD, MD, FACS
Professor and Graduate Program Director,
Department of Surgical and Hospital Dentistry,
The University of Louisville, Louisville, Kentucky

EDWARD I. LEE, MD
Fellow, Division of Plastic Surgery, Baylor
College of Medicine, Houston, Texas

JANICE S. LEE, DDS, MD, FACS
Department of Oral and Maxillofacial Surgery,
University of California, San Francisco,
San Francisco, California

KELLY R. MAGLIOCCA, DDS, MPH
Assistant Professor, Department of Pathology
and Laboratory Medicine, Emory University,
Atlanta, Georgia

DANIEL J. MEARA, MS, MD, DMD
Vice Chair, Department of Oral and
Maxillofacial Surgery and Hospital Dentistry;
Program Director, Oral and Maxillofacial
Surgery Residency; Director of Research,
Department of Oral and Maxillofacial Surgery,
Christiana Care Health System, Wilmington,
Delaware

KATHRYN S. MOFFETT, MD, FAAP
Professor of Pediatrics, Division Chief,
Pediatric Infectious Diseases, West Virginia
University, Morgantown, West Virginia

MARK MOONEY, PhD
Professor and Vice Chair, Department of Oral
Biology; Director of Student Research,
University of Pittsburgh School of Dental
Medicine; Professor, Department of
Anthropology, University of Pittsburgh;
Department of Surgery-Plastic and
Reconstructive Surgery; University of
Pittsburgh Medical Center; Department of
Orthodontics and Dentofacial Orthopedics,
University of Pittsburgh School of Dental
Medicine, Pittsburgh, Pennsylvania

CHRISTOPHER MORRIS, DDS, MD
Resident, Division of Oral and Maxillofacial
Surgery, University of Texas Southwestern
Medical Center, Dallas, Texas

BONNIE L. PADWA, DMD, MD
Associate Professor, Department of Oral and
Maxillofacial Surgery, Harvard School of Dental
Medicine; Oral Surgeon-in-Chief, Department
of Plastic and Oral Surgery, Children's Hospital
Boston, Boston, Massachusetts

PAT RICALDE, DDS, MD, FACS
Director, St Joseph's Craniofacial Center,
Tampa, Florida

REYNALDO D. RIVERA, DDS, MD
Division of Craniofacial and Cleft Surgery;
Craniofacial Surgery Fellow, Department of
Oral and Maxillofacial Surgery, University of
Pittsburgh School of Dental Medicine,
Pittsburgh, Pennsylvania

RAMON L. RUIZ, DMD, MD
Medical Director, Pediatric Craniomaxillofacial
Surgery; Vice Chair, Department of Children's
Surgery, Arnold Palmer Hospital for Children;
Associate Professor of Surgery, University of
Central Florida College of Medicine, Orlando,
Florida

SCOTT SHADFAR, MD
Department of Otolaryngology/Head and Neck
Surgery, University of North Carolina, Chapel
Hill, North Carolina

JOCELYN SHAND, MBBS(Melb), MDSc(Melb), BDS(Otago), FDSRCS(Eng), FRACDS(OMS)
Division of Plastic and Maxillofacial Surgery, Royal Children's Hospital, Parkville, Victoria, Australia

SAMUEL STAL, MD
Professor and Chief, Division of Plastic Surgery, Baylor College of Medicine, Houston, Texas

PAUL S. TIWANA, DDS, MD, MS, FACS
Associate Professor and Graduate Program Director, Chief, Pediatric Oral and Maxillofacial Surgery, Children's Medical Center, University of Texas Southwestern Medical Center, Dallas, Texas

BRADLEY V. VAUGHN, MD
Professor, Department of Neurology, University of North Carolina, Chapel Hill, North Carolina

AMY S. XUE, BS
Student, Division of Plastic Surgery, Baylor College of Medicine, Houston, Texas

CARLTON J. ZDANSKI, MD
Surgical Director, North Carolina Children's Airway Center; Associate Professor of Otolaryngology/Head and Neck Surgery, Chief, Pediatric Otolaryngology, Department of Otolaryngology/Head and Neck Surgery, University of North Carolina, Chapel Hill, North Carolina

Contents

Scott Shadfar, Amelia F. Drake, Bradley V. Vaughn, and Carlton J. Zdanski

Sleep disordered breathing syndromes in pediatric patients can lead to adverse effects in the cardiovascular system, neurocognitive function, growth, and behavior. These syndromes occur more frequently in patients with craniofacial disorders. A high index of suspicion as well as early recognition, detection, and treatment of these syndromes are considered integral to care of children with craniofacial disorders.

Bruce B. Horswell and Michael S. Jaskolka

Head injuries in children are common, comprising more than half of all injuries sustained. The mortality and morbidity associated with traumatic head injury in children is staggering, and the cumulative effect of such on the pediatric and general populations is propagated through related health care measures and subsequent socioeconomic burden. The majority of deaths due to trauma in children are caused by brain injury. This article reviews the evaluation and management of scalp injuries in the pediatric patient. The second portion addresses skull fractures, the specter of child abuse, management of acute fracture, and the phenomenon of growing skull fractures.

Christopher Morris, George M. Kushner, and Paul S. Tiwana

The management of pediatric craniomaxillofacial trauma requires the additional dimension of understanding growth and development. The surgeon must appreciate the considerable influence of the soft tissue envelope and promote function when possible. Children heal well but with an exuberant tissue response that may contribute to greater scarring, therefore, careful and prudent attention given to meticulous soft tissue repair and support is critical. Support must also be given and sought from the family of the injured child. Follow-up management of children must continue to ensure that the growth of the craniomaxillofacial skeleton continues within the normal parameters of development.

Nicholas J.V. Hogg

Injury is the most common cause of death in pediatric patients, with a large proportion related to head injury. The craniofacial region in children develops rapidly and at an early age, making the area more prominent compared with the remainder of the body, increasing the likelihood of injury. This article reviews the primary management of pediatric soft tissue injuries, including assessment, cleansing, surgical technique, anesthesia, and considerations for special wounds. The secondary management of pediatric facial injury is also discussed, including scar revision, management of scar hypertrophy/keloids, and staged surgical correction.

The purpose of craniomaxillofacial surgery is to improve function, occlusion, craniofacial balance, and aesthetics. Accurate diagnosis, assessment, and careful treatment planning are essential in achieving a successful outcome, and an understanding of the pattern of facial growth is integral in this process. Patients with craniofacial congenital dysmorphologies, posttraumatic asymmetries, or disturbances of facial balance from radiation may have functional and/or aesthetic issues that require treatment. Understanding the complexities of growth in the skull and face is a key component to appropriate treatment planning for these disorders. This article reviews growth and development in the craniofacial skeleton.

Auricular and nasal deformities can have significant social ramifications; therefore, proper repair of these deformities is critically important to a child's well-being. Moreover, the benefits of reconstruction in the pediatric population must be weighed against added concerns about potential growth restriction on the ear and the nose with any manipulation. This article reviews various methods of auricular and nasal reconstruction and discusses some of the technical pearls for improved outcome. A complete discourse on treatment of total ear and nasal reconstruction is beyond the scope of this article. Attention is focused primarily on partial to subtotal defects.

Dermoid cysts are congenital lesions that commonly arise from nondisjunction of surface ectoderm from deeper neuroectodermal structures. They tend to be found along planes of embryonic closure. Classification by site is helpful for diagnostic planning and surgical treatment. A distinction can be made between frontotemporal, orbital, frontoethmoidal, and calvarial lesions. The risk of extension into deeper tissues must be determined before surgical intervention. Simple lesions are amenable to direct excision. Deeper lesions often require a coordinated surgical approach between a neurosurgeon and craniofacial surgeon after thorough radiographic imaging. Follow-up through the developmental years is recommended for complex dermoid lesions.

Despite recent advances in the understanding of the natural history and molecular abnormalities, many questions remain surrounding the progression and management of fibrous dysplasia (FD). In the absence of comorbidities, the expected behavior of craniofacial FD (CFD) is to be slow growing and without functional consequence. Understanding of the pathophysiologic mechanisms contributing to the various phenotypes of this condition, as well as the predictors of the different behaviors of FD lesions, must be improved. Long-term follow-up of patients with CFD is vital because spontaneous recovery is unlikely, and the course of disease can be unpredictable.

The process of understanding and treating children with vascular anomalies has been hampered by confusing and occasionally incorrect terminology. The most important step when evaluating a maxillofacial vascular anomaly is to determine whether it is a tumor or a malformation. In most cases, this diagnosis can be made by history and physical examination. Selective radiographic imaging is helpful in differentiating vascular malformations or the extent of bony involvement and/or destruction. Children with vascular anomalies should be managed by an interdisciplinary team of trained providers who are committed to following, treating, and studying patients with these complex problems.

The majority of neck masses in the pediatric population are congenital or inflammatory in origin requiring a thorough understanding of embryology and anatomy of the cervical region. However, malignancy must always be ruled out as they represent 11%–15% of all neck masses in the pediatric population. The initial history and physical are of utmost important to correctly work-up and eventually diagnose the lesion. This article addresses many aspects of the workup, diagnosis and eventual proper surgical or medical management of pediatric neck masses.

Infections in children in the head and neck regions are common, leading to frequent use and overuse of antibiotics. This review includes common as well as diverse and unusual infectious diseases, such as PFAPA (Periodic Fever Aphthous stomatitis, Pharyngitis, Adenitis) syndrome, Lemierre Syndrome, Arcanobacterium infection, and tuberculous and nontuberculous adenitis, which occur in infants, children, and adolescents. In addition, the first pediatric vaccines available with the potential to prevent oropharyngeal cancers are reviewed.

Sinonasal disease is common in the pediatric population because of anatomic, environmental, and physiologic factors. Once paranasal sinusitis develops, orbital cellulitis is a concerning sequela that can result in loss of visual acuity and even intracranial disease. Thus, a clear history and physical examination in conjunction with radiographic studies are critical to a correct diagnosis and timely institution of treatment that may include hospitalization, serial ophthalmologic examinations, intravenous antibiotics, and surgery. The serious nature of orbital cellulitis in children cannot be overestimated; but, if prompt and appropriate treatment is initiated, the prognosis is excellent and long-term sequelae should be limited.

Joli C. Chou and Bruce B. Horswell

This article briefly reviews some of the most common skin lesions in the head and neck of a child. Benign "lumps and bumps" are very common in children and it is prudent for the pediatric maxillofacial surgeon to be familiar with their presentation, workup (including radiographic studies), and definitive surgical management. Inflammatory and infectious lesions require prompt treatment to avoid more serious sequelae of progressive infection and scarring.

Bruce B. Horswell and Sharon Istfan

Oral and maxillofacial surgeons are in a unique position to identify and report child abuse. In the career of any practitioner, maltreated children (both physically abused and neglected) will present for management of injuries and infections. There must be a high level of vigilance for, and understanding of, mechanisms of injury and skill in sorting out inflicted injuries or evidence of neglect. Because of this, the medical community, society, state law, and the legal system place oral and maxillofacial surgeons in a position of expertise and accountability in the care of children.

ORAL AND MAXILLOFACIAL SURGERY CLINICS OF NORTH AMERICA

THE CLINICS ARE NOW AVAILABLE ONLINE!
Access your subscription at:
www.theclinics.com

Preface
Pediatric Maxillofacial Surgery

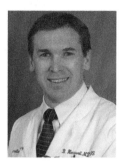 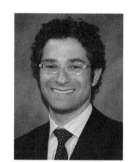

Bruce B. Horswell, MD, DDS, MS   Michael S. Jaskolka, MD, DDS
Guest Editors

Pediatric maxillofacial surgery, though not a formally recognized subspecialty by training initiatives in graduate education, is nonetheless a burgeoning area of surgical focus, clinical practice, and postresidency experience across dentistry and medicine. Children are unique in anatomy, physiology, and response to trauma and disease and, at every step in management, there is the prospect of growth and development coming to bear on our treatment proposals. Disease spectrums are changing—increased incidence of trauma among youth, evolving patterns of infections, advances in treatment of certain pathologic entities; yet it is important to be current in our understanding of common presentations of disease in children that we may see—for example, the child with a neck lump and those with dermatologic disease or vascular lesions. And, the ever-menacing prospect of abuse and neglect set amid the complexity and stress of trauma and disease requires all of our focus on behalf of those children seeking and needing our help.

We have endeavored to address these issues by inviting recognized contributors in the various fields and disciplines of pediatric management. The articles on trauma have specific focus on the uniqueness of the immature skeleton and fragile nature of the soft tissue envelope in children. Surgeons who manage trauma and deformity will encounter children with ear and nasal deformities; therefore, it is important to be well versed in the timing of surgical intervention, tissue selection, and flap design when reconstructing these complex entities. Both common and unusual pathological conditions that we may encounter in pediatric care are deftly discussed in their presentation and management. We have included an article on infections written from the pediatric infectious disease perspective, which is comprehensive and illuminating, as well as an update on sinonasal-orbital infections. It is vital that oral and maxillofacial surgeons understand the adverse influences of injury and disease on the developing craniofacial region, thus a very thorough discussion regarding assessment and management of that complex topic. Finally, all of us will at some point treat children who have been abused or neglected, and we need to be able to wisely and effectively screen for abuse and intervene, when necessary, on behalf of that child's welfare.

This issue of *Oral and Maxillofacial Surgery Clinics* is not and cannot be a comprehensive tome on all entities we may encounter in children—cleft lip and palate, cysts and tumors of the jaws in children, pain control and anesthesia,

Oral Maxillofacial Surg Clin N Am 24 (2012) xiii–xiv
doi:10.1016/j.coms.2012.05.009
1042-3699/12/$ – see front matter © 2012 Elsevier Inc. All rights reserved.

etc., all deserve mention, but those conditions represent and require special focus in a broader sense and have been deservedly published in previous *Oral and Maxillofacial Surgery Clinics*. Therefore, we deemed it wise rather to select a few areas of interest, uniqueness, commonality, and necessity within the ever-evolving practice of oral and maxillofacial surgery and the *subspecialty* of pediatric maxillofacial surgery. We trust you will agree.

Bruce B. Horswell, MD, DDS, MS
Michael S. Jaskolka, MD, DDS

Charleston Area Medical Center
830 Pennsylvania Avenue
Suite 302
Charleston, WV 25302, USA

E-mail addresses:
bruce.horswell@camc.org (B.B. Horswell)
Michael.Jaskolka@camc.org (M.S. Jaskolka)

Pediatric Airway Abnormalities
Evaluation and Management

Scott Shadfar, MD[a], Amelia F. Drake, MD[a],
Bradley V. Vaughn, MD[b], Carlton J. Zdanski, MD[c],*

KEYWORDS

- Pediatric airway • Obstructive sleep apnea • Craniofacial

KEY POINTS

- Sleep-disordered breathing occurs more frequently in patients with craniofacial disorders.
- The associated hypoxia, hypercapnia, and bradycardia associated with sleep-disordered breathing syndromes can lead to adverse effects on daytime behavior, the cardiovascular system, neurocognitive function, and growth.
- A high index of suspicion, early recognition, and detection of sleep-disordered breathing lead to more effective treatment and are considered integral to the care of all children with craniofacial disorders.
- Nocturnal signs and symptoms of sleep-disordered breathing include heavy snoring, restlessness, increased respiratory effort, posturing or positioning, and intermittent apneas or pauses in breathing.
- Airway complaints in wake and sleep of patients with craniofacial disorders should be assessed as part of their initial clinical evaluation.
- The use of formal sleep studies (polysomnography) is advocated in suspected cases of sleep-disordered breathing in children with craniofacial disorders.
- Airway obstruction is recognized as a common sequela of surgery to correct craniofacial disorders.

INTRODUCTION

The anatomy of the upper airway bears important influence on airflow and breathing cycles. The structures may limit the movement of air and also influence the dynamics of the regulation of airway reflexes and muscular tone. Many of these issues change with state. The state of sleep, in particular, is a time period in which airflow may be more disrupted, suggesting airway dysfunction. Sleep-disordered breathing (SDB) syndromes are typically divided into those related to hypoventilation and those changing the respiratory pattern, such as

apnea. Apneas are typically classified as obstructive, central, and mixed. These pauses or interruptions of breathing are commonly recognized in children with cleft lip and cleft palate (CP) and other craniofacial syndromes, with an increased incidence noted in the literature. Observed cessation of airflow at the level of the nose or mouth, whether there is partial or complete obstruction, makes continued respiratory effort against a collapsed upper airway futile. Therefore, apneas are frequently associated with poor and fragmented sleep as well as arousals. The associated hypoxia,

The authors have nothing to disclose.
[a] Department of Otolaryngology/Head and Neck Surgery, University of North Carolina, 170 Manning Drive, Chapel Hill, NC 27599, USA; [b] Department of Neurology, University of North Carolina, CB#7025, Chapel Hill, NC 27599, USA; [c] North Carolina Children's Airway Center, Pediatric Otolaryngology, Department of Otolaryngology/Head and Neck Surgery, University of North Carolina, CB#7070, PO Box, 170 Manning Drive, Chapel Hill, NC 27599, USA
* Corresponding author.
E-mail address: carlton_zdanski@med.unc.edu

Oral Maxillofacial Surg Clin N Am 24 (2012) 325–336
doi:10.1016/j.coms.2012.04.005

hypercapnia, and bradycardia can all lead to possible adverse effects on the child's daytime behavior, cardiovascular system, neurocognitive function, and growth.[1] With the possible detrimental effects of obstructive events on children, early recognition and detection lead to more effective treatment and are considered integral in any craniofacial practice.

ANATOMIC AND PHYSIOLOGIC CONSIDERATIONS

The airway can be divided into levels, beginning at the superiorly positioned area of the nose and nasopharynx, which communicate inferiorly with the oropharynx and descending into the laryngopharynx. At the level of the nose, the external and internal nasal valves are the main areas thought to provide resistance to flow. The nasal turbinates then direct flow, whether laminar or turbulent, with hypertrophy of the turbinates leading to obstruction. The upper airway is capable of collapse, and its patency is determined by its diameter; the tonic activity of muscular dilators, such as the genioglossus and tensor veli palatini; and the response to negative airway pressure generated during inspiration. During sleep, reduced tone of these dilators can lead to physiologic airway narrowing, which can result in SDB.[1] Other physiologic effects are noted as well during the apnea. Progressive increases in the drive to breathe can lead to maximal respiratory efforts against a closed airway resulting in respiratory-related decreases in blood pressure due to progressively greater negative intrathoracic pressures. The apnea is terminated by an arousal followed by a return to a deeper sleep state with normalization of blood gases. Subsequently, the airway tone becomes reduced again and the obstructive cycle begins anew (**Fig. 1**).[1]

Nasal obstruction secondary to arrhinia, pyriform aperture stenosis, septal deviation, and choanal atresia can contribute to SDB because of the increased nasal resistance to airflow, which often necessitates mouth opening and tongue retropulsion leading to further airway obstruction, narrowing, and collapse (**Fig. 2**).[1]

The clinical spectrum of SDB ranges from benign primary snoring to obstructive sleep apnea syndrome (OSAS) as the most severe.[1] The severity of the obstructions and age of presentation are often related to the degree and location of obstruction within the respiratory tract. These factors influence the severity of SDB with which a child clinically presents (**Table 1**).

The major craniofacial abnormalities associated with airway obstruction include those involving the cranium and midface (craniofacial dysostosis syndromes), those primarily involving the mandible (Nager syndrome, Stickler syndrome, and Pierre Robin sequence [PRS]), and those involving a combination of the midface and mandible (Treacher Collins syndrome, oculoauriculovertebral syndrome, and craniofacial microsomia).[2] Midface bony abnormalities are often accompanied by nasopharyngeal narrowing and oropharyngeal musculature crowding causing obstruction. In patients with mandibular abnormalities, the tongue is retropositioned, which leads to airway narrowing and obstruction (**Fig. 3**).

Enlargement of the tongue itself can also lead to airway obstruction. Beckwith-Wiedemann syndrome is a congenital disorder characterized by a unique group of physical examination findings; macroglossia is the most notable finding in the head and neck. These children can have SDB from their tongue musculature collapsing and retropulsing as well as obstruction from adenotonsillar hypertrophy necessitating surgical intervention if obstructive sleep apnea (OSA) is confirmed. In the setting of macroglossia, the differential diagnosis should also include trisomy 21, the mucopolysaccharidoses, hypothyroidism, and vascular malformations as well as tumors involving the tongue. Other less common conditions with macroglossia include hemihypertrophy syndrome, rhabdomyoma, dermoid cysts, and amyloidosis.[3]

In the child with a cleft lip and/or palate (CL/P), both anatomic and functional changes increase the risk of SDB. Cephalometric analysis of human facial skeletal morphology associated with orofacial clefting (OFC) reveals reduced midfacial and mandibular projection and development, resulting in decreased size of the pharyngeal airway.[4,5] The abnormal craniofacial relationships associated with OFC have been shown to persist beyond the period of skeletal growth. In particular, adults with a history of bilateral CL/P reveal smaller mandibular dimensions, larger vertical craniofacial dimensions, a smaller depth of the oropharynx, and an inferiorly positioned hyoid.[5,6] All of these anatomic aberrancies predispose to SDB.

Patients with bilateral CL/P have greater impairment of nasal airway caliber compared with those with unilateral CL/P or with CP alone.[5,7] Secondary palatal clefts affect the oropharyngeal musculature, with disruption resulting in abnormal airway function in addition to structural changes. The role of palatal muscle function on airway patency in the setting of CP has been reported in adult patients showing palatal musculature fulfilling an important role in maintaining the airway patency.[5,8–10]

Several studies have supported an increased incidence of SDB amongst children with CL/P, including Muntz and colleagues[11] who found

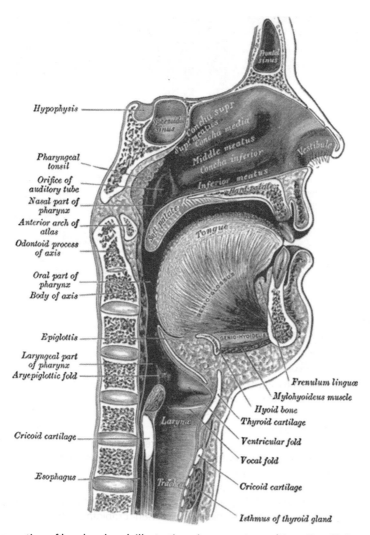

Hypophysis
Pharyngeal tonsil
Orifice of auditory tube
Nasal part of pharynx
Anterior arch of atlas
Odontoid process of axis
Oral part of pharynx
Body of axis
Epiglottis
Laryngeal part of pharynx
Aryepiglottic fold
Cricoid cartilage
Esophagus

Ethmoidal sinus
Sphenoidal sinus
Supr. meatus
Conchæ supr
Conchæ media
Middle meatus
Concha inferior
Inferior meatus
Hard palate
Soft palate
Tongue
Frontal sinus
Vestibule

Frenulum linguæ
Mylohyoideus muscle
Hyoid bone
Thyroid cartilage
Ventricular fold
Vocal fold
Cricoid cartilage
Isthmus of thyroid gland
Larynx
Trachea

Fig. 1. Sagittal cross section of head and neck illustrating airway anatomy. (*From* Gray H. Anatomy of the human body. Philadelphia: Lea and Febiger, 1918.)

symptoms of SDB in 22% of children in a retrospective review of all children presenting to a tertiary cleft and craniofacial team. MacLean and colleagues[5,11–13] have provided evidence to support the underrecognition of OSAS in children with CL/P. These studies reveal an estimated risk of SDB in children with CL/P ranging between 22% and 65%, with 28% likely to have severe SDB. The prevalence of SDB is greater in the subgroup of infants and children with syndromes as well as those with PRS.

CLINICAL PRESENTATION AND DIAGNOSIS

Nocturnal signs and symptoms of OSAS usually include heavy snoring, restlessness, increased respiratory effort, posturing or positioning, and intermittent apneas or pauses. Daytime signs and symptoms include nasal obstruction, hyponasal speech, mouth breathing, hyperactivity, and impaired memory and cognitive function. The symptoms of social withdrawal, hypersomnolence, and poor academic performance have also been reported.[14,15] Other clinical signs and symptoms include intracranial hypertension, poor growth, failure to thrive, and cardiorespiratory complications, including arrhythmias, pulmonary hypertension, cor pulmonale, and the possibility of sudden death.

The attention capacity and cognitive ability of children are adversely affected by SDB.[16,17] The ability to remain on task and attend to external stimuli play an important role in learning as well as social and academic development. The data suggest poorer sustained attention and more impulsive behavior with dose-dependent effects of SDB on memory capacity, suggesting that the

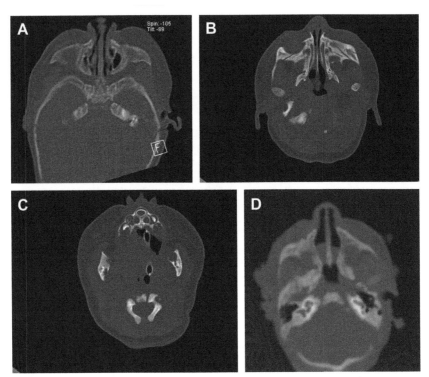

Fig. 2. Axial computed tomography illustrating (*A*) normal neonatal nose, (*B*) pyriform aperture stenosis, (*C*) central mega-incisor with pyriform aperture stenosis, and (*D*) choanal atresia.

more severe the SDB is, the poorer the child's performance will be. Some studies show these effects to be reversible with successful treatment of the upper airway obstruction.[1] Caregivers' abilities to corroborate the above-mentioned symptoms are integral in the diagnosis of SDB, hence validated questionnaires at the time of the child's visit are used as screening tools, with positive correlative results in the diagnosis of OSAS.[12]

The diagnosis of SDB in children is based on a combination of history from the caregivers, findings on physical examination, and possible adjunctive investigations. Examination should document craniofacial morphology, patency of nasal

Table 1
Age-associated findings in SDB and suggested therapies

Age	Sleep Findings	Airway Findings	Pulmonary Findings	Therapy
Infants	Obstructive and central apneas, hypoxemia	Micrognathia, glossoptosis, cleft palate, retrognathia	Inspiratory stridor, retractions, pectus excavatum	Nasopharyngeal airway, CPAP, surgery, oxygen therapy
Early childhood	Obstructive and central apnea	Micrognathia, glossoptosis, cleft palate, retrognathia, pharyngeal restriction, adenoid and tonsillar hypertrophy	Inspiratory stridor, retractions, pectus excavatum	Surgery, CPAP
Late childhood	Obstructive apnea	Tonsillar hypertrophy		Surgery, CPAP
Adolescence and adulthood	Obstructive apnea and hypoventilation	Tonsillar hypertrophy		Surgery, CPAP

Abbreviation: CPAP, continuous positive airway pressure.

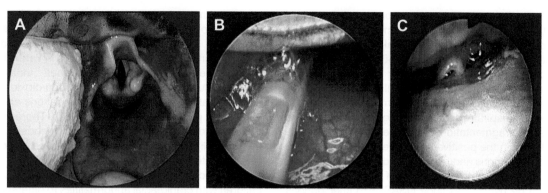

Fig. 3. Direct laryngoscopy with intubating laryngoscope illustrating (*A*) normal grade I view of larynx, (*B*) grade IV view of larynx in neonate with PRS and tongue-based airway obstruction; only the posterior pharyngeal wall and nasogastric tube are visible, and (*C*) flexible nasopharyngolaryngoscopic view of tongue base obstruction resulting from micrognathia.

airways, septal deviation, status of the palate and adenoids, and size or grade of tonsillar hypertrophy (**Fig. 4**).[18]

In addition, attention should be paid to the child's location on standardized growth charts, as well as signs of cardiorespiratory complications.

Adjunctive investigations could include lateral cephalograms, electrocardiograms, chest radiographs, and echocardiograms.

One means of diagnosis commonly used is home pulse oximetry. Arguments against the use of oximetry alone, which only measures oxygen

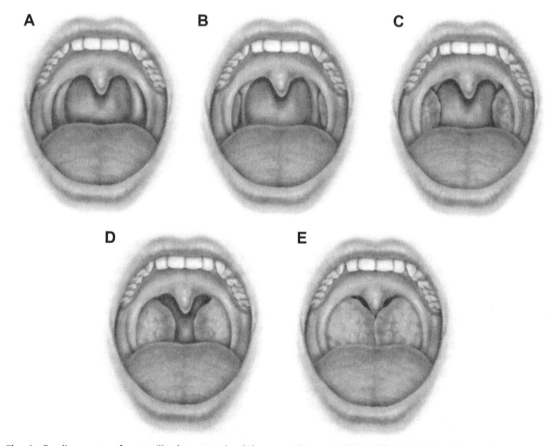

Fig. 4. Grading system for tonsillar hypertrophy. (*A*) no tonsil tissue present; (*B*) 1+; (*C*) 2+; (*D*) 3+; (*E*) 4+. (*From* Friedman M, Ibrahim H, Joseph NJ. Staging of obstructive sleep apnea/hypopnea syndrome: a guide to appropriate treatment. Laryngoscope 2004;114(3):454–9; with permission.)

saturation and pulse rate, are primarily because of the limited scope of measurement and inability to document arousals, which makes it an unreliable tool in the investigation of SDB because many patients with significant upper airway obstruction who readily arouse may be missed. Further criticism classifies oximetry as a limited sleep study in which respiratory effort, snoring, hypercapnia, and sleep fragmentation are inadequately assessed. Although the positive predictive value of observed desaturations and hypoxemia during sleep is clinically significant, the absence of desaturations cannot be used to exclude OSAS.[1,19] Other options include the use of home apnea monitors, which in the setting of young patients can be quite cumbersome for parents to configure and obtain accurate results whereas in the adult population this option has been shown to be effective.[20]

The use of formal sleep studies (polysomnography [PSG]) is advocated to evaluate the function of the airway in suspected cases of SDB in children with craniofacial abnormalities; however, not all PSG studies are alike. Most sleep studies include only temperature sensors to measure airflow. This technique has been found to be insensitive for detecting hypopneas. The American Academy of Sleep Medicine 2007 guidelines outline the importance of studies including continuous nasal pressure measurements for accurate determination of hypopneas and respiratory effort–related arousals, especially in children.[21] The American Academy of Otolaryngology-Head and Neck Surgery (AAO-HNS) recent task force assembly development panel concluded with 5 evidence-based action statements with the indications for PSG in SDB listed in **Table 2**.[22] The guidelines were admittedly limited and do not apply to children younger than 2 years, older than 18 years, to those who have already undergone tonsillectomy, to children having adenoidectomy alone, to children being considered for continuous positive airway pressure (CPAP) therapy, and to children being considered for surgical therapy other than tonsillectomy for SDB.[22] Statements in the AAO-HNS guidelines are not intended to limit or restrict care provided by clinicians, and decisions should be based on the assessment of individual patients.[22]

Questions are often raised regarding the age in which to obtain a PSG. Data in neonates are still sparse; however, the use of PSG is gaining popularity in this age group in hopes of earlier diagnosis and intervention. The general consensus is that SDB should be documented objectively, but debate exists over the type of investigation needed, how to interpret the study, who should interpret the study, and what degree of abnormality constitutes a surgically treatable disease entity.[1] Common

measures include gas exchange, respiratory effort, airflow, snoring, sleep stage, body position, limb movement, and heart rhythm. Analysis of this data aids in differentiating diagnoses as listed in **Table 3**, and indices include apnea/hypopnea index, oxygen saturation nadir, end tidal carbon dioxide, and arousals. With official recommendations and guidelines published by the American Thoracic Society and AAO-HNS, PSG is recommended in multiple clinical scenarios related to pediatric patients with craniofacial abnormalities.[22–24]

These recommendations include investigation of children with craniofacial abnormalities to differentiate benign/primary snoring from pathologic snoring and significant airway obstruction, to grade severity of OSA, and to plan medical or surgical intervention (see **Table 3**). In addition, follow-up PSG should generally be performed 12 to 18 months later in children previously diagnosed with OSA to evaluate the effectiveness of therapy, persistent symptoms after therapy, and worsening symptoms or to follow those children previously diagnosed with mild OSA. Routine clinical assessments should also be performed to ensure early detection of persistent, worsening, or recurrent OSAS.[1] It is the practice of the authors to tailor follow-up studies to the individual. Follow-up PSGs are obtained every 12 months for children using CPAP and who use mechanical ventilation and 3 months after surgical intervention. For infants and those in rapidly evolving clinical situations (eg, PRS), PSGs may be obtained more frequently. Clinical indicators and common sense should be the ultimate guide to decision making.

Additional diagnostic tools include office-based nasopharyngolaryngoscopy (NPL) and operative laryngoscopy as well as bronchoscopy to evaluate synchronous lesions including pyriform aperture stenosis, nasolacrimal cysts, choanal atresia, laryngomalacia, vocal fold paralysis, laryngeal cysts or webs, subglottic stenosis, and pathologic conditions of the trachea (**Fig. 5**).[25] Awake examination of the upper airways in the clinic setting is focused on the identification of the pathologic conditions of the nasal and nasopharyngeal regions (septal deviation, inferior turbinate hypertrophy, nasal masses, and adenoid hypertrophy), pharyngeal region (tongue base obstruction and pharyngomalacia) and laryngeal region (vocal cord paresis and masses). Children may often tolerate awake NPL; however, the individual child's age and behavior dictate the likelihood of obtaining a meaningful examination. If the examination is limited because of cooperation, or lower airway evaluation is indicated, early operative airway evaluation with appropriate diagnostic tools is advocated by the authors.

Table 2
AAO-HNS guidelines and indications for PSG

Statement	Action	Summary of Action Statements for PSG	
		Evidence	Purpose
1. Indications for PSG	Before performing tonsillectomy, the clinician should refer children with SDB for PSG if they exhibit any of the following: obesity, Down syndrome, craniofacial abnormalities, neuromuscular disorders, sickle cell disease, or mucopolysaccharidoses	Recommendation based on observational studies with a preponderance of benefit over harm	Improve diagnostic accuracy in high-risk patients and define severity of OSA to optimize perioperative treatment planning, to improve quality of life and aid in clinical treatment plans
2. Advocating for PSG	The clinician should advocate for PSG before tonsillectomy for SDB in children without any of the comorbidities listed in statement 1 for whom the need for surgery is uncertain or when there is discordance between tonsillar size on physical examination and the reported severity of SDB	Recommendation based on observational and case control studies with a preponderance of benefit over harm	Helps clinicians to encourage the use of PSG in children without any of the comorbid conditions in statement 1
3. Communication with anesthesiologist	Clinician should communicate PSG results to the anesthesiologist before induction of anesthesia for tonsillectomy in a child with SDB	Recommendation based on observational studies with a preponderance of benefit over harm	Permit early identification of a child who may require preoperative optimization and a modified approach to anesthetic management and postoperative care
4. Inpatient admission for children with OSA documented in the results of PSG	Clinician should admit children with OSA documented in results of PSG for inpatient, overnight monitoring after tonsillectomy if they are younger than 3 y or have severe OSA (apnea-hypopnea index of 10 or more obstructive events/hour, oxygen saturation nadir less than 80%, or both)	Recommendation based on observational studies with a preponderance of benefit over harm	Promote an appropriate monitored setting for children at potential risk for postoperative respiratory compromise that could necessitate medical intervention
5. Unattended PSG with portable monitoring device	In children for whom PSG is indicated to assess SDB before tonsillectomy, clinician should obtain laboratory-based PSG when available	Recommendation based on diagnostic studies with limitations and a preponderance of benefit over harm	Overnight PSG remains the gold standard for evaluating sleep-disordered breathing in children

Abbreviations: OSA, obstructive sleep apnea; PSG, polysomnography; SDB, sleep disordered breathing.
Modified from Roland PS, Rosenfeld RM, Brooks U, et al. Clinical practice guideline: polysomnography for sleep-disordered breathing prior to tonsillectomy in children. Otolaryngol Head Neck Surg 2011;145(Suppl 1):S1–15; with permission.

Table 3
Clinical spectrum of sleep-disordered breathing (SDB)

Diagnosis	AHI	Oxygen Nadir	End Tidal Carbon Dioxide	Arousal Index	Dispute Range	Therapy
Primary snoring	<1	>90	<53	<11	<1.5	Trial of nasal decongestant
UARS	<1	>90	<53	RERA>1		Nasal decongestant
Mild OSA	1.5–5	86–90	>53 or 10% of night at 50 torr	7–11	AHI 1–5 for the lower limit of therapy	No day symptoms: Nasal decongestant Day symptoms: may consider surgery, CPAP, Oxygen Therapy
Moderate OSA	5–10	75–85	>60 or 25% of night at 50 torr	>11		Consider Surgery
Severe OSA	>10	<75	>65 or 50% of night at 50 torr	>11		Consider Surgery
Central apnea	2				1.5–5.5	Respiratory stimulant, oxygen therapy, neurologic workup

Abbreviations: AHI, apnea-hypopnea index; RERA, respiratory event–related arousals; UARS, upper airway resistance syndrome.

RISKS OF SDB SECONDARY TO CORRECTIVE SURGICAL PROCEDURES

Airway obstruction in individuals with CL/P has long been recognized as a complication of the primary and secondary reconstructive surgical procedures performed to improve speech and feeding. Primary cheilorhinoplasty is rarely associated with airway compromise with only case reports alluding to increased nasal obstruction resulting in exacerbation of the underlying OSA. Increased risk of OSA has been observed after palatoplasty. Differences in techniques, age at the time of surgery, and the inclusion of syndromic children contribute to the wide variation in the estimated 6% to 40% of increased risk after palatoplasty.[5] Potential difficulties with intraoperative and postoperative airway management, particularly in an otherwise stable and thriving child, may warrant consideration for delay of palate

repair in children with syndromes, particularly PRS. The availability of pediatric specialists and appropriate facilities (ie, pediatric anesthesia and pediatric intensive care unit) are strongly advised in these situations.

Pharyngeal flap procedures used for the correction of velopharyngeal insufficiency (VPI) are well known to be associated with SDB. Both retrospective and prospective studies have shown an increased risk of SDB in the order of 3% to 96%, with older studies reporting a risk of severe airway obstruction and death.[5] A recent comparison of surgical procedures and the risk of SDB after surgical correction of CP or VPI revealed that surgical correction of VPI confers a higher risk for OSA than primary palatoplasty.[5] Syndromes, PRS, and the presence of large tonsils put children at higher risk and must be considered when choosing surgical correction and therapy.[5] The choice of technique does not seem to affect the incidence

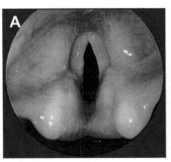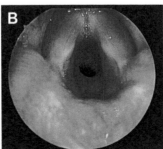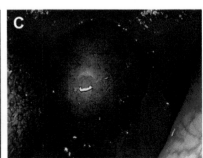

Fig. 5. Endoscopic view of (*A*) normal larynx, (*B*) grade III subglottic stenosis, and (*C*) vallecular cyst.

of OSA after surgical treatment of VPI because the use of either a pharyngeal flap or a sphincter pharyngoplasty produced relatively equivalent outcomes and complications.[26] The utility in prophylactic removal of tonsils and adenoids in patients with VPI is not advocated by the authors unless OSA is clinically present. Even then, special consideration should be given to performing tonsillectomy alone compared with total or superior pole adenoidectomy secondary to concerns for causing worse VPI postoperatively.

TREATMENT OF SDB

Treatment of SDB in children with craniofacial conditions depends on the severity of the disease, cause, age of the patient, and family/social circumstances influencing the ability to comply with treatment.[1] Treatment with early airway intervention has been shown to improve feeding, growth, breathing, and sleep. MacLean and colleagues[5] reviewed many treatment options considered for infants and children with isolated CL/P, including tonsillectomy with or without adenoidectomy, CPAP, or bilevel positive airway pressure, septoplasty, maxillary distraction, and reversal or modification of surgical procedures, which resulted in OSA.

Treatments reported in infants with PRS and micrognathia include prone sleep positioning, nasopharyngeal airways, nasal mask CPAP, tongue-lip adhesion, release of musculature of the floor of mouth, mandibular distraction, and tracheostomy.[5]

The authors advocate for early formal airway evaluation of all children with PRS and airway obstruction. The ideal paradigm for treatment does not exist, but the authors propose an algorithm in **Fig. 6**.

Nonsurgical Treatments

The use of prone positioning techniques is a noninvasive simplistic intervention, found to be valuable in infants with PRS with a 40% to 60% success rate in relieving obstruction.[5,27] In those who have failed prone positioning, some consider the use of nasopharyngeal airways to be ideal. Meyer and colleagues[27] were able to show 40% of infants who failed prone positioning were successfully managed by the use of nasopharyngeal airways in terms of relief of airway obstruction. The use of the nasopharyngeal airway allows for home care by parents, a reduction in hospital stay, increased weight gain, and no complications or readmissions.[28,29] Reported complications associated with nasopharyngeal airways include nasal regurgitation, vomiting, and nasal excoriation, which were all shown to be mild.[5,27]

An alternative effective method for the treatment of OSA is nasal CPAP, which can be used in both infants and children with CL/P. This requires regular reassessment of pressure requirements and settings in the sleep laboratory as the child grows. The risk for the development of maxillary hypoplasia from pressure of the nasal CPAP mask on

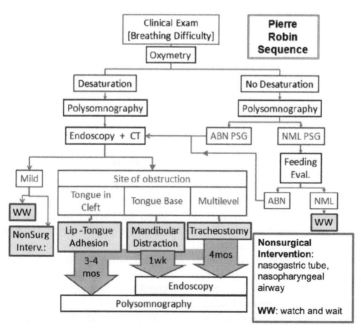

Fig. 6. Diagnosis and treatment algorithm in suspected airway abnormalities in Pierre Robin Sequence. ABN, abnormal; CT, computed tomography; NML, normal; PSG, polysomnography.

the growing midface has been debated and shown to be reversible with mask modifications.[5,30–33]

Surgical Treatments

Mandibular distraction osteogenesis (MDO) or other orthognathic procedures can be used for the improvement in airway size and patency, both in children with dentofacial deformity and children with isolated airway problems.[1] Parents must be educated regarding postoperative care and the possibility of revision surgery, particularly after initial surgery is performed in early childhood. MDO seems to offer early airway improvement with less need for revision procedures.[34,35] Recently, Scott and colleagues[36] and Sidman and colleagues[34] demonstrated improvements in airway obstruction and feeding difficulties in neonates with PRS at a mean age of 4.8 weeks after MDO. It is not clear at this time whether children who undergo MDO will require a series of distractions throughout childhood and whether mandibular growth deficiencies are the result of the surgical intervention or part of the underlying disease process.

Adenotonsillectomy is the standard initial treatment of children with SDB depending on age, physical examination, and associated conditions. The option of adenoidectomy in children with craniofacial disorders, whether complete or partial, must be carefully considered. Relative contraindications to adenoidectomy include the presence of a CP or a submucous CP because of the risk of precipitating VPI.[1,37] In these instances, consideration for tonsillectomy alone or with partial adenoidectomy can be considered.

Adenoidectomy should be considered before a trial of nasal CPAP to determine whether this is effective in reducing nasopharyngeal obstruction. Other surgical interventions include the use of septoplasty and inferior turbinate reduction techniques. Septoplasty is usually deferred until skeletal maturity has been reached unless the deviation is severe. Inferior turbinate reduction techniques (ie, radiofrequency reduction, debridement, and cautery) can also be used before formal submucous resection of the inferior turbinates in the skeletally immature child.

Modification or reversal of an intended corrective procedure such as a pharyngeal flap or pharyngoplasty can also be considered. Lesavoy and colleagues[38] reported an incidence of 10% perioperative airway obstruction after pharyngeal flap surgery, necessitating reversal.[5] Pryor and colleagues[39] found that their revisions, mainly because of the evidence of poor velopharyngeal closure and associated hypernasality, resulted from a low placement of the sphincter. They further recommended superior placement of the pharyngoplasty to reduce the need for revision surgery. Revision surgery should only be considered after an appropriate period of observation postoperatively, which is, in the authors' experience, at least 3 months. Consideration can also be given to treating OSA postoperatively with nonsurgical intervention, such as CPAP. If flap revision is required, then the extent of surgery should be tailored to the patient's pathologic condition. There is some evidence that speech benefits persist after flap division.[40]

Perkins and colleagues[41] reported as many as 60% of children with craniofacial abnormalities required airway intervention as part of their overall treatment. The incidence of tracheotomy among all children with craniofacial abnormalities range from 13% to 25% and is second only to pulmonary disease as the most common reason for tracheotomy in infants.[2,41–43] Traditionally, tracheotomy has provided the definitive airway in children with craniofacial disorders and upper airway obstruction. However, numerous other procedures, some discussed previously, have been gaining favor in the management of airway obstruction in children. This is partly because of the increasing concerns regarding morbidity including the incidence of stenosis, fistula, and bleeding, as well as high mortality rates associated with tracheotomy. The nationwide mortality rate during hospitalization for tracheotomy ranges from 5% to 7%.[40,42,44] However, close evaluation of the data reveals that the vast majority of deaths are not related to tracheotomy, but are rather due to the child's underlying chronic medical problems.[45–48] The goal of avoiding tracheotomy or achieving decannulation in children with tracheotomies may not be warranted or achievable in certain situations, such as those with multiple medical problems, multi-level airway obstruction, swallowing difficulties, aspiration, hypoventilation, neurologic impairment, and pulmonary problems. Treatment should be tailored to the individual child.[2,43]

SUMMARY

The airway complaints of patients with craniofacial disorders should be assessed in wake and sleep as part of the initial clinical evaluation to avoid the significant morbidity and mortality associated with airway obstruction. When airway obstruction is recognized, the appropriate intervention should be implemented and outcomes should be closely monitored to ensure effective management.

Regardless of the cause or severity of the airway obstruction, the treatment of children with craniofacial abnormalities and SDB requires a team approach involving individuals specializing in otolaryngology/head and neck surgery, oral and maxillofacial surgery, plastic surgery, orthodontics, sleep medicine, and pulmonology with continual reassessment of daytime and nighttime symptoms with objective measures when possible.

REFERENCES

1. Leighton S, Drake AF. Airway considerations in craniofacial patients. Oral Maxillofac Surg Clin North Am 2004;16(4):555–66.
2. Boston M, Rutter MJ. Current airway management in craniofacial anomalies. Curr Opin Otolaryngol Head Neck Surg 2003;11(6):428–32.
3. Rimell FL, Shapiro AM, Shoemaker DL, et al. Head and neck manifestations of Beckwith-Wiedemann syndrome. Otolaryngol Head Neck Surg 1995;113(3): 262–5.
4. Hermann NV, Kreiborg S, Darvann TA, et al. Early craniofacial morphology and growth in children with nonsyndromic Robin Sequence. Cleft Palate Craniofac J 2003;40(2):131–43.
5. MacLean JE, Hayward P, Fitzgerald DA, et al. Cleft lip and/or palate and breathing during sleep. Sleep Med Rev 2009;13(5):345–54.
6. Oosterkamp BC, Remmelink HJ, Pruim GJ, et al. Craniofacial, craniocervical, and pharyngeal morphology in bilateral cleft lip and palate and obstructive sleep apnea patients. Cleft Palate Craniofac J 2007; 44(1):1–7.
7. Fukushiro AP, Trindade IE. Nasal airway dimensions of adults with cleft lip and palate: differences among cleft types. Cleft Palate Craniofac J 2005;42(4): 396–402.
8. Mortimore IL, Douglas NJ. Palatal muscle EMG response to negative pressure in awake sleep apneic and control subjects. Am J Respir Crit Care Med 1997;156(3 Pt 1):867–73.
9. Malhotra A, Trinder J, Fogel R, et al. Postural effects on pharyngeal protective reflex mechanisms. Sleep 2004;27(6):1105–12.
10. Koizumi H, Kogo M, Matsuya T. Coordination between palatal and laryngeal muscle activities in response to rebreathing and lung inflation. Cleft Palate Craniofac J 1996;33(6):459–62.
11. Muntz H, Wilson M, Park A, et al. Sleep disordered breathing and obstructive sleep apnea in the cleft population. Laryngoscope 2008;118(2):348–53.
12. Maclean JE, Waters K, Fitzsimons D, et al. Screening for obstructive sleep apnea in preschool children with cleft palate. Cleft Palate Craniofac J 2009;46(2):117–23.
13. MacLean JE, Fitzsimons D, Hayward P, et al. The identification of children with cleft palate and sleep disordered breathing using a referral system. Pediatr Pulmonol 2008;43(3):245–50.
14. Gozal D. Sleep-disordered breathing and school performance in children. Pediatrics 1998;102(3 Pt 1): 616–20.
15. Urschitz MS, Guenther A, Eggebrecht E, et al. Snoring, intermittent hypoxia and academic performance in primary school children. Am J Respir Crit Care Med 2003;168(4):464–8.
16. Owens J, Spirito A, Marcotte A, et al. Neuropsychological and behavioral correlates of obstructive sleep apnea syndrome in children: a preliminary study. Sleep Breath 2000;4(2):67–78.
17. Blunden S, Lushington K, Kennedy D, et al. Behavior and neurocognitive performance in children aged 5-10 years who snore compared to controls. J Clin Exp Neuropsychol 2000;22(5):554–68.
18. Friedman M, Tanyeri H, La Rosa M, et al. Clinical predictors of obstructive sleep apnea. Laryngoscope 1999;109(12):1901–7.
19. Brouillette RT, Morielli A, Leimanis A, et al. Nocturnal pulse oximetry as an abbreviated testing modality for pediatric obstructive sleep apnea. Pediatrics 2000;105(2):405–12.
20. Akita S, Anraku K, Tanaka K, et al. Sleep disturbances detected by a sleep apnea monitor in craniofacial surgical patients. J Craniofac Surg 2006;17(1):44–9.
21. Iber C, Ancoli-Israel S, Chesson A, et al. The AASM manual for the scoring of sleep and associated event: rule, terminology and technical specifications. 1st edition. Westchester (IL): American Academy of Sleep Medicine; 2007.
22. Roland PS, Rosenfeld RM, Brooks LJ, et al. Clinical practice guideline: polysomnography for sleep-disordered breathing prior to tonsillectomy in children. Otolaryngol Head Neck Surg 2011;145(Suppl 1): S1–15.
23. Society AT. Standards and indications for cardiopulmonary sleep studies in children. American Thoracic Society. Am J Respir Crit Care Med 1996;153(2): 866–78.
24. Society AT. Cardiorespiratory sleep studies in children. Establishment of normative data and polysomnographic predictors of morbidity. American Thoracic Society. Am J Respir Crit Care Med 1999; 160(4):1381–7.
25. Daniel SJ. The upper airway: congenital malformations. Paediatr Respir Rev 2006;7(Suppl 1):S260–3.
26. Abyholm F, D'Antonio L, Davidson Ward SL, et al. Pharyngeal flap and sphincterplasty for velopharyngeal insufficiency have equal outcome at 1 year postoperatively: results of a randomized trial. Cleft Palate Craniofac J 2005;42(5):501–11.
27. Meyer AC, Lidsky ME, Sampson DE, et al. Airway interventions in children with Pierre Robin Sequence. Otolaryngol Head Neck Surg 2008;138(6):782–7.
28. Olson TS, Kearns DB, Pransky SM, et al. Early home management of patients with Pierre Robin sequence. Int J Pediatr Otorhinolaryngol 1990;20(1):45–9.

29. Anderson KD, Cole A, Chuo CB, et al. Home management of upper airway obstruction in Pierre Robin sequence using a nasopharyngeal airway. Cleft Palate Craniofac J 2007;44(3):269–73.

30. Villa MP, Pagani J, Ambrosio R, et al. Mid-face hypoplasia after long-term nasal ventilation. Am J Respir Crit Care Med 2002;166(8):1142–3.

31. Li KK, Riley RW, Guilleminault C. An unreported risk in the use of home nasal continuous positive airway pressure and home nasal ventilation in children: mid-face hypoplasia. Chest 2000;117(3):916–8.

32. Marcus CL, Rosen G, Ward SL, et al. Adherence to and effectiveness of positive airway pressure therapy in children with obstructive sleep apnea. Pediatrics 2006;117(3):e442–51.

33. Massa F, Gonsalez S, Laverty A, et al. The use of nasal continuous positive airway pressure to treat obstructive sleep apnea. Arch Dis Child 2002;87(5):438–43.

34. Sidman JD, Sampson D, Templeton B. Distraction osteogenesis of the mandible for airway obstruction in children. Laryngoscope 2001;111(7):1137–46.

35. Denny AD, Kalantarian B, Hanson PR. Rotation advancement of the midface by distraction osteogenesis. Plast Reconstr Surg 2003;111(6):1789–99 [discussion: 1800–3].

36. Scott AR, Tibesar RJ, Lander TA, et al. Mandibular distraction osteogenesis in infants younger than 3 months. Arch Facial Plast Surg 2011;13(3):173–9.

37. Saunders NC, Hartley BE, Sell D, et al. Velopharyngeal insufficiency following adenoidectomy. Clin Otolaryngol Allied Sci 2004;29(6):686–8.

38. Lesavoy MA, Borud LJ, Thorson T, et al. Upper airway obstruction after pharyngeal flap surgery. Ann Plast Surg 1996;36(1):26–30 [discussion: 31–22].

39. Pryor LS, Lehman J, Parker MG, et al. Outcomes in pharyngoplasty: a 10-year experience. Cleft Palate Craniofac J 2006;43(2):222–5.

40. Agarwal T, Sloan GM, Zajac D, et al. Speech benefits of posterior pharyngeal flap are preserved after surgical flap division for obstructive sleep apnea: experience with division of 12 flaps. J Craniofac Surg 2003;14(5):630–6.

41. Perkins JA, Sie KC, Milczuk H, et al. Airway management in children with craniofacial anomalies. Cleft Palate Craniofac J 1997;34(2):135–40.

42. Sculerati N, Gottlieb MD, Zimbler MS, et al. Airway management in children with major craniofacial anomalies. Laryngoscope 1998;108(12):1806–12.

43. Lewis CW, Carron JD, Perkins JA, et al. Tracheotomy in pediatric patients: a national perspective. Arch Otolaryngol Head Neck Surg 2003;129(5):523–9.

44. Carron JD, Derkay CS, Strope GL, et al. Pediatric tracheotomies: changing indications and outcomes. Laryngoscope 2000;110(7):1099–104.

45. Berry JG, Graham DA, Graham RJ, et al. Predictors of clinical outcomes and hospital resource use of children after tracheotomy. Pediatrics 2009;124(2):563–72.

46. Kremer B, Botos-Kremer AI, Eckel HE, et al. Indications, complications, and surgical techniques for pediatric tracheostomies–an update. J Pediatr Surg 2002;37(11):1556–62.

47. Carr MM, Poje CP, Kingston L, et al. Complications in pediatric tracheostomies. Laryngoscope 2001;111(11 Pt 1):1925–8.

48. Carter P, Benjamin B. Ten-year review of pediatric tracheotomy. Ann Otol Rhinol Laryngol 1983;92(4 Pt 1):398–400.

Pediatric Head Injuries

Bruce B. Horswell, MD, DDS, MS*, Michael S. Jaskolka, MD, DDS

KEYWORDS

- Head injuries • Children • Scalp injury • Growing skull fracture

KEY POINTS

- Scalp and head injuries are more common and more potentially life threatening in children than in adults, because of the large area of exposure relative to body size in children.
- Ischemic soft-tissue wounds will often improve with patient rewarming and correction of hypovolemia in children, resulting in salvage of complex avulsive wound flaps.
- Most avulsive scalp wounds in children that result in tissue loss will require staged reconstruction through tissue expansion.
- Initial diagnosis of pediatric skull fractures may be delayed owing to the desire to limit infant radiation exposure, making clinical follow-up critical.
- A small proportion of pediatric cranial fractures may develop into a growing skull fracture, which presents as a widening skull fracture, pulsatile mass, and neurologic symptoms.
- Computed tomography and magnetic resonance imaging are important tools in the workup of growing skull fractures, to delineate cranial and intracranial injuries.
- Patients benefit from multidisciplinary surgical care, which requires wide scalp exposure, craniotomy access, intracranial debridement, dural repair, and cranial reconstruction.

INTRODUCTION

Head injuries in children are common, estimated by the American College of Surgeons (according to data over the last 10 years in the National Trauma Data Bank) to comprise more than half of all injuries sustained by children.[1] The mortality and morbidity associated with traumatic head injury is staggering, and the cumulative effect of such on the pediatric and general populations is propagated through related health care measures and subsequent socioeconomic burden. The majority of deaths due to trauma in children are caused by brain injury.[2,3]

Many children who sustain injury to the craniofacial region will have scalp injuries and underlying skull fractures. Although there are many data that reflect the high association of traumatic brain injury with head trauma, there are few data on the percentage of those children who have associated scalp injuries.[4] And the converse is true: there are few data on the percentage of those children sustaining isolated scalp injury (no underlying fractures) who may have a brain injury. The mechanism of injury may point to the likelihood of sustaining a scalp injury in certain age groups: younger children in motor vehicle crashes and falls and older children (adolescents) in motor/recreational vehicular crashes and personal violence. Skull fractures in children are highly related to mechanism: vehicular crashes, falls, and abuse or violence.

This article reviews the evaluation and management of scalp injuries in the pediatric patient. The second portion addresses skull fractures, the specter of child abuse, management of acute fracture, and the phenomenon of growing skull fractures.

SCALP INJURIES

"I closed the scalp in 2 layers."
—Harvey Cushing. Neurosurgeon and Medical Educator

Charleston Area Medical Center, 830 Pennsylvania Avenue, Suite 302, Charleston, WV 25302, USA
* Corresponding author.
E-mail address: bruce.horswell@camc.org

Oral Maxillofacial Surg Clin N Am 24 (2012) 337–350
doi:10.1016/j.coms.2012.05.003
1042-3699/12/$ – see front matter © 2012 Elsevier Inc. All rights reserved.

The child presenting to the emergency room (ER) with a scalp injury must be fully evaluated for other injuries, particularly to the intracranial compartment. Simultaneously, attention must be given to immediate control of hemorrhage because the scalp is rich in vascularity. Scalp vasculature is derived primarily from 4 main arterial sources, as shown in **Fig. 1**. These major vessels then divide into many smaller branches that communicate with underlying arteries and arterioles running under the firm galea (aponeurosis), which tends to stent the vessels and not allow vessel constriction after injury.[5] The scalp continues to ooze, often without being attended to or noticed by medical personnel who are perhaps focused on other injuries. If the wound lies to the back of the head or has been loosely bandaged in the field, these injuries can have devastating consequences of hypovolemia and shock in the younger child. Every effort must be made to thoroughly and quickly evaluate scalp wounds in children, particularly those with complex injuries and instability. Control of hemorrhage, via either a firm dressing or actual tamponade of the vessels with instrumentation or sutures in a whip-stitch fashion, should be undertaken.

It is important to confirm and document medical status and immunization history. If there is a question as to tetanus prophylaxis in the past 5 years, a tetanus booster of Td or Tdap may be given, depending on the patient's immunization history.[6] This action is particularly important with soil or agricultural contaminant exposure. After the child has been stabilized and cleared for further management, plans for wound closure should be made in the controlled environment of the operating theater. The patient can be adequately resuscitated, if necessary, and careful monitoring undertaken. Only the simplest of scalp wounds in older children should be repaired in the ER. Many scalp wounds, once cleared of matted hair, clots, and debris, are more complex than perhaps originally thought, and a thorough evaluation through direct observation and digital exploration is necessary. Mechanisms of injury, for example, striking the pavement or a tree, may suggest the need for opening a wound even further to adequately explore, debride, and retrieve foreign bodies (**Fig. 2**). Gross contamination from soil, rotted vegetation, agricultural exposure, and so forth will necessitate a vigorous washout with pulse irrigation. The addition of antibiotics to the irrigant has not been shown to decrease the incidence of postoperative infection and wound breakdown.[7]

Initial Evaluation

When the child has been stabilized and other life-threatening injuries addressed, further evaluation can be undertaken. For any head injury in children involving a scalp wound, noncontrasted computed tomography (CT) should be obtained to rule out fractures or intracranial injury (**Fig. 3**). Because of the rich vascularity to the calvarium and scalp, there may be a great deal of swelling accompanying scalp wounds, particularly if the wound is not completely open. Particular attention should be given to infants or young children with cranial trauma and swelling, to identify possible cause of abuse and also for suspect bleeding.[8] In very

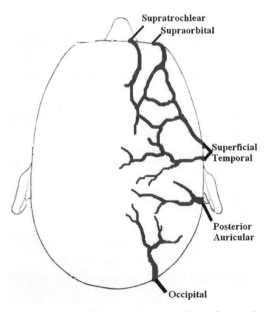

Fig. 1. Diagram of the 4 main arterial branches to the scalp. The supratrochlear and supraorbital arteries are branches of the ophthalmic artery (internal carotid); the superficial temporal, posterior auricular, and occipital arteries are branches of the external carotid.

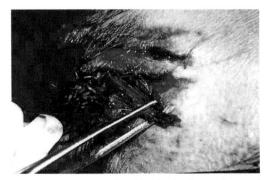

Fig. 2. Retrieving a foreign body from the scalp wound of an adolescent boy who was thrown into a wooden fence from an all-terrain vehicle.

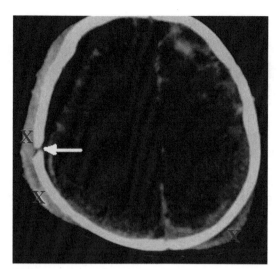

Fig. 3. CT image of skull fractures (*arrow*) and scalp (cephalo-) hematoma (X) after blunt injury.

young children with open sutures, a hematoma that crosses the suture lines is considered to be superficial to the pericranium, much like that seen in traumatic birth with caput succedaneum, whereas swelling (cephalohematoma) that is limited by the sutures is subperiosteal in nature.[9]

Once the primary and second surveys have been completed and the child stabilized, adequate exploration and management of head wounds is optimally performed in the operating theater.[8] If a small open wound suggests further exploration because of swelling or mechanism, for example, striking a tree, post, or gravel surface, the wound should be opened to allow thorough evaluation, debridement, and evacuation of contaminant or hematoma, and cleansing before closure. An evacuated hematoma or subgaleal dead space needs to be closed with either a firm dressing (preferred in young children) or small drains judiciously placed and observed.

Small Wounds

Small scalp wounds with linear or limited segmental limbs and clean margins or small stellate wounds can be washed out and closed in layers. As already noted, any extent of injury beyond the wound margin mandates further exploration and irrigation. Most of these wounds can be closed with absorbable sutures. A topical antibiotic and dressing to protect the wound can then be placed.

A puncture wound of the scalp from a dog bite requires special attention. Some dog breeds, particularly pit bulls, have a tendency to bite the head and neck region, especially in children, and can puncture the skull in young children.[10] If this is the case then CT examination is warranted and must be performed to rule out intracranial extent of injury. Dog-bite puncture wounds to the scalp with extension intracranially mandate hospitalization with intravenous antibiotics, neurosurgical consultation, and follow-up CT in 3 days to rule out early abscess formation.

Complex Wounds

Scalp wounds with various segmented or stellate limbs, macerated margins, gross contamination, or avulsive elements are considered complex. These wounds require careful attention to maintain tissue vascularity and integrity during and after repair to preserve viability of the scalp tissue. Segmented wounds with tenuous vascular integrity require immediate reorientation of the tissues to preserve viability. This intervention should be preferably addressed in the ER, as twisted pedicles will result in compromised blood flow and possible tissue loss if the segmented limbs are not correctly reoriented to their passive anatomic position and stabilized in that position. Often a small vascular pedicle in a flap of tissue will remain constricted until rehydration, patient warming, and anatomic repositioning has taken place. Children experience more heat loss through the head region, particularly after injury with open wounds, therefore every precaution should be taken to limit exposure time, maintain core temperatures, use warmed fluids for irrigation, and close wounds in a timely fashion.[3,11]

Nearly all complex wounds deserve a thorough washing out with saline solution. The addition of antibiotics has not been shown to decrease the incidence of postoperative wound infection.[7] Most complex scalp wounds need to have the surrounding hair removed to identify badly contused and macerated tissue margins and reveal areas of tissue necrosis. Proper wound cleansing and closure is made that much easier with the hair removed. Contaminated wounds that have been exposed to gross foreign-body impregnation or stagnant or soiled fluids should be thoroughly cleansed with pulse irrigation (**Fig. 4**). The mechanical dislodgment of foreign-body material and bacterial contamination through pressure irrigation has been shown to significantly reduce bacterial colonization and subsequent wound breakdown or infection.[7,12] As noted, these fluids should be warmed to decrease loss of body heat in children. Excessive pressure (<20 psi) with commercial irrigation devices should be avoided, to reduce barotrauma and shredding of compromised tissues.

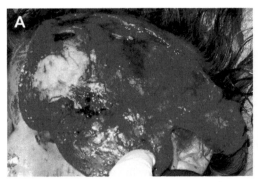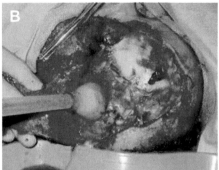

Fig. 4. (*A, B*) Pulse irrigation of contaminated avulsive scalp wounds should be undertaken before definitive wound repair.

Severely compromised, questionable, and obviously nonviable tissue should be sharply debrided under loupe magnification to obtain a precise and conservatively prepared margin for closure. There should be minimal use of electrocautery for hemostasis, as the thinner scalps of children are more prone to thermal injury of the hair follicles, leading to increased localized alopecia.[5] Simple closure of the pericranium and galea will control most bleeding points in the loose tissue, and final closure of the skin will obtain good hemostasis of the entire wound margin. In general, absorbable sutures are placed because they are well tolerated in the scalp region and will not require subsequent removal, which in very young children can be a traumatic event, particularly after injury. If pexing or mattress-type suture placement is indicated to approximate wound margins, judiciously placed permanent nylon or prolene sutures may remain in place for up to 2 weeks before significant epithelial migration and increased scarring ensues (**Fig. 5**).

Support of the wounds and obliteration of dead space under a scalp tissue flap is obtained through the careful application of a head dressing. Antibiotic ointment and xeroform or petrolatum gauze strips are applied to the wound margins, and a firm gauze dressing placed to further protect the site as well as apply light pressure to the underlying dead space to discourage hematoma formation. A mesh stockinette is used to hold the dressings in place during the immediate postoperative healing period (**Fig. 6**).

Avulsive Wounds

Scalp wounds that have small avulsive defects can usually be primarily closed with a circumferential purse-string suture to approximate the wound margins. As the fibrotic aponeurosis does not allow for much stretching of the scalp, and

because of the thin scalp in young children, full-thickness defects smaller than 2 cm^2 are generally the limit for primary closure in the author's (B.B.H.) experience without extended or additional incisions and rotational flaps. In avulsion defects of between 2 and 3 cm^2, progressive closure of the wound can take place over a short period to approximate the wound margins.[5,13] In most young children this kind of staged closure must take place under sedation or general anesthesia for reasons of patient comfort and parental anxiety associated with the procedure. Children younger than 3 years will experience further cranial vault expansion, therefore the scar will correspondingly increase in size and require final revision at a later age. The parents should be informed of this normal progression and maturation of scar.

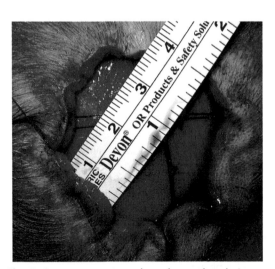

Fig. 5. Permanent sutures have been placed circumferentially at the wound periphery and across the wound to assist in serial reduction of the defect size. This procedure is performed over 2 to 4 weeks before planned definitive repair.

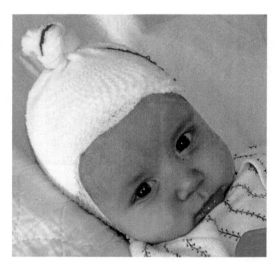

Fig. 6. Stockinette mesh is placed over protective Vaseline and sterile gauze on the wound bed to secure the dressings and prevent wound desiccation and damage.

Larger scalp wounds that have an avulsive component will require temporary tissue coverage. Underlying pericranium must be intact as a recipient site for the graft. If the avulsed portion of scalp tissue can be retrieved and adequately cleansed, it may be used as a temporary autologous free graft.[14] Preparation of the tissue necessitates thorough debridement and washing with an antibiotic solution to conceivably decrease bacterial load. Similarly, commercial decellularized dermal grafts can be used to achieve temporary coverage of a full-thickness avulsion defect.[15] Both tissue specimens are treated as temporary biological free grafts to provide for initial wound healing and stabilization. The free graft material is sutured into place providing for tie-over bolster sutures, "pie-crust" incisions are placed to allow exudative flow and discourage hematoma or seroma formation, and a firm bolster dressing of cotton and gauze placed over the graft (**Fig. 7**). After a period of 3 weeks, the bolster dressing can be removed and the wound allowed to mature for several more weeks to obtain a firm adherence of the graft (which will turn into a dermal scar) to the underlying cranial surface in preparation for tissue expansion.

Scalp Flaps

Closing defects of the scalp greater than 2 cm² may require recruitment of tissue to obtain final closure. Depending on the location of the defect, either bilobed or rotational advancement flaps or tissue expansion may be used to reconstruct the scalp defect.[15–17] In general, defects at the vertex or upper parietal and occipital regions can be closed

with rotational flaps of various designs, as demonstrated in **Fig. 8**. Flaps generated from the temporal and occipital regions have slightly increased laxity and will rotate more than those from the top of the scalp.[15,18] Rotational flaps of the scalp will require a 4- to 5-times distance in length as the width of the defect. This distance can be minimized by introducing 2 or 3 smaller rotational flaps in a circular or pinwheel fashion around the defect, as shown in **Fig. 8**. Typically some standing cones ("dog ears") will develop at the bases of the flaps, but with time these will flatten and not require excision. If there is some degree of tension at the leading border of the flap where it insets at the distalmost portion of the defect, a small back-cut incision can be made at the advancing base; however, caution should be exercised to keep this small, as it effectively reduces the width (hence vascularity) of the flap.[18]

Tissue Expansion

Patient preparation

Scalp avulsion injuries and their reconstruction in children may involve tissue expansion. In general, tissue expansion of the scalp should not be undertaken in children younger than 3 years, as the pressure exerted on the underlying cranium with potentially patent sutures may cause deformation, erosion, or remodeling.[19,20] Preoperative CT scans will confirm such anatomic features of consequence. Expanders can be placed under the galea, distant from the avulsive defect area, in children with a developed diploë, usually around age 3 or 4 years. Thorough preoperative counseling should be undertaken with the caregiver of the child so that there is no misunderstanding as to the amount of cooperation necessary, treatment duration, potential travel involved, simultaneous discomfort and need for a second surgery (and possibly more) for removal, and so forth, which attends tissue expansion. Adolescents need to fully understand what tissue expansion involves, how it addresses treatment goals in reconstruction of their injury, and the necessity for strict adherence to expansion protocols and hygiene measures in caring for the expansion site. Time spent before implementation of tissue expansion will go a long way in preventing future frustration or misunderstanding on the patient's part during the expansion process which, in the author's (B.B.H.) experience, is inevitable.

Expander selection

The skin of the scalp region is thick and variable in texture compared with other body regions, even in children, therefore tissue expansion is slightly more prolonged and uncomfortable. Because of

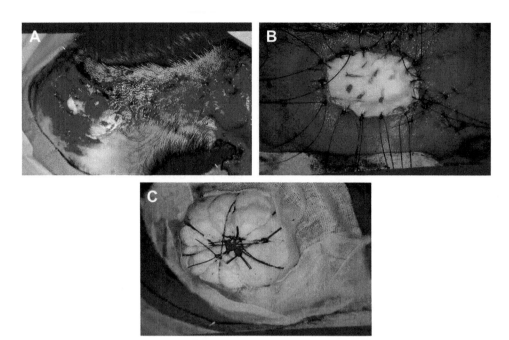

Fig. 7. Series of photos of an adolescent girl who was thrown from her bicycle and struck her head on the pavement. (*A*) Avulsive scalp wound with full-thickness tissue loss. (*B*) After several weeks of wound-bed preparation (calvarial perforations were placed to encourage granulation tissue formation), a full-thickness skin graft is placed. (*C*) Tie-over bolster dressing in place for 3 weeks.

variable characteristics of scalp tissue, the tissue reservoir from which to recruit, and the defect to be reconstructed, there are several commercially available expanders of a variety of shapes and volumes. Rectangular, round, and crescent-shaped expanders (see **Fig. 9**) are available, but the most popular for scalp reconstruction is the crescent in 100- to 200-mL volumes.[21] Studies have confirmed that an expander can be safely overinflated several times that of their reservoir volume, should that be necessary.

One must consider the area to be reconstructed and from where tissue recruitment will derive.

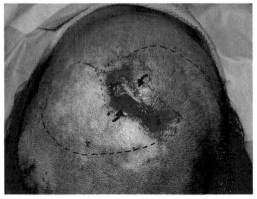

Fig. 8. Smaller scalp defects can be closed with circular rotational flaps.

Round or elliptical defects are most easily reconstructed with crescent-shaped expanders, and typically 2 are arranged at some proximity to the defect. The borders of the defect or the peripheral scar margin will be incorporated in the advancing expanded scalp and subsequently excised at advancement and inset of the flap. Gibney[22] and van Rappard and colleagues[23] have confirmed that the expander base should be roughly 2 to 3 times the area of the defect to be reconstructed.

Technique

Access incisions for insertion of the expander should be made near the junction of the defect (confirm that the scar is mature and not thin) and uninvolved scalp tissue. If the incision is made in thin or atrophic tissue, the possibility of dehiscence is greater, thereby jeopardizing exposure of the expander with subsequent infection and loss. The expander is placed in a well-dissected pocket in the subgaleal plane and above the pericranium. Great care should be exercised not to thin or perforate the overlying scalp during preparation of the expander pocket, which in young children is easy to do. If this occurs, a delay in expansion is necessary to allow for sufficient healing of the perforated tissue.

Placement of the injection port can usually be made through the expander access site if the port is to be buried. It is important to place the

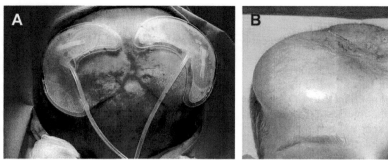
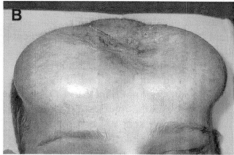

Fig. 9. (*A*) Midline scalp and forehead defect with plans for placement of bilateral crescent-shaped (250 mL) expanders. (*B*) Defect reconstructed with bilateral crescent-shaped expanders after four weeks of expansion.

port a sufficient distance from the expander to allow for ease in identification and safe needle placement during expansion. Buried ports are desirable in older children (adolescents), who may be more active and will tolerate needle placement for expansion. Younger children (<10–12 years) will do better with external ports, which can be accessed easily and kept protected under a head or scalp dressing or clean garment during the expansion process. There are no reports of external ports being more prone than buried ports to infection,[21] and this has been the author's (B.B.H.) experience as well. After expander placement, confirmation of position and contour of the expander is done with injection of normal saline; this also obliterates any dead space around the reservoir and achieves some degree of hemostasis by pressure. Some initial expansion can be done on the table, but blanching of the overlying scalp skin should be avoided to ensure vascularity. Permanent sutures are placed to firmly hold the access incision during the expansion process.

Expansion can begin about 2 weeks after initial expansion, and is accomplished with a 23-gauge needle placed through the injection port at right angles to avoid cutting or tearing the hub and increase chances of leakage from the port. Tissue expansion proceeds at 1- to 2-week intervals depending on the amount of expansion accomplished and the tolerance of the patient. Usually smaller injection amounts done on a weekly basis for younger children is better tolerated. The parents can administer an appropriate dose of acetaminophen or ibuprofen before the visit, which helps to alleviate any discomfort. Also, oral midazolam may be administered for the very frightened or anxious child. For patients living some distance from the surgeon's office, the parents can be instructed on fluid administration if there is an external port, and the entire procedure can be monitored nowadays via cell-phone video capture and immediate e-mail. After each expansion procedure the overlying skin must be confirmed to be viable, with adequate capillary refill; this is

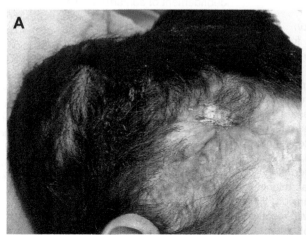
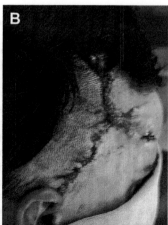

Fig. 10. Temporal scalp defect in an adolescent boy. (*A*) At final expansion of parietal and vertex scalp. (*B*) Reconstruction of temporal defect and reestablishment of hairline after removal of expanders and flap advancement.

documented should there arise any question as to vascular compromise to the overlying skin with subsequent ischemia and tissue loss. Expansion will typically take about 4 to 8 weeks.

Site preparation for the expanded tissue necessitates excising the scar or tissue bed of the defect down to pericranium. It is important to try to integrate hair-bearing scalp with the margin of the recipient site. Obliteration of the scar will be enhanced by creating a geometric or w-plasty type margin at the leading edge of the flap, which will inset into a similar recipient margin. At removal of the expanders there will typically be a large amount of redundant tissue or folds of tissue, which will remain after the flap(s) has been inset (**Fig. 10**). These folds will settle with time. To assist in obliteration of the dead space under an advanced flap, a small drain and a pressure dressing should be placed and left in position for several days. All sutures should be absorbable, to avoid the messiness of removal from a tangle of matted hair in an anxious child.

Histologic changes

Tissue expansion has been shown to increase skin thickness through increased basal layer activity and net gain in donor tissue.[24] The deeper dermis decreases in thickness, and this is directly related to the rate and degree (amount) of expansion: the faster the rate and amount, the thinner the dermis becomes. Collagen bundles in the reticular interstitium become more parallel and thin as well.[24] Hair follicles become more sparsely spaced but the actual numbers remain the same. If there is rapid expansion, the phenomenon of hair shock may occur, with loss of hair, but the follicles remain viable and hair regrows after cessation of expansion. Lastly, expansion may stimulate melanocytic activity, resulting in hyperpigmentation of the overlying skin, particularly in darker pigmented children.[21]

Pitfalls and complications of expansion

Postoperative hematoma or seroma formation may be seen following expander placement. This shortcoming will usually be avoided if expander inflation is undertaken at the time of placement to sufficiently obliterate dead space and achieve some small measure of skin pressure and mechanical vascular compression, albeit minimal.

The underlying calvarium is prone to thinning under an expander in younger children, therefore less expansion volume should be undertaken at each visit if possible. Usually cortical thinning occurs with rapid and aggressive expansion.[19,20] Any "cupping" under an expander will resolve with time on removal. A plain radiograph taken at right angles to the expander will demonstrate any undue cortical thinning (risk of perforation); should

this occur, expansion should be halted for a period of time before reinflation.

A capsule nearly always forms around tissue expanders. The longer the expansion process, the greater the chance of capsule formation and the more dense it will become. If a capsule forms, this should be minimally excised at the base or periphery of the expander but not overlying the expander, as this may compromise the flap vascularity. Most capsules will flatten and remodel with time.[21]

Erosion of the overlying expanded skin is the most common complication of tissue expansion, either in the access incision site or through scarred and atrophic overlying tissue.[22] Exposure of the expander can usually be managed by withdrawing some fluid, placement of reinforcement or bolster sutures, and allowing a period of initial healing before reinflation, now at a slower pace. If this occurs late in the expansion process, the surgeon can proceed with plans to remove the expander and complete the reconstruction of the defect. Exposure of the implant reservoir early in the process will necessitate removal of the expander; after allowing for a period of healing, one then proceeds with another expander, probably in an area distant from the perforation. Undoubtedly this latter event and complication is the one that should be thoroughly reviewed with the parents before undertaking expansion, as the delay in reconstruction and prolongation of treatment is a discomfiture to all involved. Exposure of a buried injection port is of no worrisome consequence; with excellent hygiene measures expansion can take place accordingly, now through an external port.

Summary

Scalp repair and reconstruction in children is optimally addressed through careful and meticulous debridement of contaminated wounds, appropriate tissue cleansing, and approximation of wound margins, and the proper closure of the scalp in 2 layers with postoperative support dressings. Many avulsive scalp wounds also have a closed head injury component, and this needs to be addressed in the triage of the injured child. It is important to decompress an avulsive or degloving type of scalp wound to prevent hematoma/seroma formation and provide for tissue viability. For wounds that cannot be primarily closed the wound bed should be prepared for future tissue expansion, which will restore hair-bearing scalp in a normal pattern and appearance for the child.

PEDIATRIC SKULL FRACTURES

Infants and children are relatively more susceptible to head trauma than are adults, because of the disproportionate size of the cranium compared with the remainder of the facial skeleton. The cephalocaudal growth pattern of the face combines with the pneumatization of the sinuses and dental development to reverse this ratio in adulthood.[25] The overall number of pediatric craniofacial injuries is fewer than adult injuries, due to the normal sheltered environment that children live within. However, many of the most common causes are similar to those in the adult population and include falls, traffic accidents, violence, and play/sports-related injuries.[26] More obscure causes include intrauterine events, forceps or delivery trauma, and iatrogenic development following cranial surgery.

Growing Skull Fractures

Growing skull fracture (GSF), first described by John Howship in 1816,[27] is a rare complication following head trauma and consists of a widening fracture with associated neurologic sequelae. Development traditionally occurs as a result of significant cranial trauma with a resultant skull fracture, underlying dural tear, and intracranial injury.[28] However, GSFs can also occur less commonly following minor closed head injuries with minimally displaced linear fractures.[29] Reported incidence in the literature ranges from 0.05% to 1.6% of all skull fractures. This figure likely underestimates the occurrence rate when exclusively considering the pediatric population, as 90% of GSFs occur before age 3 years, and more than 50% occur before 12 months of age.[30]

The nature of the injury implies delayed presentation, which may involve several different health care providers, often several months following head trauma. High-risk patients who sustain clinically apparent fractures or immediate neurologic deficit are likely to undergo a period of initial hospitalization and radiographic evaluation. Following stabilization and resolution of cerebral edema, surgical exploration may be undertaken with dural repair, in the hope of preventing the development of a GSF.[31] Whether surgery has been undertaken or not, these patients are likely to be closely followed after hospital discharge, both clinically and radiographically, for development of complications.

In pediatric patients who have sustained less obvious trauma and are thought to be at low risk, the initial workup in the ER can be obfuscated by a limited neurologic examination and the general desire to limit radiation exposure. Vignes and colleagues[29] recommend that patients younger than 3 months with a presenting scalp hematoma undergo plain skull radiographic evaluation. Ultrasonography may also be an additional noninvasive adjunct for early diagnosis,[32] but its role has yet to be thoroughly delineated in the literature.

A triad of clinical and radiographic signs has been proposed by Thompson and colleagues[33] to include localized swelling, neurologic deficit, and fracture diastasis greater than 4 mm. The parietal region is the most common site of fracture.[28] Often a previously diagnosed scalp hematoma does not resolve, or slowly increases in size. In retrospect, a cephalohematoma with an underlying skull fracture was likely misdiagnosed. The presenting mass is normally pulsatile, and a cranial defect can normally be palpated; however, depression is also reported in the literature (**Fig. 11**).[28] Neurologic complications are commonly part of the presenting symptoms and include, but are not limited to, hemiparesis, seizure activity, and developmental delay.[34]

Plain skull radiographs may indicate an area of fracture diastases with scalloped edges if compared with prior images. CT imaging provides a more thorough evaluation. Demonstration of fracture maturation includes rounding of the edges as well as cranial erosion (**Fig. 12**). The presence of a leptomeningeal cyst or herniation of cerebral tissue, encephalomalacia, and ipsilateral ventricular dilation and porencephaly may also be detected. Magnetic resonance imaging (MRI) evaluation has helped to further delineate the underlying cerebral contusion and atrophy as well as demonstrate abnormal cerebrospinal fluid (CSF) flow and collection in the subcutaneous tissues that may be indirect evidence of dural tear (**Fig. 13**).[35]

Pathophysiology
The understanding of the pathophysiology of GSF has developed over time. In 1937, Dyke[36] first described a leptomeningeal cyst at the site of an expanding skull fracture. In 1953, Taveras and

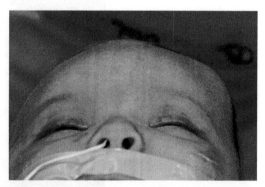

Fig.11. Preoperative photograph of an 8-month-old female child who previously fell from a changing table. She presented on referral from her pediatrician for evaluation of a left frontoparietal mass.

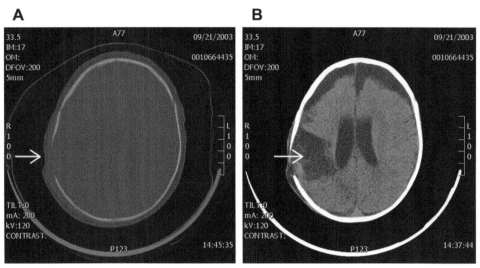

Fig. 12. Cranial CT images (*A*) bone windows demonstrating a widened skull fracture (*arrow*); (*B*) intracranial injury (*arrow*).

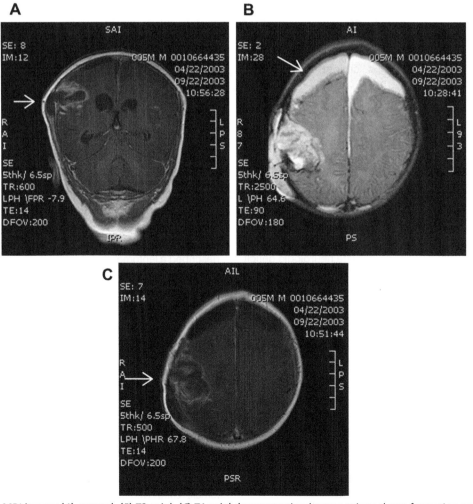

Fig. 13. MRI images (*A*) coronal, (*B*) T2 axial, (*C*) T1 axial demonstrating leptomeningeal cyst formation and cerebrospinal fluid collection (*arrows*).

Ransohoff[37] further suggested that the cyst formation was a result of CSF entrapment within arachnoid tissue at the fracture through a ball-valve mechanism. In 1970, Rosenthal and colleagues[38] definitively disproved this theory with the use of a canine model by using India ink injections to demonstrate a lack of communication between the cystic fluid and the CSF compartment. Furthermore, clinical observation has revealed the regular absence of associated cysts and the common presence of herniated brain tissue at the site of fracture.

Experimental studies have demonstrated that a tear in the dura is a requisite for formation of a GSF, and injury to the underlying pia and arachnoid increase the likelihood of development.[39,40] Although increased intracranial pressure has been suggested as an additional causative factor in the development and progression of GSF, contemporary MRI evaluation has cast doubt on this supposition because of the absence of radiographic indicators of increased intracranial pressure (transependymal flow, mass effect, and basilar cistern effacement). Physiologic CSF pulsations appear to produce a change in the normal flow patterns and subsequent pressure imbalance between the brain and skull caused by fracture. Rapid brain and skull growth appear to be predisposing characteristics, making the highest incidence of GSF found in pediatric patients; however, numerous case reports are found in the literature that cite occurrence in adult patients. Although there is some suggestion that these injuries may grow to a certain point and become stable,[41] this has generally been refuted by the findings of continued cranial asymmetry, fracture expansion, and neurologic deficit.

Neurologic injury is thought to be bimodal. Initial trauma is often associated with parenchymal contusion and bleeding. However, continued damage occurs secondary to changes in intracranial pressure distribution, cerebral herniation, leptomeningeal cyst formation, changes in CSF and blood flow dynamics, and surface trauma secondary to continued brain pulsation against the fractured skull edge.

Surgical treatment

The management of GSFs should be undertaken expeditiously after diagnosis, because of the likelihood of continued expansion. Treatment consists of surgical exploration, debridement of cystic tissue, management of herniated cerebral tissue, dural repair, and cranioplasty.[34]

Wide exposure is best carried out through incision away from the underlying mass (**Fig. 14**). Ideal exposure is completed with a partial or complete coronal incision modified in anterior-posterior location based on the location of the fracture. Detailed description of the recommended surgical technique is well delineated by Ruiz and colleagues.[42] Special

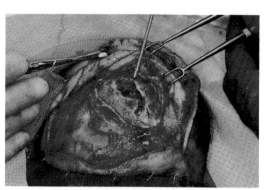

Fig. 14. Wide dissection away from and around the area of skull injury affords excellent exposure and reduces possible injury to the underlying dura and brain. Note the supraperiosteal and subperiosteal dissection. This approach also provides for access to uninvolved calvarium to obtain split grafts for reconstruction.

attention must be given to the dissection of the scalp directly over the skull defect, as cystic or herniated cerebral tissue may be directly adherent, especially in long-standing injuries.[43] Consideration of the desired plane of dissection should be based on the planned use of free or vascularized pericranial tissue for dural repair and coverage. Supraperiosteal dissection directly around the fracture margins is necessary to delineate the fracture anatomy. In general, there are areas of erosion and thinning surrounded by thicker sclerotic bone. This dissection should be continued circumferentially in a wide margin to provide enough exposure for the surrounding craniotomy. Burr holes should be placed at a distance from the fracture margin, and a wide bone flap is then turned to expose the edges of the retracted underlying dura (**Fig. 15**). Tissue protruding through the dural laceration may be cystic or herniated brain. Limited debridement and cauterization, especially of noted gliotic or granulated tissue, should be carried out to prevent

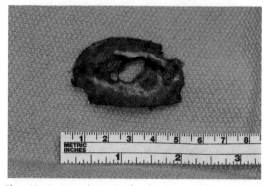

Fig. 15. Resected area of calvarium with expanded skull fracture. Note the areas of thickened and sclerotic margins at the fracture site.

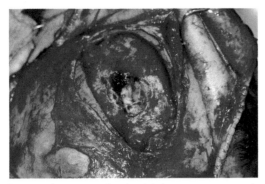

Fig. 16. The resected calvarial fracture exposes the underlying dural defect and injured brain tissue, which will be excised before definitive repair. Careful attention must be given to ensuring hemostasis after excision.

recurrence and rebleeding (**Fig. 16**). Intraoperative use of mannitol or furosemide may assist with brain decompression. Dural patching and closure is critical to success. Reconstruction can be carried out with autogenous pericranial tissue or allograft such as bovine pericardium (**Fig. 17**). Dural tacking sutures to the skull help to prevent epidural fluid collection and also help to stabilize the repair.

Skull reconstruction can be carried out in several ways depending on the size of the fracture,

extent of erosion, and age of the patient.[44] Because of the demographics of injury, treatment of GSF is commonly undertaken in young children, making the normal growth patterns of the brain, dura, and skull relevant in determining the reconstructive approach. Autogenous bone is the gold standard and split calvarial grafting remains the technique of choice. Bone graft can be obtained either by splitting a full-thickness bone flap or through removal of a portion of the outer cortex in situ. Both techniques may be challenging in children younger than 3 years, as there is limited bicortical development by this age. Semirigid fixation with biodegradable screws and mesh is easily accomplished, with minimal complications (**Fig. 18**). Because of the osteogenic potential of the dura in young children, small defects will likely heal but, at a minimum, the area of dural reconstruction should be completely covered (**Fig. 19**). Once children have reached the age of 7 years, the cranium is 95% developed and alloplastic materials may be used.

Perioperative CSF diversion may be helpful in the management of large fractures with significant herniation of the brain or tenuous dural reconstruction, but is not normally indicated in small fractures. The standardized use of perioperative antibiotics is recommended to minimize surgical-site infection and postoperative meningitis. A prolonged course may be considered in cases requiring significant reconstruction or implantation

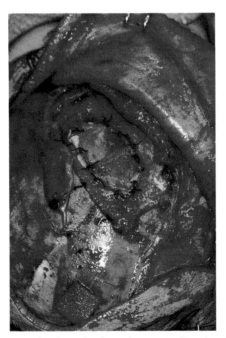

Fig. 17. A dural patch of autologous pericranium has been placed over the excised brain tissue and carefully sutured to the native dura to ensure a watertight closure and dural integrity. Note that the dura has been tacked to the undersurface of the calvarium to prevent fluid accumulation.

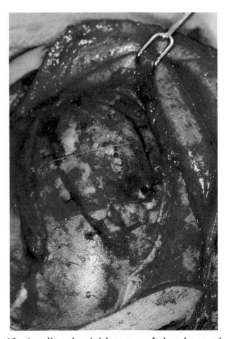

Fig. 18. A split calvarial bone graft has been placed over the defect and fixated with resorbable mesh plate.

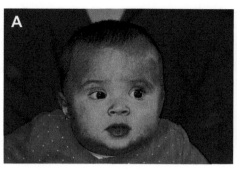
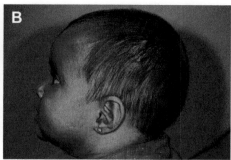

Fig. 19. Frontal (*A*) and lateral (*B*) postoperative photographs taken 2 months after surgical treatment. Note the postauricular position of the coronal incision used for exposure.

of alloplastic hardware and materials. Steroid use is also suggested to assist in the limitation of intracranial and extracranial edema. Seizure prophylaxis is not normally indicated, but may be considered based on the preoperative history as well as the extent of debridement of brain tissue.

Recurrence of GSF following contemporary treatment is rarely reported, but is thought to be associated with incomplete duraplasty.[45] Reoperation may be necessary for persistent cranial defects, removal of alloplastic materials, or residual cosmetic deformities of the bone or scalp. General improvement in neurologic symptoms is reported in pediatric patients following early diagnosis and surgical treatment of GSF.[46] However, the majority of the literature comprises highly variable surgical case studies without detailed preoperative and postoperative neurologic documentation, making prognosis difficult to predict.

Summary

GSF is an uncommon complication of head trauma primarily found in young children. Delayed presentation of a widening fracture, a pulsatile mass, and neurologic symptoms are highly suggestive. CT and MRI are important adjunctive tools in the evaluation of this process. Treatment is undertaken shortly after diagnosis to prevent further progression, and involves wide craniotomy exposure, cerebral debridement, dural repair or reconstruction, and primary autologous cranioplasty.

ACKNOWLEDGMENTS

The authors thank Ramon L. Ruiz, DMD, MD, Greg Olavarria, MD, and John H. Schmidt III, MD, FACS.

REFERENCES

1. NTDB Annual Pediatric Report. 2010. American College of Surgeons. Available at: www.facs.org/trauma/AnnPedReport2010. Accessed January 5, 2012.

2. Available at: http://cdc.gov/ncipc/factsheet/children.htm. Accessed January 5, 2012.

3. Smith JL. Treatment of severe pediatric head injury: evidence-based practice. In: Wesson DE, editor. Pediatric trauma. Pathophysiology, diagnosis and treatment. New York: Taylor and Francis; 2006. p. 211.

4. DaDalt L, Marchi AG, Laudizi L, et al. Predictors of intracranial injuries in children after blunt head trauma. Eur J Pediatr 2006;165(3):142–8.

5. Hoffman JF. Management of scalp defects. Otolaryngol Clin North Am 2001;34:571–9.

6. CDC. Updated recommendations for use of tetanus toxoid reduced diphtheria toxoid and Tdap from the Advisory Committee on Immunization Practices. 2010. MMWR Morb Mortal Wkly Rep 2011;60:13–5.

7. Matthaiou D, Peppas G, Falagas ME. Meta-analysis on surgical infections. Infect Dis Clin North Am 2009; 23(2):405–30.

8. Cox SC Jr. Trauma from child abuse. In: Wesson DE, editor. Pediatric trauma. Pathophysiology, diagnosis and treatment. New York: Taylor and Francis; 2006. p. 73–82.

9. Billmire ME, Myers PA. Serious head injury in infants: accident or abuse? Pediatrics 1985;75:340–2.

10. Mason AC, Zabel DD, Manders EK. Occult craniocerebral injuries from dog bites in young children. Ann Plast Surg 2000;45(5):531–4.

11. Hutchinson J, Guergueria AM. Head trauma: medical management. In: Mikrogianakis A, Valani R, editors. Manual of pediatric trauma. The Hospital for Sick Children. New York: Lippincott, Williams and Wilkins; 2008. p. 61–8.

12. Hespenthal DR, Green AD, Crouch HK, et al. Infection prevention and control in deployed military medical facilities. J Trauma 2011;71(Suppl 2): S290–8.

13. Lee S, Rafii A, Sykes J. Advances in scalp reconstruction. Curr Opin Otolaryngol Head Neck Surg 2006;14(4):249–53.

14. Dickson L, Kattan A, Thoma A. Two-technique reconstruction following traumatic scalp avulsion: Replantation and composite graft. Plast Reconstr Surg 2010;125(4):151e–2e.

15. Earnest LM, Byrne PJ. Scalp reconstruction. Facial Plast Surg Clin North Am 2005;13(2):345–53.

16. Iida N, Ohsumi N, Tonegawa M, et al. Reconstruction of scalp defects using simple designed bilobed flap. Aesthetic Plast Surg 2000;24(2):137–40.

17. Seline PC, Siegle RJ. Scalp reconstruction. Dermatol Clin 2005;23:13–21.

18. Hoffman JF. Reconstruction of the scalp. In: Baker SR, editor. Local flaps in facial reconstruction. Philadelphia: Elsevier. Mosby; 2007. p. 637–63.

19. Schmelzeisen R, Schimming R, Schwipper V, et al. Influence of tissue expanders on the growing craniofacial skeleton. J Craniomaxillofac Surg 1999;27:153–9.

20. Keith AH, Heather R, John GM. Pediatric cervicofacial tissue expansion. Int J Pediatr Otorhinolaryngol 2005;69:21–5.

21. Swanson RW. Controlled tissue expansion in facial reconstruction. In: Baker SR, editor. Local flaps in facial reconstruction. Philadelphia: Elsevier. Mosby; 2007. p. 667–89.

22. Gibney J. Tissue expansion in reconstructive surgery. ASPRS Annual Scientific Meeting. Las Vegas, May 7-10, 1984.

23. van Rappard JH, Sonneveld GJ, Borghouts JM. Geometric planning and the shape of the expander. Facial Plast Surg 1988;5:280–7.

24. van Rappard JH, Molenaar J, van Doorn K, et al. Surface area increase in tissue expansion. Plast Reconstr Surg 1988;82(5):833–9.

25. Chan J, Putnam MA, Feustel PJ, et al. The age dependent relationship between facial fractures and skull fractures. Int J Pediatr Otorhinolaryngol 2004;68(7):877–81.

26. Eggensperger NM, Holzle A, Zachariou Z, et al. Pediatric craniofacial trauma. J Oral Maxillofac Surg 2008; 66(1):58–64.

27. Howship J. Practical observations in surgery and morbid anatomy. London: Longman; 1816.

28. Muhonen MG, Piper JG, Menezes AH. Pathogenesis and treatment of growing skull fractures. Surg Neurol 1995;43(4):367–72 [discussion: 372–3].

29. Vignes JR, Jeelani NU, Jeelani A, et al. Growing skull fracture after minor closed-head injury. J Pediatr 2007;151(3):316–8.

30. Lende RA, Erickson TC. Growing skull fractures of childhood. J Neurosurg 1961;18:479–89.

31. Sanford RA. Prevention of growing skull fractures: report of 2 cases. J Neurosurg Pediatr 2010;5(2):213–8.

32. Djientcheu V, Njamnshi AK, Ongolo-Zogo P, et al. Growing skull fractures. Childs Nerv Syst 2006; 22(7):721–5.

33. Thompson JB, Mason TH, Haines GL, et al. Surgical management of diastatic linear skull fractures in infants. J Neurosurg 1973;39:493–7.

34. Yu M, Schmidt J, Trenton BA, et al. Growing skull fracture in a 5-month old child: a case report. W V Med J 2010;106(2):12–6.

35. Husson B, Pariente D, Tammam S, et al. The value of MRI in the early diagnosis of growing skull fracture. Pediatr Radiol 1996;26(10):744–7.

36. Dyke CG. The roentgen ray diagnosis of diseases of the skull and intracranial contents. In: Golden W, editor. Diagnostic roentgenology. Baltimore (MD): Williams and Wilkins; 1938. p. 1–34.

37. Taveras J, Ransohoff J. Leptomeningeal cysts of the brain following trauma with erosion of the skull: a study of seven cases treated by surgery. J Neurosurg 1953;10:233–41.

38. Rosenthal SA, Grieshop J, Freeman LM, et al. Experimental observations on enlarging skull fractures. J Neurosurg 1970;32(4):431–4.

39. Keener EB. An experimental study of reactions of the dura matter to wounding and loss of substance. J Neurosurg 1959;16:424–47.

40. Goldstein F, Sakoda T, Kepes JJ, et al. Enlarging skull fractures: an experimental study. J Neurosurg 1967;27:541–50.

41. Ramamurthi B, Kalyanaraman S. Rationale for surgery in growing fractures of the skull. J Neurosurg 1970;32:427–30.

42. Ruiz RL, Pattisapu JV, Costello BJ, et al. The coronal scalp flap: surgical technique. Atlas Oral Maxillofac Surg Clin North Am 2010;18(2):69–75.

43. Singhal A, Steinbok P. Operative management of growing skull fractures: a technical note. Childs Nerv Syst 2008;24(5):605–7.

44. Jaskolka MS, Olavarria G. Reconstruction of skull defects. Atlas Oral Maxillofac Surg Clin North Am 2010;18(2):139–49.

45. Naim-Ur-Rahman, Jamjoom Z, Jamjoom A, et al. Growing skull fractures: classification and management. Br J Neurosurg 1994;8(6):667–79.

46. Pezzotta S, Silvani V, Gaetani P, et al. Growing skull fractures of childhood. Case report and review of 132 cases. J Neurosurg Sci 1985; 29(2):129–35.

Facial Skeletal Trauma in the Growing Patient

Christopher Morris, DDS, MD[a],
George M. Kushner, DMD, MD[b],
Paul S. Tiwana, DDS, MD, MS[c],*

KEYWORDS

- Pediatric • Skeletal facial trauma • Rehabilitative physiotherapy • Craniofacial trauma

KEY POINTS

- Appreciate the anatomy and physiology unique to pediatric patients.
- Understand the potential implications of surgical insult on future growth and development.
- Emphasize the importance of early rehabilitative physiotherapy on future growth and function.

INTRODUCTION

The management of maxillofacial trauma has changed over time. These changes are caused by the evolving complexity of injuries secondary to higher-impact mechanisms and advances in imaging, instrumentation, and fixation. The greatest influence on surgical management of pediatric craniomaxillofacial disease likely came from the contribution of Dr Paul Tessier[1] in his principles of cranio-orbital surgery first introduced in 1967.[1] Others have additionally provided the many operative principles of maxillofacial trauma used today, such as the sequencing of panfacial injuries, autogenous bone grafting, and the important role of rigid fixation in re-establishing facial height, width, and projection.[1–3] These principles have provided the fundamental underpinnings of modern facial fracture treatment. More recently, these principles that work so well in adult patients have been applied in the management of pediatric maxillofacial trauma. Posnick and Kaban[4–7] have more clearly described the epidemiology and further clarified the advantages of rigid internal fixation for these injuries.[1,4–7]

The current understanding of complex facial injuries has primarily been through the observation of adult patients. However, one must recognize that the treatment of pediatric patients requires additional considerations and that the application of adult-type treatment can be inappropriate in many circumstances. There is still a place for conservatism in the treatment of craniomaxillofacial injuries in children.

The maxillofacial trauma surgeon will best serve pediatric patients with a combination of age-appropriate sensitivity and a fundamental understanding of the complex issues surrounding the growth of the craniofacial skeleton and the potential for traumatic and surgical injury to negatively alter it.

GENERAL CONSIDERATIONS
Craniofacial Growth and Development

The role of the human face is significant, both functionally and esthetically. This role is secondary to the highly evolved and specialized functions of the face in vision, breathing, mastication, speech, smell, and hearing, among others. Indeed, it is the culmination of an extremely complex process of growth and development that provides the functional and aesthetic framework of the human face. Interruption of this process, such as insult from maxillofacial injury, may produce deleterious

[a] Division of Oral & Maxillofacial Surgery, UT Southwestern Medical Center, Dallas, TX, USA; [b] Department of Surgical & Hospital Dentistry, The University of Louisville, Louisville, KY, USA; [c] Pediatric Oral & Maxillofacial Surgery, Children's Medical Center, UT Southwestern Medical Center, Dallas, TX, USA
* Corresponding author.
E-mail address: paul.tiwana@utsouthwestern.edu

Oral Maxillofacial Surg Clin N Am 24 (2012) 351–364
doi:10.1016/j.coms.2012.05.005
1042-3699/12/$ – see front matter © 2012 Elsevier Inc. All rights reserved.

alterations of the facial framework resulting in aesthetic and functional deficits. For the surgeon who treats pediatric facial fractures, an understanding of this process becomes crucial in developing and exercising sound surgical judgment.[8–10]

The cranial vault at birth is comprised of flat plates of intramembranous bone separated by connective tissue. The interposing areas or sutures allow for the deformation of the head through the pelvis during delivery and then to accommodate rapid brain growth during the first year of life. This process is largely accomplished through the apposition of bone at the sutural areas and, to a lesser degree, remodeling of the inner and outer cortex of the skull. Head circumference reaches greater than 90% of its adult size between 3 and 5 years of age. In contrast, the bones of the skull base are formed from areas of endochondral ossification. In between these areas of ossification, synchondroses are formed that continue to allow for growth through the replacement of cartilage with bone. The orbit, although comprised of numerous bones, reaches skeletal maturity between the ages of 5 and 7 years. This growth mirrors the growth of the soft tissue orbital contents. The midface is comprised of intramembranous bone and its growth vector is downward and forward, which is propelled by the apposition of bone at the cranial base and deep sutures of the maxilla and remodeling of the surface of the midface. The mandible, on the other hand, has both a component of endochondral ossification at the temporomandibular joint regions bilaterally and remodeling and apposition of bone in the corpus. The mandibular body and alveolus again follows the downward and forward vector of movement the midface takes, but the rami and condyles grow upward and backward to maintain contact with the skull base. Vertical height is gained at the condyle through endochondral replacement and length is added through an active remodeling of the ramus. Skeletal maturity of the maxilla and mandible is reached by approximately 14 to 16 years of age in girls and 16 to 18 years of age in boys.[11,12]

The functional matrix concept of growth first proposed by Moss has gained general acceptance.[13–16] This theory postulates that growth occurs as a result of expanding functional requirements of the cranial, nasal, and oral cavities and that these requirements are transmitted to the bone and cartilage by the soft tissue envelope of the face. The bones grow in response to the expansion of the cranial and facial capsule. The nasal septum and mandibular condyles *react* to growth requirements and, therefore, should not be considered the primary centers of growth. Therefore, surgical attention in managing injuries of the

mandibular condyle, for example, should be directed at preserving as scar-free an envelope of soft tissue as possible and promoting function of the joint. The application of this theory to other craniofacial problems leads to similar conclusions. A classic example of the influence of the soft tissue envelope on growth resides in patients with cleft palates. Maxillary growth restriction in these patients is the result of scarring from palatal surgery. The cleft palate itself, if left unoperated until skeletal maturity, would have little to no effect on maxillary growth.[17] The importance of understanding the deleterious effects of scar tissue, traumatically or surgically induced, and the restricted function on growth and development is fundamental to the management of children with facial fractures.

Surgical Anatomy

Critical examination of the stages of gross anatomic craniofacial development leads to several particular issues that have an impact on the epidemiology and management of facial bone injuries in children (**Fig. 1**). First, during infancy and early childhood, rapid brain and ocular growth causes a significant increase in cranio-orbital dimensions as noted in the previous discussion regarding growth and development. This increase provides for the characteristic appearance of the prominent forehead and orbits seen in infancy and early childhood. The later-maturing lower facial skeleton remains protected behind a prominent forehead during this period, therefore, this region is more exposed and prone to injury. During the early years of development, bone has a high osteogenic potential and is characterized by a thick medullary space and thin bony cortices that tend to greenstick fracture. Unerupted teeth also tend to buttress fractures and prevent fracture displacement. In addition, the eruption of the permanent teeth in conjunction with loose exfoliating primary teeth makes maxillomandibular wiring and fracture reduction and stabilization more difficult. The paranasal sinuses also continue to pneumatize and expand, which may alter fracture patterns in the midfacial skeleton secondary to decreased bone bulk and brittleness (**Fig. 2**).[18] As the permanent dentition erupts at about 12 years of age and growth continues into adolescence, the craniofacial skeleton becomes more adultlike. During this stage of development, adultlike surgical management becomes increasingly more appropriate.

Epidemiology

It has been estimated that 11.3% of all pediatric emergency department visits are the result of pediatric maxillofacial injury.[19] Overall, children

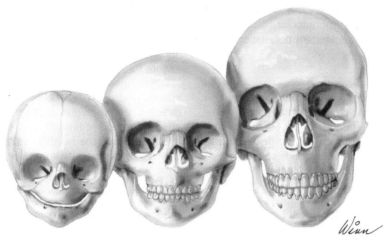

Fig. 1. Growth of the facial skeleton from early childhood to adulthood.

have a lower incidence of facial injury than adults. For the most part, they reside in a protective social environment. In the early years of life, parental supervision and a child-friendly environment mitigate the likelihood of serious injury. Although falls during these years are common, a low center of gravity ensures that little harmful force is generated that might cause injury. As they reach the later childhood years, children become involved in numerous activities, such as school and play with other peers. Participation in athletic activity later in life is also a cause of facial injury proximate to a developing neuromuscular coordination system and decreased situational awareness.

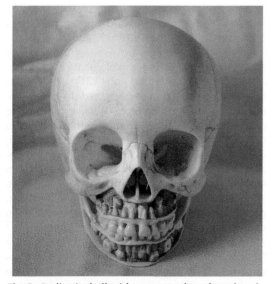

Fig. 2. Pediatric skull with unerupted teeth and undeveloped paranasal sinuses.

Balls, hockey pucks and sticks, lacrosse sticks, bats, elbows, and knees are all commonly cited as the cause of pediatric facial injuries during athletic events, especially when the appropriate personal protective equipment is not worn.

There have been several excellent studies regarding the epidemiology of pediatric facial trauma. Posnick and colleagues[6,7,20] reviewed 137 pediatric patients with facial fractures; most of the patients were boys, and the largest group of patients was found in the 6- to 12-year age range. The most common cause of trauma was motor-vehicle related, followed by falls, sports injuries, and interpersonal violence. Mandibular fractures composed most of the injuries (55%), followed by orbital fractures (30%), dentoalveolar fractures (23%), midface fractures (17%), nasal fractures (15%), complex fractures (14%), and cranial fractures (6%). Among the reported mandibular fractures, condyle fractures were the most common, followed by the symphyseal region, the body, and the angle of the mandible.[6,7,20] However, the incidence will naturally vary geographically depending on multiple factors. In addition, many more minor injuries, such as nasal and dentoalveolar fractures, are likely underreported because they can be commonly managed on an outpatient basis. There were no cervical spine injuries in this study. In a recent, large, epidemiologic study of more than 12,000 pediatric fractures over 4 years, Imahara and colleagues[21] recorded in the National Trauma Data Bank the common mechanisms of injury as motor vehicle collision (55.1%), violence (11.8%), and falls (8.6%). The most common fractures were the mandible (32.7%), nasal bones (30.2%), and maxillary bones/zygoma (28.6%). Toddlers and infants are more likely to experience midfacial and cranial injuries, and mandibular fractures are more common in the adolescent population.

Prevention

As previously noted, children are ensconced in a well-protected social environment with close adult supervision during their early years. However, as they begin to engage in social and athletic activity, their exposure to situations in which injury might occur heightens. The use of personal protective equipment is critical to lowering the incidence of facial injuries in children. Specifically included is the use of helmets, face shields, and mouth guards during sports play. Protective equipment during noncontact activities, such as bicycling and skateboarding, is equally important. Recently, there has been significant social momentum to change the composition of playground equipment and the surfaces of athletic fields to further lessen the chance of injury. Adults supervising children, either indirectly or directly, engaged in these activities must assume the responsibility of ensuring that appropriate safety equipment is used.

Perhaps the single most important factor in reducing the incidence of pediatric trauma overall is the correct mandatory use of seat belts and safety seats in vehicles for infants and children. According to recommendations from the National Highway Traffic Safety Administration (NHTSA), a rear-facing seat in the back seat of a vehicle should be used until 1 year of age and the attainment of at least 20 pounds. Car seats facing forward in the back should then be used until 4 years of age and the attainment of 40 pounds. Newer recommendations with a campaign for public awareness from the NHTSA have been advocated for children aged 4 to 8 years and at least 4 ft 9 in tall to be secured in a booster seat with a seat belt in the rear of the vehicle. The common use of air bag restraint systems in the modern vehicle is a concern for any child younger than 10 years of age seated in the front seat. Deployed air bags during a collision may apply tremendous forces to the cervical and chest regions of young children, with reports of severe injuries and fatalities sustained after being struck by an air bag.[22]

All-terrain vehicles (ATV), especially in rural areas, also represent a significant potential for maxillofacial injury in the pediatric population.[23] Little federal or state regulation exists for the operation of these motorized vehicles, and older children with little to no experience and questionable judgment are often operating these vehicles. Risk-taking behavior in youth, particularly adolescent boys, places them at an increased risk for serious injury with ATV and motorcycle use. Close adult supervision and responsibility is critical to ensure that safety measures are followed.

Other areas of focus regarding prevention include the alarming incidence of gun violence directed at or involving children.[24] Educational efforts directed at firearm safety in the home and at schools and the heightened awareness of the public to this issue are important.

Perioperative Management

A meticulous treatment plan must be designed for the examination, resuscitation, and intraoperative and postoperative care of pediatric patients with maxillofacial injuries. Children in general have tremendous resiliency to stress from surgical procedures but they are not tolerant of inappropriate fluid and drug administration. Delays in the evaluation and management of major trauma are thought to contribute to approximately 30% of early deaths in seriously injured children, making thorough and expedient triage and management crucial.[25]

Surgical preoperative management begins with the initial examination. The physical examination and history is not significantly different than in adult patients with the exception that much of the history must be obtained from the parents or other caretakers. Gaining cooperation for the physical examination can be difficult, especially with children shortly after experiencing a traumatic injury. Gentle examination with encouragement from the child's parents is usually sufficient. Examination under general anesthesia or sedation should be approached with caution during initial management because this may obfuscate neurologic injury. In addition, because of the difficulty with movement during radiological procedures, such as computed tomography (CT) scans, sedation or anesthesia maybe necessary to ensure the diagnostic value of the study obtained. In severe pediatric maxillofacial trauma, particularly when central nervous system involvement is suspected, CT is the preferred method of radiographic evaluation.[26] In the management of the injured child in extremis, adherence to the prescribed trauma life support algorithm is mandatory. In addition, specific pediatric protocols exist for the evaluation of possible cervical spine injury in children.[27,28] Although airway embarrassment secondary to craniomaxillofacial trauma in children is uncommon, airway preservation with adequate respiratory exchange must be maintained. Intubation is preferred if there is any question of airway integrity. Also, cricothyroidotomy for surgical maintenance of the airway is contraindicated in children less than 12 years of age because of the risk of subglottic stenosis.[29,30]

Hypothermia in trauma resuscitation of children is common, therefore, elevated room temperature, patient warming devices, and warmed normal saline is recommended for the initial resuscitation. Rapid intravenous access can be challenging in pediatric patients making intraosseous or central access more commonplace. In situations with major volume loss, the surgeon should seek to resuscitate the child with 20 mL/kg boluses of appropriate crystalloid fluids in a 3 mL to 1 mL ratio to blood loss. If subsequent blood transfusions are required, these are generally administered in 10- to 20-mL/kg increments. In addition, as a result of the smaller amount of intravascular volume, the surgeon should be cognizant that coagulopathy is more likely with massive transfusion. Acidosis is a particularly ominous sign in children that reflects inadequate tissue perfusion and should be managed early and aggressively. Maintenance intravenous fluids should be calculated using the 4-2-1 rule: 4 mL/kg/h for the first 10 kg of weight, 2 mL/kg/h for the second 11 to 20 kg of weight, followed by 1 mL/kg/h for each additional kilogram of weight thereafter. Maintenance fluids in babies and toddlers are usually given as one-quarter normal saline with dextrose; one-half normal saline should be reserved for older children and teenagers. Urine output is normally 1 to 2 mL/kg/h in the child and should be recorded to ensure adequate volume. The importance of weight-based administration and monitoring of fluids and medications in pediatric patients cannot be overemphasized.

CRANIOFACIAL FRACTURES
Frontal Bone and Superior Orbital Fractures

As a result of rapid brain growth in infancy, the upper third of the facial skeleton remains prominent in early childhood. For this reason, injury to this anatomic region is a common fracture pattern. Neurosurgical and ophthalmologic concerns must come first before the management of the facial bone injuries. Operative intervention for neurologic injury, such as repair of dural tears, should be viewed by the craniomaxillofacial trauma surgeon as an opportunity to collaborate with the neurosurgeon and simultaneously reduce and stabilize the fractured segments. In the absence of a cerebrospinal fluid (CSF) leak and significant displacement of the fractured segments, frontal bone injuries can be conservatively managed in a closed fashion without significant functional or aesthetic sequelae.

As a rule of thumb, the displacement of the anterior cranial vault or superior orbital rim by the full-thickness width of the bone involved is a reasonable indication that there will be postinjury aesthetic concerns prompting the need for operative intervention. Growing skull fracture is a unique entity of calvarial fracture in young children, which is caused by the herniation of the leptomeninges or brain at the site of dural tears. Despite normal intracranial pressure, brain swelling and subsequent growth and CSF pulsations allow calvarial displacement along the fracture (or sutural) seam. Formal cranioplasty may be necessary for the repair of the defect, and definitive neurosurgical care is required for management of herniated brain tissue.

The disruption of the orbital roof causing direct contact of the dura with the periorbita is a significant concern. If left untreated, this may cause orbital pulsations and potentially increase intraorbital pressure. The roof itself is thin, especially in the young child, and is often not amenable to fixation even with a large fracture segment. Reconstruction of the roof with split calvarial grafts (children with a developed diploe) remains the gold standard for treatment.

Frontal Sinus and Fronto-Basilar Injuries

The frontal sinus, which begins as a cephalic evagination of the middle meatus, develops around 1 to 2 years of age. Radiographically, it becomes visible around 6 to 7 years of age and continues to expand into early adulthood. The management of these injuries in children when the sinus is present is similar to adult patients and is most often dictated by neurosurgical concerns. For posterior table fractures with dural tears, cranialization is the treatment of choice. Every effort must be made to seal the anterior cranial fossa at the conclusion of these craniofacial approaches to prevent a CSF leak and minimize the risk of postoperative meningitis. The placement of a pericranial flap with autogenous bone as necessary and fibrin glue on the anterior skull base is an effective maneuver to isolate the anterior fossa from the ethmoids and nasal cavity (**Fig. 3**). Osteomyelitis of the skull in children is a rare postoperative complication but can have devastating consequences. Maintaining the sterility and integrity of the operative field is of paramount importance. For anterior table fractures, simple elevation and stabilization is appropriate. Sinus preservation is preferred in children, therefore, sinus obliteration is generally not undertaken, particularly with the advent of the endoscopic control of sinus disease should that eventuate

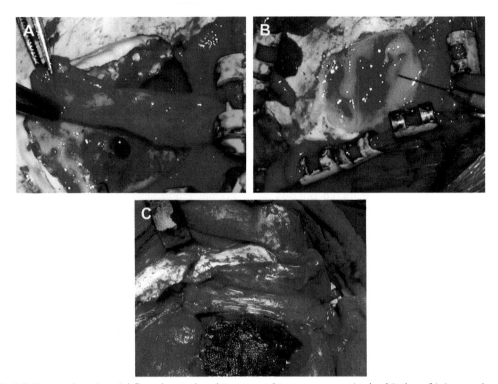

Fig. 3. (*A*) Temporal pericranial flap elevated and transposed to cover a repaired orbital roof injury and cranialized frontal sinus. (*B*) Fibrin tissue glue placed over the pericranial flap and repaired dura. (*C*) Temporal pericranial flap secured in place before closure.

after injury. The follow-up with serial CT scans to rule out pathologic conditions and demonstrate sinus function is mandatory.

Naso-Orbito-Ethmoid Fractures

The management of naso-orbito-ethmoid (NOE) fractures in children is similar to adult patients. Ophthalmology consultation is essential to rule out injury to the globe and assess vision. Sedation or assessment in the operating theater may be necessary to adequately evaluate lacrimal integrity. If the fractures extend into the anterior cranial fossa, neurosurgical consultation should also be obtained. If sinus drainage is compromised by bone displacement, the reduction and restoration of nasofrontal drainage is necessary. For the most part, when there is minimal displacement of the medial canthus and medial orbital fractures, NOE fractures in children can be managed in a closed fashion with one caveat: the nasal reduction must be stable. If the nose can be reduced, but will not stay elevated or cannot be reduced, internal fixation is necessary. If the nasal reduction is stable, the use of a nasal cast to compress the tissues medially and maintain the nasal reduction

is usually all that is required. Rarely, the reduction of the impacted fractures will allow for CSF leakage from the previously injured anterior cranial fossa and will necessitate open reduction.

Open reduction and internal fixation of NOE fractures should be performed through a coronal incision or through an overlying laceration. Severe comminution of the nose is uncommon but, when present, requires strut bone grafts harvested from the calvarium or ribs and placed on the dorsum to help prevent posttraumatic saddle nose deformity. It is unusual to see avulsion of the medial canthal tendon because usually it is attached to a significant fragment of bone. Care must be taken not to strip the canthal attachment from the fragment. This practice will allow the surgeon to reduce and plate the fracture and, thus, reposition the tendon. Many have found that recreating the pretrauma contour of this region is extremely difficult and it becomes even more troublesome if formal wire canthopexy is performed. Meticulous attention should be paid to the anatomic reduction of the fracture segment. Even when internal fixation is used for operative treatment, the placement of a nasal cast to compress the overlying stripped soft tissues in place is helpful in controlling nasal width and recreating contour of the soft tissue in the region between the nose and the lacrimal lake on each side.

Orbital Fractures

Fractures of the orbit are common in children because of its anterior projection and size. Ophthalmologic consultation is recommended to rule out ocular injury and assess vision. Vision, pupillary responses, and movement should be recorded and rechecked. Proper intraocular examination of the globe in children requires specialty-level skill and experience for accurate diagnosis. CT scans (axial, coronal, and sagittal views) is required to properly evaluate the extent of fractures, particularly those that extend posteriorly to the orbital apex. Fractures that seem to approach the optic canal should be studied with 1-mm coronal cuts to properly evaluate canal integrity and possible optic neurovascular compromise. If there are fractures involving the optic canal area and visual compromise is recorded, neurosurgical consultation with a view toward canal decompression or administration of corticosteroids or acetazolamide to control swelling and decrease intracranial/orbital pressure should be given consideration.

Surgical access to the orbit is the same as adult patients. Overlying lacerations, if present and appropriately positioned, should be used if possible. From an aesthetic standpoint, a transconjunctival approach to the orbit remains particularly appealing. If the treatment of the orbital fracture is combined with other upper facial fractures, access to the superior, medial, and lateral walls can be achieved through the coronal incision. Blow-in fractures of the orbit may result in increased intraocular pressure and cause permanent visual compromise. In addition, sharp fragments of bone protruding into the periorbital tissue should be identified and removed. The exploration and reduction of these fractures should proceed as rapidly as possible.[31] Blowout orbital fractures in children should be managed conservatively and nonoperatively in the case of minimal displacement, excellent globe mobility, and no ophthalmologic indications. Late enophthalmos rarely occurs in children with minimal orbital wall blowout. In the setting of significant disruption of the orbital floor or inferior orbital rim, the exploration and reduction of the fractures is necessary. The rare instance of true muscle entrapment should be regarded as a surgical emergency in children (**Fig. 4**). Bony entrapment of the inferior rectus muscle can cause scarring, and shortening of the muscle leads to permanent restriction of ocular motility. Eye muscle repair of

this problem is extremely difficult and has limited success. As in adults, the correction of late enophthalmos is challenging and requires overcorrection with orbital grafts, which is generally undertaken as soon as the condition is diagnosed.

The reconstruction of the skeletally immature orbit should be performed with autogenous bone grafts. Although somewhat controversial, resorbable mesh can also be used to restore orbital volume, with or without bone grafts (**Fig. 5**). After 7 years of age, the orbit is generally of adult size and development and reconstruction can be achieved with the use of several different materials, including autogenous bone; titanium mesh; or implants, such as porous polyethylene.

Zygomaticomaxillary Complex Fractures

Fractures of the malar or zygomaticomaxillary (ZMC) complex are uncommon in children but increase in adolescence because of sports and violence. High-velocity injuries generally result in the ZMC unit being fractured or comminuted. Minimally displaced fractures with little or no loss of facial projection and no ophthalmologic concerns should be conservatively managed. Fractures that require reduction and fixation may be accessed through inferior and superior orbital incisions and transconjunctival and transoral approaches. From an aesthetic viewpoint, the transconjunctival and upper blepharoplasty approaches are preferred. Less commonly, access through a coronal incision is required for severely comminuted fractures. Coronal access also provides for calvarial harvest if desired.

Fixation at 2 points is usually adequate for stabilization in children with ZMC fractures (**Fig. 6**). Caution must be exercised when placing internal fixation at the zygomaticomaxillary buttress area in younger children to prevent screw placement in unerupted teeth. In addition, wide stripping of the periosteal envelope should be limited in the immature skeleton to avoid possible adverse consequences of periosteal scarring and inhibition of future growth.

Nasal Fractures

Nasal fractures in children are fairly common. Their incidence is underreported because a significant number of parents seek outpatient care through direct referral at the time of injury. Plain film radiographic examination of the fracture may be all that is necessary if there is no suspicion of additional fractures or a lack of unusual findings on clinical examination. Intranasal inspection with a speculum must be performed to rule out the deviation or distortion of the nasal septum, with a particular

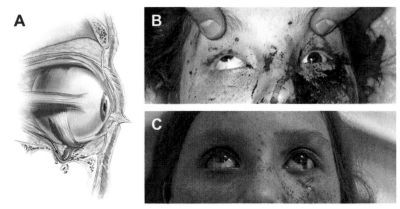

Fig. 4. (*A*) Blowout fracture of the orbital floor demonstrating entrapment. (*B*) Child with orbital floor fracture in central gaze. (*C*) Upward elevation reveals entrapment on the left side. (*From* Fonseca RJ, Marciani RD, Turvey TA. Oral and Maxillofacial Surgery, 2nd edition. Figure 20–4. p. 360; with permission [*A*].)

focus on the identification of a septal hematoma if present. Hematomas must be evacuated and the septum stabilized with compressive stents to support the cartilage, eliminate dead space and blood reaccumulation, and provide for perichondrial healing (**Fig. 7**). The nose is inspected for symmetry and projection; if displacement is present, closed reduction is performed. The surgeon should alert the parents to the possibility of growth disturbance of the midface and the potential for nasal stenosis or obstruction and emphasize the need for long-term follow up.

As mentioned previously, most pediatric nasal fractures are managed in a closed fashion with nasal splints or cast. Unfortunately, for many surgeons, closed reductions of nasal fractures in children are perfunctory procedures and consequently have less-than-ideal outcomes. The aesthetic component becomes extremely important to self-esteem as the child moves into adolescence and the management of these injuries requires strict attention to detail. A custom-molded splint or cast is indispensable in properly supporting the reduced nose and stabilizing the fracture. If the reduction is not adequate and there is residual deformity after healing, selected

and focused nasal surgery may be undertaken during growth; however, most nasal deformities should be deferred to adolescence when formal rhinoplasty can be performed more safely.

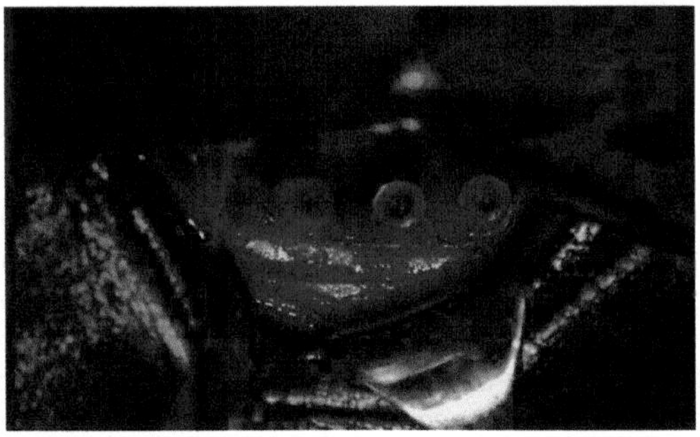

Midface Fractures

Facial fractures in children that involve the midface are uncommon. In early childhood, the midface is protected by a prominent forehead, it is small compared with the other skeletal units, and there is little sinus development. The sinuses begin to accelerate their development after 6 years of age, with the further downward and forward growth of the maxilla as the mixed dentition erupts.

The treatment of minimally displaced midface fractures in children is closed reduction with maxillomandibular fixation. Fractures with significant malocclusion or displacement are often associated with other injuries and usually require open reduction with rigid or semirigid internal fixation. The surgeon must be careful to not injure the developing dentition with screw placement at the Le Fort I level when internal fixation is used. In extreme cases of buttress comminution and facial foreshortening, bone grafts may need to be placed to assist in restoring facial height and projection.

MANDIBULAR AND DENTOALVEOLAR FRACTURES
Dentoalveolar Fractures

Fractures of the alveolar segment represent a true bony fracture of the jaws and must be considered as such even though teeth are contained in the mobile segment.[32,33] These fractures remain common in children and, like nasal fractures, are likely underreported because they are usually managed in the emergency department or dental office as outpatients.

Fig. 5. Resorbable mesh used to treat an orbital floor blowout fracture.

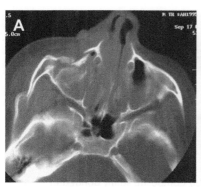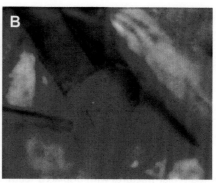

Fig. 6. (*A*) Axial CT image of fractured and displaced right ZMC. (*B*) Placement of resorbable plate at zygomatic buttress to stabilize malar fracture.

The clinical presentation usually reveals gingival hemorrhage combined with gross mobility of at least a 2-tooth segment. The teeth are usually displaced in a palatal or lingual direction leading to a malocclusion (**Fig. 8**). Loose or exfoliating teeth can be misleading in evaluating alveolar component injuries in children, therefore, detailed radiographic examination may be prudent. Missing teeth that cannot be accounted for may necessitate a chest or abdominal radiograph to rule out aspiration or ingestion.

The debridement of the comminuted and open dentoalveolar injury of clot, very loose primary teeth, and nonviable bone is necessary. The displaced segment is then gently reduced into position. The patient's occlusion is checked for appropriate contact. Care should be exercised to minimize the stripping of gingival tissue from the mobile segment because this may contribute to avascular necrosis. Next, the segment is stabilized with the application of a semirigid wire splint (Risdon cable) or arch bar for approximately 4 to 6 weeks. The preferred method today is a composite bonded wire splint that does not impinge on the gingiva (**Fig. 9**). Although arch bar and wire stabilization are more likely to be applied in an

emergency department or operating room, this can be changed to wire and composite later in an office environment with facilities and equipment for bonding. The affected dentition is monitored for the possibility of pulpal necrosis, and root canal therapy is instituted should this occur. Sometimes adequate reduction and stabilization of the fragments are not possible, therefore, open reduction and internal fixation are necessary, which typically requires minimal access for the placement of microplates and screws.

Symphyseal and Parasymphyseal Mandibular Fractures

Mandibular fractures in children require thoughtful consideration in management to avoid further injury to the developing dentition and significant growth disturbance. Older compliant children are more amenable to closed reduction with maxillomandibular fixation (MMF) or the use of lingual splints with skeletal fixation. Increased osseous metabolism and remodeling provide for rapid healing and improved occlusion even when discrepancies in alignment are noted after fixation. Infants with mandibular fractures should be treated with observation. Dietary modification is not usually necessary in this age group.

For anterior mandibular fractures in young children, closed reduction is the preferred treatment. However, in fractures whereby proper alignment cannot be gained with MMF alone or condyle fractures require jaw function and physiotherapy, 2 alternative options exist. Construction of a lingual splint from dental models is an elegant but time-consuming technique for reduction and fixation (**Fig. 10**). Its use requires dental impressions, generally obtained in the operating theater, followed by the fabrication of stone models. Often an additional general anesthetic is required for application with the use of interdental and

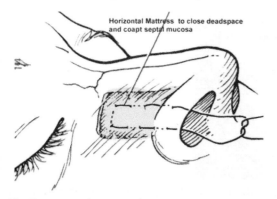

Horizontal Mattress to close deadspace and coapt septal mucosa

Fig. 7. Intranasal compressive stent.

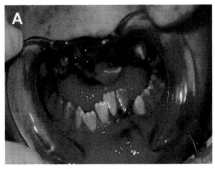
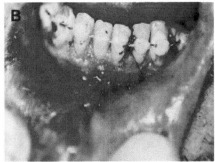

Fig. 8. (*A*) Dentoalveolar fractures with displaced teeth. (*B*) Composite splint bonded in place.

circumandibular wires to further secure the splint. This type of fixation allows for anatomic stabilization of the fracture and facilitates mandibular mobility for condylar fracture rehabilitation.

The second treatment is the placement of MMF and a transoral monocortical miniplate placed at the *inferior* border of the mandible. This combination of internal fixation and arch wire or bar superiorly allows adequate stability and postoperative function with guiding elastics if desirable. The importance of placing the plate at the very inferior aspect of the mandible is emphasized. In the young child with unerupted teeth, the risk of screw placement and injury to teeth is higher (**Fig. 11**).

Mandibular Body and Angle Fractures

Mandibular body and angle fractures can usually be treated with some form of MMF with or without simple fracture segment approximation. Sagittal fractures of the mandibular body may also benefit from the placement of a circumandibular wire or suture to aid in fracture reduction. These fractures are easily approximated and fixated with a single monocortical fixation plate in children with erupted first permanent molars and 7 to 10 days of elastic MMF. Older children may be managed similar to the adult condition.

Mandibular Condyle Fractures

Condyle fractures are insidious in children for 2 reasons: First, a significant number of these injuries remain undiagnosed. Second, whether diagnosed or not, condyle fractures can cause significant lower facial asymmetry as growth ensues. The mandible is one of the last bones to reach skeletal maturity and, as such, is vulnerable

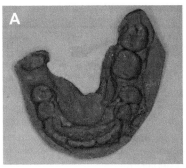
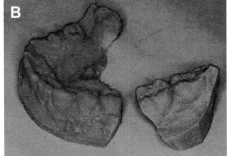
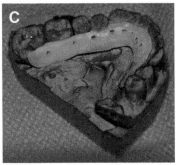

Fig. 9. (*A*) Dental model of displaced left mandibular body fracture. (*B*) Separated fractured mandibular segments before realignment. (*C*) Fabrication of acrylic splint to maintain proper alignment.

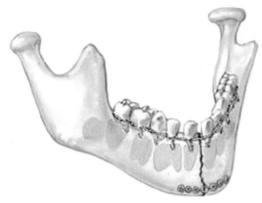

Fig. 10. Fracture reduction with wire and bonding technique.

to growth perturbations after injury to the condyles. The fracture pattern is also different than that observed in adults. Children have a propensity to fracture through the condylar head rather than the low-neck pattern seen in adults because children have a relatively thick and short condylar neck. Compression injuries of the fossa and condylar head and medial pole fractures are more common in children.

Classically caused by a fall and commonly heralded by a laceration in the submental region, condyle fractures are characterized by the shortening of the ramus on the affected side causing deviation of the chin to the affected side. On the unaffected side, open bite and flattening of the body of the mandible are seen. In bilateral fractures of the condyle, posterior displacement of the mandible is seen with anterior open bite. Occasionally, the child will be able to hold projection, symmetry, and occlusion in the mandible without difficulty. In such cases, observation with diet modification is usually sufficient for treatment.

Closed treatment of condylar fractures in children remains the standard treatment today.

Advocacy for closed treatment is biologically based by Walker[34] who confirmed adequate growth and development in primate juvenile models of fractures treated with closed reduction. Others corroborated his observations in the human population.[34–37] Although in adult patients closed treatment results in forced adaptation to the altered anatomy, in children, rapid and progressive remodeling of the condylar unit is common. Dramatic evidence of extensive remodeling is seen with long-term postoperative CT scans of injured children (**Fig. 12**). Although closed treatment of condyle fractures with a *brief* period of MMF followed by physiotherapy and training elastics is not time or technically demanding, this type of management requires serial appointments and long-term follow-up. Although ankylosis following condylar fracture is uncommon in North America, children with these injuries should be followed at regular intervals until the completion of mandibular growth. The assistance of an orthodontist who is familiar with functional appliance therapy for growth modification is invaluable should asymmetry begin to develop in the early postinjury phase. The single most important guideline in managing condylar fractures in children is to provide function with achievable occlusion through initial tight elastic MMF and converting to function with elastic guidance by 1 to 2 weeks. Proffit and colleagues[38] has reported that up to 10% of patients in the dentofacial-deformity population have evidence of previously undiagnosed condyle fractures.

Given the well-documented capacity for rapid bone healing and the important relationship of the functional soft tissue envelope on bone in growing patients, rapid return to function seems biologically sound. In instances when there are accompanying fractures of the mandibular corpus, treatment with a lingual splint or inferior border monocortical plate still allows immediate

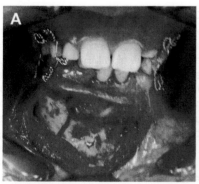
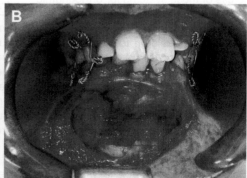

Fig. 11. (*A*) Ivy loop fixation prior to plate placement of parasymphysis fracture of the mandible. (*B*) Single "ladder" type resorbable plate with monocortial screw fixation.

A   **B**

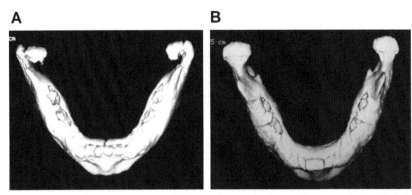

Fig. 12. (*A*) Three-dimensional (3D) CT image of bilateral fractured condyles in a child. (*B*) A 3D CT image of remodeled condyles several years after fracture displacement.

mandibular function. This point is particularly important in lateral or superolateral displacement of the condylar segment because contact with the zygoma is likely responsible for the development of ankylosis.[39] For the surgeon managing pediatric maxillofacial trauma, an in-depth understanding of these fractures is essential for good outcomes. The maintenance of mandibular projection, symmetry, and a functional occlusion through the closed technique remains the cornerstone in the treatment of condyle fractures in children.

SPECIAL CONSIDERATIONS
The Role and Use of Rigid Internal Fixation in Children

For the most part, as detailed extensively in this article, there is little indication for the generalized use of plate and screw-type internal fixation as in adult craniomaxillofacial trauma. However, there are some key considerations if internal fixation is used for fracture stabilization.

Biodegradable bone plates and screws have been regarded by some as excellent materials for pediatric facial bone surgery.[40,41] In addition, Turvey and colleagues[42] have extensively documented the use of these systems for orthognathic surgery in the mandible and maxilla. The systems remain bulky and oversized in relation to the bones of the pediatric facial skeleton to maintain some rigidity. In addition, aggressive degradation of the plates and screws has been noted to cause sterile abscesses that may further complicate healing.

One must first carefully consider several factors before using this type of fixation. First, if the bone that requires fixation has reached skeletal maturity, then plate and screw migration is not a concern. Second, and especially in the mandible, is rigid fixation desirable for rapid return to function? If the use of the biodegradable system does not offer the appropriate amount of rigidity

for stabilization, particularly for older children, or a period of closed reduction is necessary, then the advantage of using rigid internal fixation to allow immediate function is diminished. Certainly for cranial vault fractures in the growing child, the advent of biodegradable systems has been useful. Although titanium plate and screw migration has not been shown to cause neurologic injury, resorbable plates and screws have eliminated this concern and there is less need for rigidity in fixation in the cranial vault. In other areas of the facial skeleton, the desirability for open reduction with internal fixation should guide the use of these systems by the surgeon. If titanium fixation systems are used, adequate stabilization of the fracture can be achieved with low-profile plates and monocortical screw placement. Consideration can be given to the removal of the internal-fixation hardware once union has been achieved, which generally means a return to the operating theater. Sufficient healing and osseous maturity is achieved by 6 to 8 weeks in the growing child to permit the removal of any internal-fixation appliance.

The Risdon Cable in Pediatric Maxillofacial Trauma

The primary and early mixed dentitions have numerous anatomic challenges associated with the placement of MMF devices. The crowns of the teeth are short, squatty, and bulbous and can be loose. In addition, the replacement of teeth as a normal process of the dentition leads to edentulous areas awaiting full eruption. Various types of arch bars are universally used in the application of MMF during trauma and elective reconstruction of the maxillofacial skeleton. Unfortunately, the design and bulk of these arch bars do not fit the pediatric dentition well. As a result, the circumdental ligature wires loosen and slide off, on occasion, before patients have left the recovery room. To overcome these shortcomings, many advocate the use of skeletal fixation, such circummandibular, circumzygomatic, and pyriform aperture wires to hold the arch bars in place. This procedure only adds further steps to achieve solid MMF appliances; with the soft nature of the bone in children, the wires can saw through the bone if diligence is not exercised during placement.

The use of a modified Risdon cable in the primary and early mixed dentition is efficient in its application, provides excellent stability for elastic fixation, and does not require the additional placement of skeletal fixation. As the name implies, it was first described by Risdon, an otolaryngologist, in 1938.[43] In essence, the bar is replaced by a cable of twisted 24-gauge stainless steel wire taken from one side of the dental arch to the other and secured to each tooth with a circumdental 24-gauge stainless steel wire (**Fig. 13**). Alternatively, the cable can be started posteriorly on both sides of the same arch and tied together in the midline for added compression of anterior mandibular fractures. The fundamental advantage is that the cable is thin enough and contoured easily to allow for adequate engagement of the circumdental wires. The circumdental wires are then twisted into loops for holding elastics for MMF or guiding functions. Application is rapid in both arches, and very tight MMF can be achieved with elastics alone.

SUMMARY

The successful management of pediatric craniomaxillofacial trauma requires the additional dimension of understanding growth and development. The surgeon must appreciate the considerable influence of the soft tissue envelope and promote function when possible. Children heal well but with an exuberant tissue response that may contribute to greater scarring, therefore, careful and prudent attention given to meticulous soft tissue repair and support is critical.

Support must also be given and sought from the families of the injured children to engage them in the treatment and sequelae of the facial injuries and to encourage compliance with postoperative care. The follow-up management of children must continue long after the parents and children have forgotten about the initial injuries to ensure that the growth of the craniomaxillofacial skeleton continues within the normal parameters of development. For the most part, conservative management leads to excellent results in the long term.

REFERENCES

1. Tessier P. Total facial osteotomy. Crouzon's syndrome, Apert's syndrome: oxycephaly, scaphocephaly, turricephaly. Ann Chir Plast 1967;12:273 [in French].
2. Gruss JS, Mackinnon SE, Kassel EE, et al. The role of primary bone grafting in complex craniomaxillofacial trauma. Plast Reconstr Surg 1985;75:17.
3. Manson PN, Crawley WA, Yaremchuk MJ, et al. Midface fractures: advantages of immediate extended open reduction and bone grafting. Plast Reconstr Surg 1985;76:1.
4. Kaban LB. Diagnosis and treatment of fractures of the facial bones in children 1943-1993. J Oral Maxillofac Surg 1993;51:722.
5. Posnick JC. The role of plate and screw fixation in the treatment of pediatric facial fractures. In: Yaremchuk MJ, Gruss JS, Manson PN, editors. Rigid fixation of the craniomaxillofacial skeleton. Stoneham (MA): Butterworth-Heinemann; 1992. p. 396.
6. Posnick JC. Management of facial fractures in children and adolescents. Ann Plast Surg 1994;33:442.
7. Posnick JC. Craniomaxillofacial fractures in children. Oral Maxillofac Clin North Am 1994;1:169.
8. Farkas LG, Posnick JC. Growth and development of regional units in the head and face based on anthropometric measurements. Cleft Palate Craniofac J 1992;29:301.

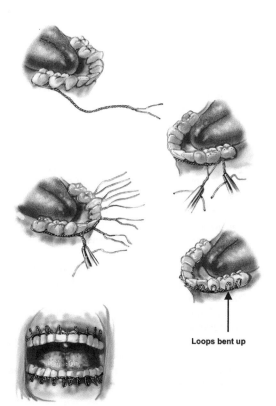

Loops bent up

Fig. 13. Risdon cable application.

9. Farkas LG, Posnick JC, Hreczko TM. Anthropometric growth study of the head. Cleft Palate Craniofac J 1992;29:303.

10. Farkas LG, Posnick JC, Hreczko TM, et al. Growth patterns in the orbital region: a morphometric study. Cleft Palate Craniofac J 1992;29:315.

11. Enlow DH, Hans MG. Essentials of facial growth. Philadelphia: WB Saunders; 1996.

12. Proffitt WR, Fields HW. Contemporary orthodontics. St Louis (MO): Mosby; 2000.

13. Moss ML. The functional matrix hypothesis revisited. 4. The epigenetic antithesis and the resolving synthesis. Am J Orthod Dentofacial Orthop 1997; 112:410.

14. Moss ML. The functional matrix hypothesis revisited. 3. The genomic thesis. Am J Orthod Dentofacial Orthop 1997;112:338.

15. Moss ML. The functional matrix hypothesis revisited. 2. The role of an osseous connected cellular network. Am J Orthod Dentofacial Orthop 1997;112:221.

16. Moss ML. The functional matrix hypothesis revisited. 1. The role of mechanotransduction. Am J Orthod Dentofacial Orthop 1997;112:8.

17. Bishara SE. Cephalometric evaluation of facial growth in operated and non-operated individuals with isolated clefts of the palate. Cleft Palate J 1973;10:239.

18. Hollishead WH. Anatomy for surgeons. 3rd edition. Philadelphia: JB Lippincott; 1982.

19. National Hospital Ambulatory Medical Care Survey (NHAMCS). Atlanta (GA): Center for Disease Control and Prevention; 1999.

20. Posnick JC, Wells M, Pron GE. Pediatric facial fractures: evolving patterns of treatment. J Oral Maxillofac Surg 1993;51:836.

21. Imahara SD, Hopper RA, Wang J, et al. Patterns and outcomes of pediatric facial fractures in the United States: a survey of the National Trauma Data Bank. J Am Coll Surg 2008;207:710.

22. Occupant protection for children safety information. National Highway Traffic Safety Administration; 2004. DOT HS 809 231.

23. Prigozen JM, Horswell BB, Flaherty SK, et al. All-terrain vehicle-related maxillofacial trauma in the pediatric population. J Oral Maxillofac Surg 2006; 64:1333.

24. Hepburn L, Azrael D, Miller M, et al. The effect of child access prevention laws on unintentional child firearm fatalities, 1979-2000. J Trauma 2006;61:423.

25. Browne GJ, Cocks AJ, McCaskill ME. Current trends in the management of major paediatric trauma. Emerg Med (Fremantle) 2001;13:418.

26. Alcala-Galiano A, Arribas-Garcia IJ, Martin-Perez MA, et al. Pediatric facial fractures: children are not just small adults. Radiographics 2008;28:441.

27. Smith JL, Ackerman LL. Management of cervical spine injuries in young children: lessons learned. J Neurosurg Pediatr 2009;4(1):64–73.

28. Kreykes NS, Letton RW Jr. Current issues in the diagnosis of pediatric cervical spine injury. Semin Pediatr Surg 2010;19(4):257–64.

29. Guzetta PC, Anderson KD, Altman RP, et al. Pediatric surgery. In: Schwartz SI, editor. Principles of surgery. New York: McGraw Hill; 1999. p. 1715.

30. Nakayama DK, Bose CL, Chescheir NC, et al. Critical care of the surgical newborn. Armonk (NY): Futura Publishing; 1997.

31. Antonyshyn O, Gruss JS, Kassel EE. Blow-in fractures of the orbit. Plast Reconstr Surg 1989;84:10.

32. Baumann A, Troulis MJ, Kaban LB. Dentoalveolar injuries and mandibular fractures. In: Kaban LB, Troulis MJ, editors. Pediatric oral & maxillofacial surgery. Philadelphia: Saunders; 2004. p. 441.

33. Ellis EE, Assael LA. Soft tissue and dentoalveolar injuries. In: Peterson LJ, editor. Contemporary oral & maxillofacial surgery. 2nd edition. Philadelphia: Mosby; 1993. p. 557.

34. Walker RV. Traumatic mandibular condyle fracture dislocations, effect on growth in the Macaca rhesus monkey. Am J Surg 1960;100:850.

35. Gilhuus-Moe O. Fractures of the mandibular condyle in the growth period. Acta Odontol Scand 1971;29:53.

36. Lindahl L. Condylar fractures of the mandible. IV. Function of the masticatory system. Int J Oral Surg 1977;6:195–203.

37. Lund K. Mandibular growth and remodeling process after condyle fracture, a longitudinal roentgencephalometric study. Acta Odontol Scand 1974; 32(Suppl 64):3–117.

38. Proffit WR, Vig KW, Turvey TA. Early fracture of the mandibular condyles: frequently an unsuspected cause of growth disturbances. Am J Orthod 1980; 78:1.

39. He D, Ellis E 3rd, Zhang Y. Etiology of temporomandibular joint ankylosis secondary to condylar fractures: the role of concomitant mandibular fractures. J Oral Maxillofac Surg 2008;66:77.

40. Bell RB, Kindsfater CS. The use of biodegradable plates and screws to stabilize facial fractures. J Oral Maxillofac Surg 2006;64:31.

41. Eppley BL. Use of resorbable plates and screws in pediatric facial fractures. J Oral Maxillofac Surg 2005;63:385.

42. Turvey TA, Bell RB, Phillips C, et al. Self-reinforced biodegradable screw fixation compared with titanium screw fixation in mandibular advancement. J Oral Maxillofac Surg 2006;64:40.

43. Risdon F. The surgical treatment of facial injuries. Can Med Assoc J 1938;38:33.

Primary and Secondary Management of Pediatric Soft Tissue Injuries

Nicholas J.V. Hogg, MD, DDS

KEYWORDS

- Pediatric facial injuries • Soft tissue repair • Soft tissue management • Dog and human bites
- Nerve and duct injuries • Avulsive defects

KEY POINTS

- Pediatric facial injuries are common due to multiple factors.
- Identification of the type and severity of the wound aids in the application of management strategies.
- Anesthesia plays an important role in the accurate repair of soft tissue injuries in children.
- Wound support and daily cleansing of wounds as well as measures to decrease wound tension help decrease scar formation.
- Hypertrophic scars require special management and despite best intentions some scars require secondary revision.
- The use of serial staged surgeries may be used to provide good functional and esthetic outcomes for pediatric patients with complex soft tissue injuries.

INTRODUCTION

Trauma remains the number one cause of mortality and morbidity in children. Although some safety measures have decreased the incidence of fatal head injuries, there has been a concomitant increase in nonfatal injuries.[1] The popularity of manual high-speed wheeled devices, such as bicycles, skateboards, and scooters, in the pediatric population also contributes to the increased rate of injury.[2] Additionally, the use of motorized vehicles, such as dirt bikes, go-karts, and all terrain vehicles, is implicated in high-velocity injuries, resulting in amplified peripheral damage.[3] Engaging in sporting activities, whether on a playground or in a supervised environment, is also a common cause of pediatric injuries. Prevention is key: the use of helmets, protective gear, and restraints reduces but does not eliminate the occurrence of facial injury in users.

Injury is still the most common cause of death in pediatric patients, with a large proportion of trauma related to head injury.[3] The craniofacial region in children develops rapidly and at an early age, making the area much more prominent in comparison to the remainder of the body; this increases the likelihood of injury to this area of the body. Craniofacial soft tissue injuries are commonly encountered by surgeons who are providing pediatric facial trauma coverage.[4,5]

In this article, the primary management of pediatric soft tissue injuries is reviewed, including assessment, cleansing, surgical technique, anesthesia, and considerations for special wounds. The secondary management of pediatric facial injury is also discussed, including scar revision, management of scar hypertrophy/keloids, and staged surgical correction.

PRIMARY SURGICAL MANAGEMENT

Soft tissue facial injuries are common in pediatric patients due to the prominence and relative size of the head in young children. Facial fractures

Private Practice, 843 Dundas Street, London, Ontario, Canada N5W 2Z8
E-mail address: drhogg@drnicholashogg.com

Oral Maxillofacial Surg Clin N Am 24 (2012) 365–375
doi:10.1016/j.coms.2012.04.007
1042-3699/12/$ – see front matter © 2012 Elsevier Inc. All rights reserved.

are less frequent because of the elastic nature of the craniofacial skeleton in the pediatric population. The history of injury is often taken from a witness or caregiver who should be queried on the time, mechanism, and details of the injury (eg, striking objects, trees, or pavement; sharp or blunt injury; or loss of consciousness). This information helps give an indication of the type, extent, and severity of soft tissue injuries that may be encountered. This history may also help predict wound progression and guide management, particularly in older and contaminated wounds. For open wounds, the tetanus status of the child should be determined and early treatment should be initiated.[6]

Initial evaluation can begin once a patient has been stabilized and a complete injury list has been determined. Pediatric patients with facial injuries often have concomitant injuries that require a multidisciplinary approach to management.[7] Visual inspection is often initiated in the presence of the parents; thus, it is important to remain calm and positive during this initial encounter with a patient's caregivers.[8] They can provide information that is important in predicting the esthetic outcome of the scar healing and they become important members of the wound management team.

Physical examination of the head and neck proceeds from top to bottom. Visual inspection of the scalp is often made difficult by the presence of hair matted in blood. A superficial cleansing with removal of hair helps detect scalp lacerations. Care must be taken to visually inspect all aspects of the scalp due to its extensive vascularity, which can result in profound blood loss. An oft-neglected and commonly injured area is the posterior scalp. Although sometimes difficult to visualize, it is important to inspect, identify, and control any prominent bleeding vessels. A cranial pressure dressing may need to be applied to stabilize patients before definitive treatment (**Fig. 1**).

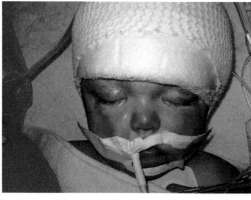

Fig. 1. Cranial pressure dressing to support tissues and prevent hematoma formation.

Once the scalp and cranium have been thoroughly evaluated, inspection of the remainder of the face and neck can be completed. Careful attention should be given to the soft tissue coverage and integrity of the cartilage of the nose and ear. Examination of the periorbital region should include the eyelids, conjunctiva, cornea, and globe. Signs of globe injury—asymmetric pupils, hyphema, torn bulbar conjunctiva, corneal damage, and so forth—should prompt immediate evaluation by an ophthalmologist.[9,10]

PRINCIPLES OF SOFT TISSUE REPAIR IN CHILDREN

The sequence and timing of the various stages of surgical management are important and may depend on a multitude of factors, including the extent of other injuries to the patient. In general, a more predictable result is obtained if the repair is undertaken closer to the time of injury.[11] Due to the extensive collateral circulation that is present in the vessels of the head and neck, however, some soft tissue injuries can wait up to 24 hours. Waiting beyond this point to repair wounds may compromise the final result because accumulation of edema, reduced tissue compliance, and difficulty in accurately approximating the wound edges all interact unfavorably.

Principles of soft tissue repair in children must take into account the differences in wound healing response in children, which is intense and more accelerated.[12] If not managed properly, this can result in hypertrophy and scarring. Children are more apt to heal quickly and more predictably because most children are free of systemic disease and habits that impair wound healing, such as alcohol use and tobacco smoking.[13]

Initially wounds should be thoroughly cleansed with copious amounts of irrigating solution to reduce the bacterial load and the excessive inflammatory wound responses that can be the result of the presence of wound contaminants. Consideration can be made for use of an antibiotic cleansing solution. This eases the identification and removal of foreign bodies, which can tattoo adjacent skin, if a wound is inadequately rinsed and debrided (**Fig. 2**). This is particularly true for pigmented and petroleum-related materials.

Suturing of the skin is most predictable if the skin is sutured below the skin. Suture choices can include the use of monofilament sutures; however, braided resorbable or nonresorbable nylon sutures are also popular. Care should be taken in suture choice depending on skin type and the likelihood of patients prone to keloid formation. Surface skin sutures should be avoided

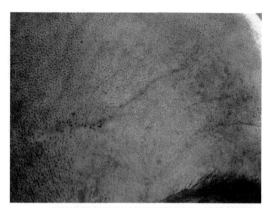

Fig. 2. Scar with tattoo from insufficient removal of road tar after injury.

if possible in children due to the potential for inflammation and infection and the difficulty in removing skin sutures. If some skin closure is necessary, the use of fast resorbing skin sutures is recommended, which are exfoliated quickly within 3 to 5 days and do not necessitate removal.[14] Cyanoacrylate glues or skin tapes, which are better tolerated by young patients, are commonly used in many emergency departments.[15–17] If a wound is leaky or moist, however, these may not adhere to the skin sufficiently. Also, skin glue should not be relied on to approximate wounds that are under tension (**Fig. 3**). Another choice is the use of over-the-counter adhesive dressings in infants because of the reduced cost and the lower concentrations of potential inflammatory chemicals.

Wounds need to be securely and adequately dressed to protect from subsequent injury. Wounds should be protected from excessive or intense drying or moisture as well as from widely fluctuant temperature variations. Parents or

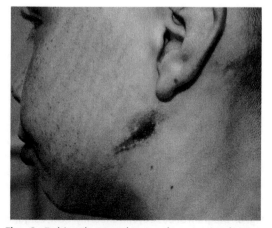

Fig. 3. Dehisced wound secondary to inadequate closure with skin glue.

caregivers need to be actively involved in postoperative wound care. Frequent cleansing of the wounds with removal of debris and scabs provides a better result as does appropriate dressing changes and scar management. Some children are pickers; therefore, attention must be directed to protecting wounds from constant irritation and scratching. Also, children with atopic dermatitits or eczema do not tolerate well a healing wound, which may become intensely pruritic. Consideration should be given to the use of topical corticosteroids and antihistamines, which may help in reducing the dermatitic response and itching during wound healing and prevent further inflammation, infection, or scarring. In these patients it is important to avoid cyclic changes in skin temperatures, hydration, topical dressings, and lotions, which may trigger increased skin sensitivity.[18]

ANESTHESIA

A combination of sedation and local anesthesia can be useful when suturing facial lacerations in children. Midazolam syrup is helpful even when used in subtherapeutic doses. The addition of inhalational agents, such as nitrous oxide and/or sevoflurane, alone or in combination with oral agents can be helpful adjuncts during stimulating portions of the surgical repair, such as administration of local anesthesia or tissue advancement under tension. Intravenous benzodiazepines, opioids, or general anesthetic agents, such as propofol, can be used in an infusion or small bolus doses to deepen the sedation at appropriate points during the surgical repair. This advanced level of sedation necessitates increased levels of monitoring and airway support as well as increased support staff. Consideration should be made to complete more complex procedures in an operating room environment depending on the training and level of comfort of the surgical and the anesthesia support teams.[8]

Under some circumstances, general anesthesia is required to accomplish diagnostic and surgical goals. Any periorbital work requires a general anesthetic to prevent movement of the patient, which can result in corneal abrasion or more severe globe injury. Nerve or duct repair is often completed under the use magnification in an operating room environment.

SPECIAL WOUNDS

Special wounds, such as those involving either eyelid or ear and nasal cartilage, require thorough cleansing and removal of any foreign bodies whose presence in a contaminated wound can lead to cartilage necrosis and loss of tissue support. Once the wounds have been cleansed, then meticulous closure of skin and cartilage is required. Consideration to the use of tissue support, including the possible use of acrylic supports or bolster dressing, should be made. Cartilage requires less oxygen than bone but it needs complete soft tissue coverage and some support or bolster dressing to prevent hematoma or seroma formation (**Figs. 4** and **5**). Bolster dressings can be removed in 7 to 14 days. Patients and parents should be informed of the possibility of growth disturbances or deformity as a result of cartilaginous disruption. This is particularly true for pediatric nasoseptal injury, which may result in the late development of nasoseptal deviation and deformity.[19,20]

Injuries to the eyelids require an ophthalmologic assessment to rule out injuries to the globe before surgical closure. Any significant injury to the periorbital area necessitates ophthalmologic evaluation, including the use of pupillary dilation and slit lamp examination to rule out significant or penetrating injury. Staining with fluorescein dye can reveal corneal and lacrimal injuries. If the canaliculi or punctum has been torn or bruised, then obstruction, stasis, and infection can result. Most children do not tolerate a thorough lacrimal and canalicular evaluation, so a detailed evaluation is often completed under general anesthesia. Canalicular injury requires intubation of the lacrimal and

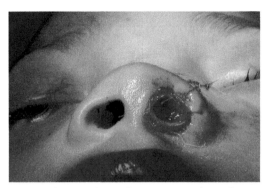

Fig. 5. Bolster and nasal stent sutured in place to support torn cartilage and prevent collapse.

canalicular system with silicone tubes. These tubes remain in place for 6 to 8 weeks until the lacrimal system has redeveloped and re-epithelialized.[21]

The eyelids are composed of anatomic layers called lamellae: the anterior lamella—skin and muscle; the middle lamella—includes the tarsal plate and either the levator (upper lid) or depressor (lower lid) aponeurosis; and the posterior lamella—conjunctiva (**Fig. 6**). Each lamaella should be addressed by ensuring that either direct repair or support has been provided to regain full function of the eyelids.

Surgical repair of the eyelids is completed under general anesthesia in the operating room with the patient paralyzed to prevent movement during the detailed and meticulous repair of the eyelids and related structures. The tissue must be irrigated thoroughly and any loose flaps of tissue carefully debrided and retained if possible. A lubricated pediatric corneal shield should be placed preoperatively to prevent corneal abrasion, which is an extremely painful postoperative complication (**Fig. 7**). The eyelid is sutured in a layered fashion

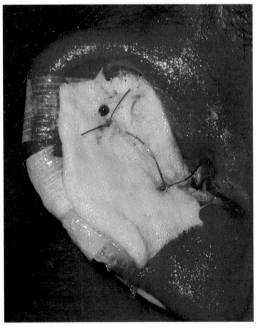

Fig. 4. Bolster dressing on ear wound to support injured cartilage and prevent hematoma formation.

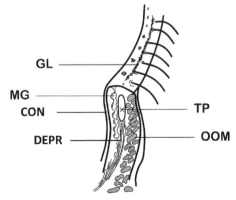

Fig. 6. Diagram of basic eyelid anatomy. CON, conjunctiva; DEPR, depressors; GL, gray line; MG, meibomian gland; OOM, orbicularis oculi muscle; TP, tarsal plate.

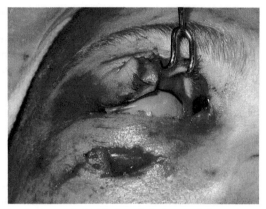

Fig. 7. Corneal shield placed during eyelid repair.

lead to excessive pressure on the globe and optic nerve with consequent blindness. Postoperative ophthalmologic evaluation should be performed routinely with evaluation for pain, proptosis, and pupillary function, which can be indicative of an evolving hematoma or ocular contusion. Emergent treatment includes release of sutures and/or canthotomy to evacuate clot, relieve pressure, and prevent permanent optic nerve damage. Although controversial, use of perioperative intravenous steroids is thought to decrease the progression of intraorbital edema and pressure.[23] In summary, expedient and expert maxillofacial care is necessary for management of pediatric orbital soft tissue injuries if a good result is to be obtained.

Nerve and Duct Injuries

During evaluation, particular attention should be given to the wounds that may involve the facial nerve. Grossly, wounds may evidence depth of injury if the fat is exposed in young children, indicating high likelihood of facial nerve injury (**Fig. 9**). Preoperative clinical assessment may reveal facial nerve paralysis, although in a young or disconsolate and uncooperative child this may be unreliable. A line drawn from the lateral canthus to the midbody of the mandible gives an indication of potential for nerve regeneration after injury. As a general rule, lacerations proximal to this line, depending on their depth and length, require exploration under magnification and microsurgical repair to regain function.[24]

Injuries that extend into the subcutaneous fat of the cheek in the parotid region should be evaluated for injury to Stensen duct. A small-gauge lacrimal probe or small intravenous catheter can be useful in exploring the continuity of the parotid duct (**Fig. 10**). This can be introduced transorally via the parotid papilla to reveal any injury or

using anatomic landmarks for closure. The gray line is carefully coapted to ensure lid alignment. This can be accomplished with inverted 7-0 or 8-0 Vicryl passed through meibomian gland orifices or everted suture with the tails left long to stabilize away from the conjunctiva (**Fig. 8**).[22] The tarsal plate is then repaired because this structure provides the supportive element of the eyelid. If the septum has been violated, then the periorbital fat may be seen protruding. The septum must be reapproximated to prevent orbital fat herniation, which can result in deformity, dysfunction, and possibly diplopia.

When treating periorbital lacerations, which communicate intraorbitally, hemostasis must be rigorously achieved. Subsequent bleeding can result in a retrobulbar hematoma, which may

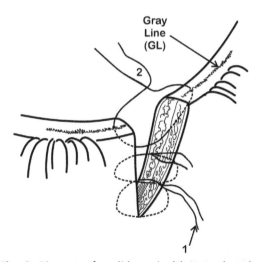

Fig. 8. Diagram of eyelid repair. (1) Note that the suture tails are left long to tape to the skin and out of harm's way. (2) A suture is passed in a buried manner through the meibomian gland orifice to help align the gray line (GL).

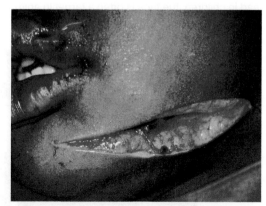

Fig. 9. Toddler with depth of injury likely involving the facial nerve (mandibular branch).

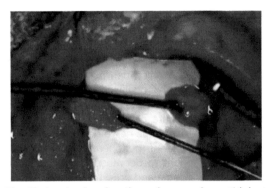

Fig. 10. Lacrimal probes through severed parotid duct before microsurgical repair.

interruption of the proximal duct within the wound bed.[25]

Ductal injury may require microsurgical repair with permanent sutures or repair over a temporary stent.[26] Repaired parotid ducts, which have been stented, should be monitored until epithelial continuity of the lumen of the duct has been achieved. This can take up to 2 to 4 weeks and the stent should be left in place until ductal continuity and integrity have been restored.[25,26] Both types of repairs may result in temporary salivary stasis at the site of repair; therefore, consideration should be given to 1 to 2 weeks of antibiotics. Parents should be alerted to the possible development of prolonged stasis and parotid enlargement. Salivary stimulation, through the use of sugar-free lozenges or gum, is recommended to increase saliva production and the resultant increased flow.

Bites

Children are eager to play with family pets as well as other animals and pets they encounter. Young children should not be left unsupervised in the presence of any animal for any length of time. Due to small stature and the prominence of the head in children, the face is often a target in animal attacks. Animal bites require prompt confirmation of rabies status and identification and quarantine of the animal. Initial surgical treatment involves thorough wound exploration and irrigation with closure of the linear aspects of the wound (**Figs. 11 and 12**). Puncture wounds should be irrigated to their depth, kept open, and frequently inspected to detect the occurrence of infection.[27] Animal bites result in intense inflammation that may last 2 to 3 days, but this eventually subsides. Particular attention should be given to attack dog (pit bull breeds) bites to the head in young children because penetrating skull injuries have been reported with late development of intracranial abscess and meningitis.[28]

Human bites to the face are more problematic and are often associated with *Eikenella corrodens*, *Streptococcus*, and *Staphylococcus*, which are more virulent and resistant organisms.[6,29] The infectious status (hepatis, HIV, and so forth) of the offending person should be ascertained and appropriate documentation obtained. In children, bite wounds are mostly inflicted at play or fighting and directed to the limbs of another child. Bite wounds of the face should be thoroughly cleansed and debrided and a decision made to repair the wound based on the status of the wound. An open wound with nonmacerated margins may be closed immediately; wounds with questionable viable components should be left open and dressed, to be closed later.[30,31] An exception is that puncture wounds should be left open for daily cleansing and to see patients on frequent recall.[32] After a wound has declared itself as noninfected, revision and primary closure may be performed, if desirable.[31]

Antibiotic prophylaxis is advisable for both human and animal bites. Amoxicillin/clavulanate provides excellent coverage for most bite pathogens in both animals and humans. The choice of antibiotics in penicillin-allergic patients is controversial. Clindamycin or azithromycin alone or in

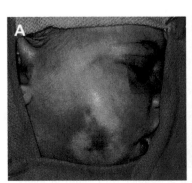
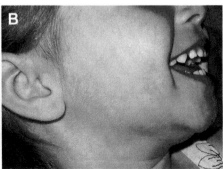

Fig. 11. (*A*) Repair of puncture-type dog-bite wound in 2-year-old girl. (*B*) Scar result 1 year later.

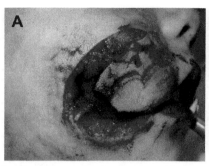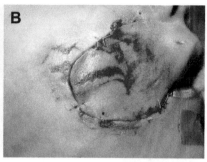

Fig. 12. Avulsive dog bite to cheek of 4-year-old. (*A*) Avulsive wound. (*B*) Immediate closure with venous stasis evident.

combination with trimethoprim/sulfamethoxazole can be an appropriate choice in children. Bite wounds typically result in an intense inflammatory response but this does not suggest infection; rather, it is the host response to foreign microorganisms. This response should subside in 2 to 3 days. Increasing erythema and pain beyond 3 days suggest infection. A recall appointment to check the wound is important.

Avulsive Wounds

High-velocity recreational activities can result in avulsive wounds of the craniofacial region. Bicycles, skateboards, and motorized off-road vehicles, such as dirt bikes and all-terrain vehicles, are commonly implicated in these injuries. Under general anesthesia in an operating room, careful exploration is performed under magnification. Pulse irrigation with an antibiotic-containing solution is completed before identification and débridement of poorly vascularized flaps of tissue (**Fig. 13**). If the tissue cannot be approximated, local or regional flaps may be required and in larger defects vascularized or nonvascularized tissue may be required to close the defect.[33] Passive or active suction drains are used to prevent hematoma formation. Pressure dressings

are applied with careful attention to allow both arterial inflow and venous outflow. Leech therapy may be necessary in distal portions of compromised tissue flaps (see **Fig. 13**C).

Wounds with extensive loss of tissue require a staged approach to reconstruction. The initial effort is to cleanse and debride wounds to prevent infection and further tissue loss. Serial wound debridement and dressing changes may be required in the first 2 weeks after injury (**Fig. 14**). Vacuum-assisted drainage can be helpful in evacuation of debris, circumferential diminishment of wounds, and stimulation of the wound vascular bed in preparation for final repair.[34]

Frequent inspection of wounds is necessary to preserve viable tissue. If tissue viability is a concern, care is taken for enhanced wound support and drainage and early suture removal may be undertaken if necessary. Hyperbaric oxygen may be beneficial for hypoxic wounds with portions of tissue that area marginally viable.[35]

SECONDARY SURGICAL MANAGEMENT

The final surgical result is dependent on the quality of the postoperative care as much as on the initial surgical treatment. Children heal well but have a tendency to heal with increased scarring or

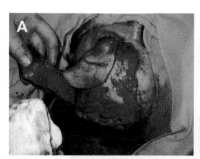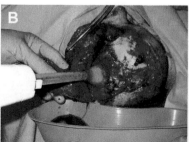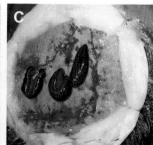

Fig. 13. Avulsive scalp wound. (*A*) Preservation of vascular pedicle and inspection of wound. (*B*) Pulse irrigation of wound bed. (*C*) Leech therapy for venous outflow insufficiency in distal portion of avulsed tissue.

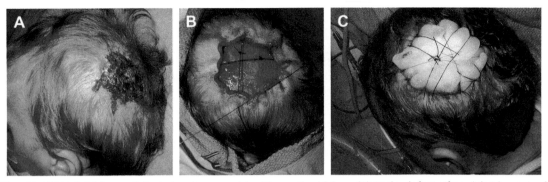

Fig. 14. (A) Full-thickness, infected scalp wound in 15-month-old boy. (B) Scalp defect after debridement of necrotic tissue and placement of pexing sutures. (C) Placement of a cranial dressing for preparation of the wound bed before staged reconstruction.

possibly hypertrophic scars. In order to manage this, it is important to supervise healing and guide wounds during active healing.[36] The initial sutures can be removed earlier in children and an attempt to do this should be made during the first 3 to 5 days. Wound support dressings, such as surgical tapes or skin glue, should be applied for the first 10 to 14 days to prevent tension from developing in the wound bed, which can cause an increase in collagen deposition. Frequent inspection of wounds is necessary (cell phone imaging is useful whereby a parent can relay daily images to the surgeon for inspection) to identify if there is latent skin reaction to dressings. Any pathologic influences on a wound should be removed and any crusts should be gently removed daily, both of which can cause an increased inflammatory response. Wounds should be kept moist and uncovered at 2 weeks postoperatively and any antibiotic ointment should be discontinued to prevent increased tissue reactivity, irritation, and unfavorable scar maturation.

Once a wound is well epithelialized, silcone sheets or topical gels can be applied to flatten and positively influence the maturation and healing of the scar.[36] Silicone sheeting can be applied for

several weeks to maintain continued mild pressure on the scar and surrounding tissue, which help reduce the amount of collagen deposition into the scar. It is important to avoid excessive wetting, drying, heat, or irritating agents during the postoperative healing period, which can result in exacerbation of the inflammatory response. Use of sunblock with a high level of sun protection factor is crucial during the healing period to avoid ultraviolet stimulation of melanocytes in the wound bed, which can result in hyperpigmentation. Use of a wide-brimmed hat, occlusive agent, or sunblock is recommended for up to 1 year's time to achieve the best scar result.

Children are more likely to develop hypertrophic scars or keloids and to have adverse pigment changes in which the scar bed does not match the surrounding skin. Monitoring wounds is recommended for early detection of adverse wound healing in which a scar extends beyond the initial wound margins, which may indicate hypertrophic scar formation or keloid formation (**Fig. 15**). Early treatment with topical hydrocortisone for mild hypertrophy may be effective. For more aggressive keloid formation, injectable steroids, such as triamcinolone in combination with silastic

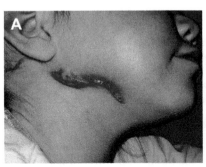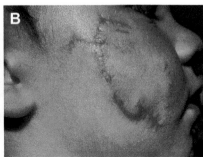

Fig. 15. (A) Inflamed hypertrophic scar in a young girl. (B) Mature hypertrophic scar from a dog bite.

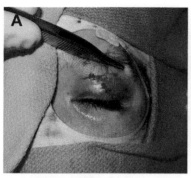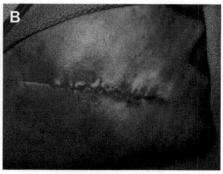

Fig. 16. (*A*) Z-plasty for lid lengthening in an eyelid repair for a dog-bite injury in a 3-year-old boy. (*B*) A cheek scar perpendicular to the resting skin tension lines is camouflaged using a W-plasty technique in a 9-year-old girl.

sheeting, are recommended.[36] Injection is performed under high pressure directly into the keloid via small-caliber needle (31 gauge), which can be uncomfortable. Low-dose radiation may also be effective for treatment for persistent keloids. As a final resort, re-excision with more vigilant supervision and the serial application of pressure dressings is indicated. This should be deferred until final maturation is completed which can take up to 12 months. Scars with uneven coloration or dyspigmentation can be carefully tattooed with permanent medical grade pigment to match the surrounding skin.

Scars that do not lie in the resting skin tension lines or have prominence of an unesthetic nature can be realigned or camouflaged with scar realignment. This can be accomplished with Z-plasty or W-plasty (**Fig. 16**). Other camouflage techniques include random pattern or irregular scar excision/reconstruction. Dermabrasion can also be used to flatten or diffuse prominent scars with irregular or uneven edges (**Fig. 17**).

STAGED SURGERIES

When tissue loss is extensive, as is the case in avulsive wounds, it can be difficult if not impossible to close these wounds primarily at the time of the initial surgery. In cases like this, serial wound debridement can result in tissue defects that can be treated by secondary reconstruction. When considering scalp reconstruction, staged surgeries may be necessary to provide enough local tissue to reconstruct the avulsive area anatomically with the correct amount and appropriate kind of tissue. Wound expansion can be completed over the course of 6 to 8 weeks (see article on scalp injuries for more detail elsewhere in this issue).

An initial surgery is necessary to implant a balloon expander with a remote access port

that is used to inflate the bladder of the tissue expansion device (**Fig. 18**A). The size of the expander should be twice that of the amount of tissue needed to close the defect. Small amounts of saline are injected into the self-sealing access port using small 10 mL to 20 mL aliquots at a time. This may be accompanied by some discomfort and oral sedation may be warranted to perform expansion on a weekly or biweekly basis. Tissue blanching gives an indication of the amount of expansion that is generated at each expansion appointment. The expansion appointments are arranged approximately every 7 to 10 days apart and the rest period can be extended if signs of tissue necrosis are observed. At the definitive surgery, the tissue expanders are removed, flaps are elevated and advanced, and incisions closed (see **Fig. 18**B–D). This technique can be used to close a defect not possible otherwise or when patients are not amenable to

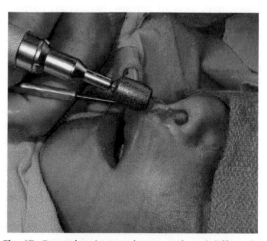

Fig. 17. Dermabrasion used to smooth and diffuse the pronounced edges of a lip scar.

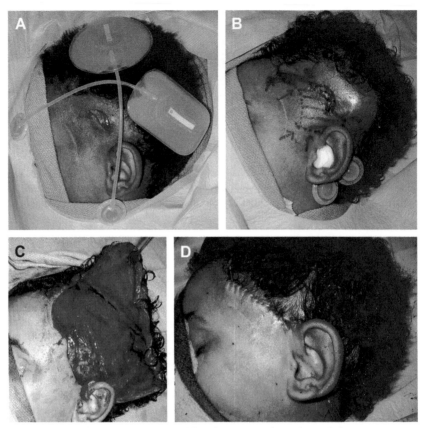

Fig. 18. (*A*) Tissue expanders placed to reconstruct a hair-bearing scalp avulsion defect in an 8-year-old boy. (*B–D*) Secondary scalp reconstruction 6 weeks after expansion with advancement of the scalp flap and restoration of the hairline.

treatment at the time due to more severe and potentially life-threatening injuries.

SUMMARY

Pediatric facial injuries are common due to children's high level of activity, decreased parental supervision, and a tendency toward risk-taking behavior. Identification of the type and severity of the injury is important in developing a strategic approach to cleansing, débridement, and repair. Prioritizing soft tissue wounds is important; identifying and maintaining tissue viability is paramount, as is early diagnosis and repair of nerve and ductal integrity. Anesthesia plays an important role in the repair of soft tissue injuries in children. Involving the parent in postoperative wound maintenance is important in determining the long-term outcome of the scar. Wound support and daily cleansing of wounds, as well as measures to decrease tension, help decrease scar formation. Children heal well but they heal with scars. These can become hypertrophic and require special management. Despite the best intentions, some injuries and scars require secondary management. Using a staged approach, surgeons can provide good functional and aesthetic outcomes for pediatric patients with significant soft tissue injuries.

REFERENCES

1. Guice KS, Cassidy LD, Oldham KT. Traumatic injury and children: a national assessment. J Trauma 2007; 63(Suppl 6):S68–80 [discussion: S81–6].
2. Munante-Cardenas JL, Olate S, Apirino L, et al. Pattern and treatment of facial trauma in pediatric patients. J Craniofac Surg 2011;22(4):1251–5.
3. Horswell BB, Flaherty SK, Henderson JM, et al. All-terrain vehicle-related maxillofacial trauma in the pediatric population. J Oral Maxillofac Surg 2004; 62:399–407.
4. Haug RH, Foss J. Maxillofacial injuries in the pediatric patient. Oral Surg Oral Med Oral Pathol 2000; 90(2):126–34.
5. Gassner R, Tuli T, Hachl O, et al. Craniomaxillofacial trauma in children: a review of 3,385 cases with 6060 injuries in 10 years. J Oral Maxillofac Surg 2004;62(4):399–407.

6. Stephanopoulos PK, Tarantzopoulou AD. Facial bite wounds: management update. Int J Oral Maxillofac Surg 2005;34(5):464–72.

7. Thoren H, Schaller B, Suominen AL, et al. Occurrence and severity of concomitant injuries in other areas than the face in children with mandibular and midfacial fractures. J Oral Maxillofac Surg 2012;70(1):92–6.

8. Vasconez HC, Buseman JL, Cunningham LL. Management of facial soft tissue injuries in children. J Craniofac Surg 2011;22(4):1320–6.

9. El-Sebaity DM, Soliman W, Soliman AM, et al. Pediatric eye injuries in upper Egypt. Clin Ophthalmol 2011;5:1417–23.

10. Ryan ML, Thorson CM, Otero CA, et al. Pediatric facial trauma: a review of guidelines for assessment, evaluation, and management in the emergency department. J Craniofac Surg 2011;22(4):1183–9.

11. Costello BJ, Papadopoulos H, Ruiz R. Pediatric craniomaxillofacial trauma. Clin Ped Emerg Med 2005; 6:32–40.

12. Pajulo OT, Pulkki KJ, Alanen MS, et al. Duration of surgery and patient age affect wound healing in children. Wound Repair Regen 2000;8(3):174–8.

13. Hogg NJV, Horswell BB. Soft tissue pediatric facial trauma: a review. J Can Dent Assoc 2006;72:549–52.

14. Luck RP, Flood R, Eyal D, et al. Cosmetic outcomes of absorbable sutures in pediatric facial lacerations. Pediatr Emerg Care 2009;24(3):137–42.

15. Beam JW. Tissue adhesives for simple traumatic lacerations. J Athl Train 2008;43(20):222–4.

16. Singer AJ, Kinariwala M, Lirov R, et al. Patterns of use of topical skin adhesives in the emergency department. Acad Emerg Med 2010;17(6):670–2.

17. Zempsky WT, Parrotti D, Grem C, et al. Randomized controlled comparison of cosmetic outcomes of simple facial lacerations closed with steri strip skin closures or dermabond tissue adhesive. Pediatr Emerg Care 2004;20(8):519–24.

18. Krakowski AC, Eichenfield LF, Dohil MA. Management of atopic dermatitis in the pediatric population. Pediatrics 2008;122(4):812–24.

19. Wright RJ, Murakami CS, Ambro BT. Pediatric nasal injuries and management. Facial Plast Surg 2011; 27(5):483–90.

20. Hogg NJ, Horswell BB. Hard tissue pediatric facial trauma: a review. J Can Dent Assoc 2006;72: 555–8.

21. Jordan DR, Gilberg S, Mawn LA. The round-tipped, eyed pigtail probe for canalicular intubation: a review of 228 patients. Ophthal Plast Reconstr Surg 2008; 24:176–80.

22. Perry JD, Aguilar CL, Kuchtey R. Modified vertical mattress technique for eyelid margin repair. Dermatol Surg 2004;30(12):1580–2.

23. Assimes TL, Lessard ML. The use of perioperative corticosteroids in craniomaxillofacial surgery. Plast Reconstr Surg 1999;103(1):313–21.

24. Evans AK, Licameli G, Brietzke S, et al. Pediatric facial nerve paralysis: patients, management and outcomes. Int J Pediatr Otorhinolaryngol 2005; 69(11):1521–8.

25. Steinberg MJ, Herrera AF. Management of parotid duct injuries. Oral Surg Oral Med Oral Pathol 2005; 99(2):136–41.

26. Van Sickels JA. Management of parotid gland and duct injuries. Oral Maxillofac Surg Clin North Am 2009;21(2):243–6.

27. Wu PS, Beres A, Tashjian DB, et al. Primary repair of facial dog bite injuries in children. Pediatr Emerg Care 2011;27(9):801–3.

28. Mason AC, Zabel DD, Sanders EK. Occult craniocerebral injuries from dog bites in young children. Ann Plast Surg 2000;45(5):531–4.

29. Brook I. Microbiology of human and animal bite wounds in children. Pediatr Infect Dis J 1987;6:29–39.

30. Broder J, Jerrard D, Olshaker J, et al. Low risk of infection in selected human bites treated without antibiotics. Am J Emerg Med 2004;22(1):10–3.

31. Stucker FJ, Shaw GY, Boyd S, et al. Management of animal and human bites in the head and neck. Arch Otolaryngol Head Neck Surg 1990;116:789–93.

32. Schweich P, Fleisher G. Human bites in children. Pediatr Emerg Care 1985;1(2):51–3.

33. Bilkay U, Tiftikcioglu YO, Temiz G, et al. Free-tissue transfers for reconstruction of oromandibular area in children. Microsurgery 2008;28(2):91–8.

34. Avery C, Pereira J, Moody A, et al. Clinical experience with the negative pressure wound dressing. Br J Oral Maxillofac Surg 2000;38(4):343–5.

35. MacFarlane C, Cronje FJ. Hyperbaric oxygen and surgery. S Afr J Surg 2001;39(4):117–21.

36. Tsao SS, Dover JS, Arndt KA. Scar management: keloid, hypertrophic, atrophic and acne scars. Semin Cutan Med Surg 2002;21:46–55.

Growth and Development Considerations for Craniomaxillofacial Surgery

Bernard J. Costello, DMD, MD[a,b,c,*], Reynaldo D. Rivera, DDS, MD[a,b],
Jocelyn Shand, MBBS(Melb), MDSc(Melb), BDS(Otago), FDSRCS(Eng), FRACDS(OMS)[d],
Mark Mooney, PhD[e,f,g,h]

KEYWORDS

• Craniomaxillofacial surgery • Growth • Development • Dysmorphology

KEY POINTS

• Dysmorphologies may result from congenital malformations, trauma, radiation, or iatrogenic disturbances.
• Most orbital growth is completed by 5 to 7 years of age, making it the optimal time to reconstruct deformities in this area for a more definitive result. Growth of the zygoma and maxilla is initially slower than the cranial-orbital region; however, most growth is complete by 7 years.
• Malposition of the mandible is usually reserved until cessation of growth; however, a surgeon may consider mandibular advancement in a growing patient with severe airway obstruction or obstructive sleep apnea, to improve the overall growth vector of the face and for psychological reasons.
• Risk factors for relapse after surgical mandibular intervention in a growing patient include high mandibular plane angles, preexisting condylar disorders, and advancements of 10 mm or greater.
• After surgical intervention for vertical maxillary excess in the growing patient, the vertical growth of the maxilla may continue, with a high risk for clockwise mandibular rotation, relapse, and development of an anterior open bite.

INTRODUCTION

The goals of craniomaxillofacial surgery include establishing a stable morphology and improving facial aesthetics. Dysmorphologies or deformities may result from congenital malformations, radiation, or iatrogenic growth disturbances. The surgical treatment designed to treat these disorders may necessitate manipulation of the soft tissues or bony structures based on the particular

[a] Division of Craniofacial and Cleft Surgery, University of Pittsburgh School of Dental Medicine, 3501 Terrace Street, Pittsburgh, PA 15261, USA; [b] Department of Oral and Maxillofacial Surgery, University of Pittsburgh School of Dental Medicine, 3501 Terrace Street, Pittsburgh, PA 15261, USA; [c] Pediatric Oral and Maxillofacial Surgery, Children's Hospital of Pittsburgh, 4401 Penn Avenue, Pittsburgh, PA 15224, USA; [d] Division of Plastic and Maxillofacial Surgery, Royal Children's Hospital, Flemington Road, Parkville, Victoria 3052, Australia; [e] Department of Oral Biology, University of Pittsburgh School of Dental Medicine, 3501 Terrace Street, Pittsburgh, PA 15261, USA; [f] Department of Anthropology, University of Pittsburgh, 3302 WWPH, Pittsburgh, PA 15260, USA; [g] Department of Surgery-Plastic and Reconstructive Surgery, University of Pittsburgh Medical Center, 200 Lothrop Street, Pittsburgh, PA 15213, USA; [h] Department of Orthodontics and Dentofacial Orthopedics, University of Pittsburgh School of Dental Medicine, 3501 Terrace Street, Pittsburgh, PA 15261, USA
* Corresponding author. Department of Oral and Maxillofacial Surgery, University of Pittsburgh Medical Center, 3471 Fifth Avenue, Suite 1112, Pittsburgh, PA 15213.
E-mail address: bjcl@pitt.edu

Oral Maxillofacial Surg Clin N Am 24 (2012) 377–396
doi:10.1016/j.coms.2012.05.007

deformity or dysmorphology. For example, the failure of fusion that creates facial clefting is usually repaired in infancy during the growth phase. Just repairing these soft tissues in key growth areas may have negative consequences later in life. Radiation or trauma at an early age may cause hypoplasias and asymmetries that require treatment at different stages of growth. The interplay between the different growth areas of the facial structures highlights the possible biologic consequences of early intervention during the growth phase.

When skeletal discrepancies exceed the envelope of those that can be appropriately treated with orthopedic growth modification and/or orthodontic compensation techniques, surgical repositioning of the craniofacial structures may be indicated.[1] In many instances, patients with skeletal deformities benefit from surgical correction following the completion of facial growth. This approach allows a definitive treatment that is highly predictable and stable in most cases.[2] In contrast, surgical treatment performed before skeletal maturity is less predictable and may require reoperation following skeletal maturation. However, early intervention may be warranted for functional or aesthetic reasons, but the hoped-for advantage of early surgical interventions to unlock growth has not been realized, and, in most cases, there are no clear benefits to early operative intervention.[3,4] These common issues emphasize the importance of considering growth when planning surgical treatment.

This article reviews the concepts of growth and development in the craniofacial skeleton as they relate to the treatment of soft tissue and skeletal dysmorphologies. The basic principles of craniofacial growth are reviewed, and the specific patterns of craniofacial dysmorphologies are discussed with regard to potential early and/or staged intervention. A balanced approach to treatment planning is presented with growth as the primary factor to consider. However, functional aspects of the airway and occlusion are of considerable importance in some patients. Certain clinical situations require intervention, even at the cost of iatrogenic disruption of growth potential, when there is a significant benefit perceived. In addition, aesthetic concerns in patients with severe deformity often require early intervention for psychosocial reasons.

GROWTH DISCREPANCY AND THE CRANIOFACIAL SKELETON

Growth discrepancies involving the craniofacial skeleton are common, and many of these discrepancies can be managed with orthopedic growth modification and/or orthodontics alone if they are not severe.[1] In particular, congenital craniofacial malformations, deformities, and pathologic or traumatic disruptions may have severe skeletal dysmorphologies and discrepancies. For example, deformational plagiocephaly causes cranial and possibly orbital asymmetry that, when diagnosed early, is treated with a form of growth modification using custom-molding helmets or bands. In instances when the discrepancy is particularly large or other deformities of the cranio-orbital region are encountered, surgery may be helpful to dismantle the craniofacial components and reposition them in a more normal conformation. There are several examples of skeletal and soft tissue discrepancies that occur in childhood requiring treatment. Deciding when to intervene is important to optimize the long-term results for these clinical challenges.

Growth abnormalities and dysmorphology of the lower face are the most commonly encountered clinical problems for the craniomaxillofacial surgeon. When these discrepancies involve the teeth, most minor discrepancies are treated with orthodontic compensation. However, some are beyond the envelope of orthodontic compensation techniques and may benefit from surgical repositioning of skeletal components. Orthognathic surgery for the treatment of skeletal discrepancy and malocclusion has traditionally been undertaken following the completion of growth, and there is substantial literature regarding the effects and stability of these procedures. However, there are only a limited number of studies that have investigated the outcome following orthognathic, craniofacial, or other types of maxillofacial surgery performed in the growing child.[5–12] The supposition that surgical intervention before skeletal maturation may inhibit the future growth potential of the involved bone is long-standing. This concept is, in part, based on studies of patients with cleft lip and palate deformities, Robin sequence, craniofacial microsomia, Treacher Collins syndrome, and a range of other conditions in those who had undergone surgical procedures during growth.[13] Data regarding growth consequences are lacking in areas of posttraumatic and radiation deformity. Empirical evidence reveals that many patients suffer asymmetry caused by soft tissue scarring and bone growth abnormalities associated with significant trauma or radiation. The results and observations from these studies provide information about growth potential; however, is it important to recognize that these patients also have underlying dysmorphologies or disorders that may influence facial growth, independently of surgical correction. In the assessment of subsequent facial growth problems, it is difficult to delineate between that related to the preexisting condition with its aberrant growth pattern and that potentially caused by the surgical osteotomy or other manipulations. Early surgery has usually been reserved for individuals with marked skeletal dysmorphologies and/or severe functional concerns (eg, intracranial pressure increases, choanal atresia, or severe obstructive sleep apnea). The presence of severe functional problems or implications for the psychosocial development of the child may become important when considering early surgery. A firm understanding of the patterns of facial growth is essential when planning surgical reconstruction.[14]

There is some predictability to the growth of the cranium and face, but individual variation and pathologic conditions must be considered.[15,16] Common growth variations (eg, vertical maxillary excess with mandibular hypoplasia) and pathologic clinical situations (eg, maxillary hypoplasia in the patient with a cleft palate) should be recognized, and treatment planned and then staged with these issues in mind. Clinicians must be aware of these early discrepancies, not to force early intervention in most cases but to develop a diagnosis and stage the reconstruction for the most predictable result. Treatment plans can then be formulated based on the best estimation of the expected pattern of growth.

CONCEPTS OF CRANIOFACIAL SKELETAL GROWTH AND DEVELOPMENT

Craniofacial development, growth, and remodeling are a complex interplay of structure and function beginning in the embryo and continuing throughout adult life. The delicate equilibrium that exists between various parts of the craniofacial skeleton is stimulated by genes and local function that coordinate complex biomechanical and molecular signaling to yield a composite skeletal form.[17] Problems can occur at anytime during this process and negatively affect the development and growth

process. Understanding the basic biology of craniomaxillofacial growth is essential when planning treatment of malformations, disruptions, and deformities. The basic definitions of growth are important to understand when discussing the biology of growth and development (**Table 1**).

In general, there is a cephalocaudal growth vector that occurs throughout early life and facial development that is thought to be closely linked to the functional demands of each region (**Fig. 1**). Enlow[18,19] discussed the concepts of growth in detail and outlined the 2 main morphologic events that direct craniofacial growth. These include (1) basal cranium growth and (2) development of the pharyngeal and facial airway structures. This vector of cephalocaudal growth is directly related to the changes seen in the proportions of the head and face during early life. In the early phase, this is reflected in the relative importance of cranial growth as a response to the rapid growth of the brain tissues. This response occurs in the neurocranium, which houses the structures of the brain, orbits, and olfactory system, and this region comprises the cranium and upper third of the face. The remainder of the facial tissues accelerate their growth at a later phase as the airway and muscles of mastication increase their function. This region represents the viscerocranium (**Table 2**).

The bones of the craniofacial skeleton grow and develop by remodeling and displacement throughout young life. Remodeling occurs as a result of local factors that result in the change in the size and shape of various components of the facial skeleton. Displacement occurs by bones that move apart at the joint, suture, or articular regions.[18,19] This displacement occurs away from the articular surfaces (ie, cranial sutures, temporomandibular joints, or maxillary sutures). Bone growth is modulated through this process by augmenting or diminishing various regions in response

Table 1 Definitions	
Term	**Definition**
Dysmorphology	Abnormal morphology of tissues
Malformation	Formation of tissue is poor as a result of an intrinsic problem with development
Disruption	A breakdown in normal tissue development causing abnormal morphology
Deformation	Changes in morphology caused by external forces on normal tissue
Growth	Increase in cell size (plasia) or cell number (trophy)
Remodeling	Compensatory or adaptive changes of tissue
Development	Increase in complexity
Hypertrophy	Increase in the size of the cells
Hyperplasia	Increase in the number of cells

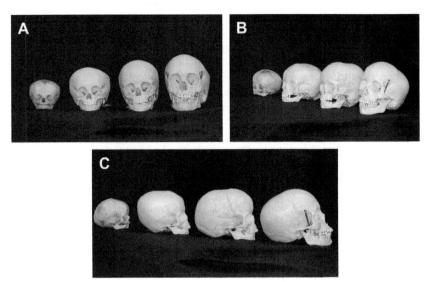

Fig. 1. (A–C) Multiple views of skulls from infancy to adolescence show the progression of craniofacial bone growth. The general progression is from superior to inferior with a downward and forward growth vector.

to the functional needs and the timing of gene expression. The 2 processes of remodeling and displacement should occur in a coordinated and interdependent fashion. If the processes are balanced, the skeleton develops appropriately. In contrast, if the balance is disturbed, such as by nasal obstruction or prenatal cranial suture fusion, the skeleton develops outside the envelope of equilibrium, resulting in a skeletal discrepancy.[1]

Local signaling seems to occur between the bony components of the face to develop each area in response to the increasing functional demands of mastication and breathing. The orbits, maxilla, and mandible are dependent on one another early in this phase, whereas the cranial base has a more intrinsic or genetically based control mechanism.[18,19] The cranium and orbits develop in response to the rapid growth of the brain and globes, which occurs during the first year of life, and hence the cranio-orbital complex is much larger than the maxillomandibular complex in infancy. The early developing neuro-cranial complex creates a craniocaudal growth vector that is clockwise in direction when viewing the right lateral skull. Later, the functional demands of mastication and deglutition on the mandible become more significant, and the nature of the equilibrium balance with the maxilla is also altered in response to the growth and development of the airway and the functional needs of mastication and speech development. Constant modifications to this process are made throughout growth and development to obtain a functional state of equilibrium. This interplay drives the growth process from cephalad to caudad.

The equilibrium of the craniofacial complex is altered following a series of normal developmental events:

1. Central neurologic development
2. Optic pathway development
3. Speech and swallowing development
4. Airway and pharyngeal development
5. Facial expression and muscular changes
6. Tooth development and exfoliation.

Each region has a unique growth curve, and there are various peaks of growth velocity that alter craniofacial equilibrium and result in skeletal

Table 2 Average percent growth completion of various craniofacial dimensions			
	Average Adult % Completed by Age 1 y	Average Adult % Completed by Age 5 y	Average Age at Maturity (y)
Cranium	84–86	90–94	Boys, 14 Girls, 16
Orbits	84–86	88–93	Variable
Zygoma	72	83	Boys, 15 Girls, 13
Maxilla	75–80	85	Boys, 15 Girls, 14
Mandible	60–70	74–85	Boys, 16 Girls, 14

Data from Refs.[18–23]

growth changes to restore this equilibrium. It is essential to have an understanding of each region when deciding the timing of various reconstructive efforts. In general, more definitive corrections are performed later in the growth phase and, ideally, should be undertaken at the completion of growth because earlier intervention may alter the growth curve and disrupt the equilibrium. Relapse toward the original deformity or dysmorphology is more likely to occur when the body attempts to restore the balance that has been altered by surgical intervention performed before skeletal maturation.[18,19]

REGIONS OF CRANIOFACIAL GROWTH AND DEVELOPMENT
Cranium

The cranium is made up of the chondrocranium and the neurocranium. The chondrocranium, or cranial base, develops initially in cartilage derived from occipital somites and then becomes bone by endochondral ossification. These ossification centers form the bones of the base of the skull, (ie, the occipital, sphenoid, temporal, and ethmoid bones). Growth of the cranial base bones occurs interstitially at articulations called synchondroses. Although most of the growth is occurring at the synchondroses, once ossified, the inner and outer surfaces of each bone can also remodel via appositional growth.

The neurocranium, or cranial vault, is made up of large and small curved, flat bones that are formed intramembranously, most of which are derived from neural crest cells. The growth of these bones occurs interstitially at the fibrous articulations (ie, the sutures) and appositionally on the endocortical and ectocortical surfaces. The cranial vault grows rapidly in the first year of life, and the velocity of growth plateaus in the following 5 years. A diploic space is present between 2 clear cortices of bone in most children between the ages of 2 and 5 years. Most growth in this area is complete by ages 5 to 7 years.[3,4] At 1 year of age, the width of the head is 84% of its adult size, and, at 5 years of age, the head width increases to 93%.[20–23] Head circumference is similar, with 86% of the growth complete by 1 year of age and 94% of growth completed by 5 years of age. The maturation age of the cranium width is 14 years in girls and 15 years in boys. The large amount of growth within the first 5 years of life reflects the neurodevelopment that occurs during this time.[20–23]

Craniosynostosis is the premature fusion of cranial vault sutures, which is generally an antenatal event that causes growth restriction perpendicular to the affected suture. Craniosynostosis is most often seen with only 1 suture. However, craniofacial dysostosis syndromes occur when the cranial base synchondroses (primarily the presphenoethmoid synchondroses) and, to a lesser extent, the cranial vault sutures are affected to varying degrees. The alteration of the midface occurs in craniofacial dysostosis syndromes, such as Apert, Pfeiffer, and Crouzon syndromes. These syndromes are characterized by a restriction of growth in the anterior cranial vault and cranial base that results in severe orbital and midfacial hypoplasia and class III malocclusion. In addition, when the brain and cranial base components do not form in their normal fashion (eg, Binder sequence and Down syndrome), the development of the midfacial complex and the balance is also distorted.[24–26]

Treatment of dysmorphology in the cranial vault and orbits is usually more definitive after 1 year of age because most growth in the cranium is complete at this time. In the case of craniosynostosis, surgical treatment is necessary earlier to allow appropriate volume for brain growth. For patients with craniofacial dysostosis in which skull base fusion has also affected the orbits and midface, this is treated at a later stage (**Fig. 2**).

Orbits

The orbits consist of bones from the cranio-orbital and nasomaxillary complexes, and most of the growth in the orbit region occurs at the sutures between these bones. The orbits grow rapidly in the first year of life in association with the globe, optic nerves, and neurocranial development, and the velocity decreases over the next 5 years. Most of the growth in this area is completed by 5 years of age.[3,4] The intercanthal width at age 5 years is, on average, 30 mm, which is approximately 93% of the adult value. Intercanthal width is fully mature in boys at 11 years of age and in girls at 8 years of age. Orbital height grows at a more gradual rate compared with the other orbital dimensions. The impressive growth of this region before 5 years of age is a result of the rapidly developing globes and optic neurologic system.[3,4]

Orbital dysmorphology is seen in unicoronal craniosynostosis, the craniofacial dysostosis syndromes, and also in patients who fail to obliterate the foramen cecum during development with midline lesions, such as gliomas, dermoids, or encephaloceles. The delicate balance is disturbed, and the tissues adapt based on the pathologic condition that is present. Most treatments are best performed after the age of 5 years (**Fig. 3**).

Zygoma

The zygomatic bones grow rapidly in the first year of life and level off in velocity over the next 5 to 7

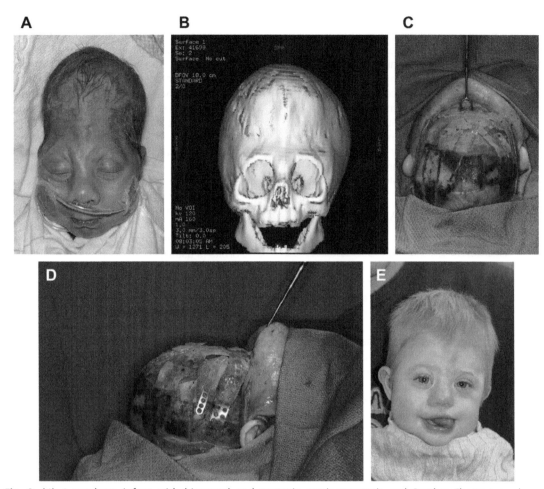

Fig. 2. (*A*) A newborn infant with bicoronal and metopic craniosynostosis and Saethre-Chotzen syndrome. Constriction of growth perpendicular to the sutures is evident, with the resultant dysmorphology and small cranial vault requiring expansion. (*B*) Three-dimensional computed tomography (CT) scan showing the cranial vault constriction associated with craniosynostosis. (*C and D*) Cranial vault reshaping has been performed by disassembling the dysmorphic bones, advancing the cranio-orbital complex, and reshaping the bones to a more normal conformation and expanded volume to accommodate the brain at this critical time of growth. (*E*) Postoperative result showing improved cranial vault and orbital morphology. (*From* Fonseca RJ, Marciani RD, Turvey TA. Oral and maxillofacial surgery. 2nd edition. Saunders; 2009. Figure 43-2, p. 852; with permission.)

years. Growth in this area is initially more gradual compared with the cranium and orbits, but most of the growth in this area is similarly complete by age 5 to 7 years. The bizygomatic width is 83% of the mature adult size by the age of 5 years, and the width of the face is mature at 15 years in boys and 13 years in girls.[3,4]

Zygomatic deformities are seen in Treacher Collins syndrome, craniofacial dysostosis syndromes, Down syndrome, achondroplasia, cretinism, and other growth restrictions of the cranial base. The hypoplasia is also evident in the maxilla and nasal complex. Definitive treatment in this area can usually be performed after the age of 5 years (**Fig. 4**).

Maxilla

Much like the cranium, the maxilla develops by intramembranous ossification of neural crest cells. Maxillary growth is a result of early nasal septal growth and later by sutural growth and surface remodeling with a forward and downward displacement relative to the cranial base. Midfacial height (nasion to gnathion) reaches maturity at 13 years in girls and 15 years in boys.[3,4] The most active times of growth are from the ages of 1 to 2 years and 3 to 5 years. The height of the midface (nasion to stomion) matures slightly earlier in boys at 14 years and 12 years in girls. Midfacial projection (tragus to stomion) reaches maturity at 14 years in boys and 13 years in girls.[3,4]

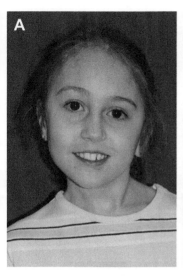 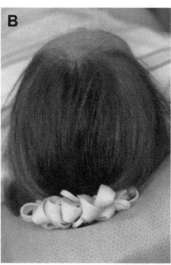

Fig. 3. (*A* and *B*) The effects of naso-maxillary injury in this young girl with a history of long-standing torti-collis that exhibits facial asymmetry and cranial asymmetry. The cranial vault asymmetry has the typical conformation associated with skull molding or positional plagiocephaly. The compensatory changes in the orbit and lower face can be addressed at different times based on future facial growth velocities and presumed completion of growth. (*From* Fonseca RJ, Marciani RD, Turvey TA. Oral and maxillofacial surgery. 2nd edition. Saunders; 2009. Figure 43-3, p. 853; with permission.)

The midfacial hypoplasia seen in craniofacial dysostosis syndromes, achondroplasia, and other disorders is impressive, often in all 3 dimensions.[27] Nasomaxillary trauma in early childhood can also result in significant midface hypoplasia.[28–30] Patients may develop severe anterior-posterior maxillary hypoplasia, transverse discrepancies, and anterior open bites. For these reasons, definitive correction of maxillary dysmorphology is usually reserved for after the ages of 14 years in girls and 16 years in boys once skeletal maturity has been achieved. When these deformities are particularly severe, early intervention is entertained, which may include attempts at growth modification (ie, reverse-pull headgear) or early midfacial advancement with osteotomies (**Figs. 5** and **6**).

Mandible

There is a classic notion that the condyle is the independent growth center of the mandible.

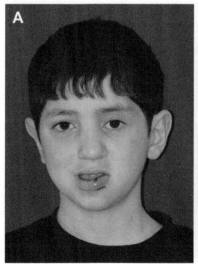 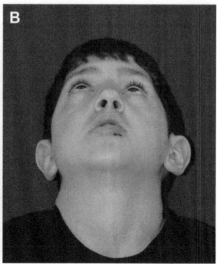

Fig. 4. (*A* and *B*) This young boy had a skull base procedure in infancy for a skull base tumor and postoperative radiation therapy to the left orbit, zygoma, and skull base. At the original procedure, symmetry was good, but, as the child grew during the following decade, facial asymmetry developed, including lower orbital and zygomatic hypoplasia. (*From* Fonseca RJ, Marciani RD, Turvey TA. Oral and maxillofacial surgery. 2nd edition. Saunders; 2009. Figure 43-4, p. 853; with permission.)

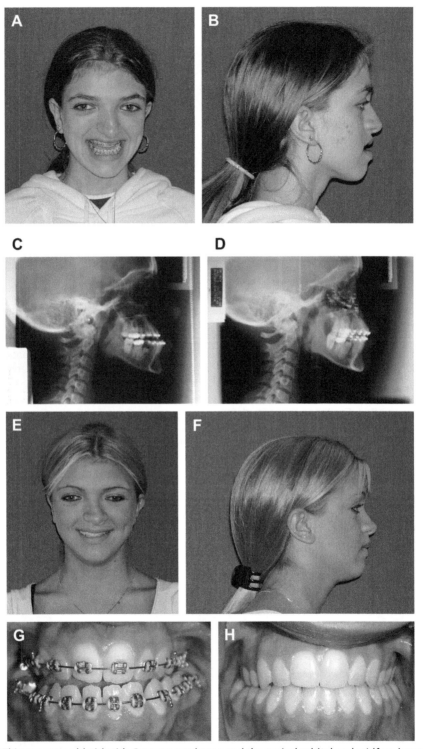

Fig. 5. (A–H) Thirteen-year-old girl with Crouzon syndrome and the typical orbital and midface hypoplasia resulting in a class III skeletal-dental relationship. She underwent a modified Le Fort III procedure advancing her zygomas and maxilla to provide her with positive overbite and overjet. Because the procedure was performed at the near completion of growth, her result has remained stable without a recurrent class III relationship. (*From* Fonseca RJ, Marciani RD, Turvey TA. Oral and maxillofacial surgery. 2nd edition. Saunders; 2009. Figure 43-5, p. 854–5; with permission.)

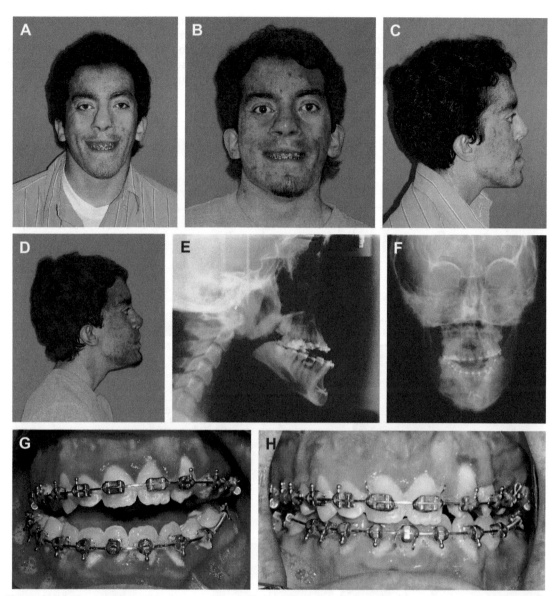

Fig. 6. (*A–H*) This young man underwent distraction osteogenesis advancement via a Le Fort I osteotomy with a genioplasty setback by another surgeon when he was 9 years of age. The treatment was complicated by difficulty with vector control and an anterior open bite after surgery. He subsequently underwent traditional orthognathic surgery, repositioning the maxilla and mandible at skeletal maturity for his definitive treatment.

Although the condyle is important in the growth and development equilibrium, the mandible develops by displacement and remodeling in all regions, not just the condyle. Periosteal apposition (eg, posterior ramus region), resorption (eg, anterior coronoid and ramus), and endochondral growth occur in the mandible. The coordinated apposition and resorption results in an inferior and anterior displacement of the mandible throughout the growth phase. Mandibular width is nearly 93% complete by the age of 5 years; however, it does not mature until 13 years in boys and 12 in girls.[3,4] Mandibular depth (tragus to gnathion) is 85% complete at age 5 years; however, it does not reach the mature dimension until 15 years in boys and 13 years in girls. Mandibular height is 67% complete by 1 year and 88% complete by 5 years. Mandibular height is mature at 12 years in girls and 15 years in boys.[3,4,31]

Marked alterations in the development of the mandible are found in Cornelia de Lange syndrome, Nager syndrome, Treacher Collins syndrome, and craniofacial microsomia (**Figs. 7** and **8**). There is frequently severe mandibular hypoplasia yielding a class II malocclusion and a high mandibular plane angle, and there may be anomalies of the temporomandibular joint complex. In contrast, class III malocclusion and mandibular hyperplasia, particularly in the ascending ramus, is seen in syndromes such as acromegaly.[32] Treatment of mandibular deformities is usually reserved until after the ages of 16 years in girls and 18 years in boys. Early

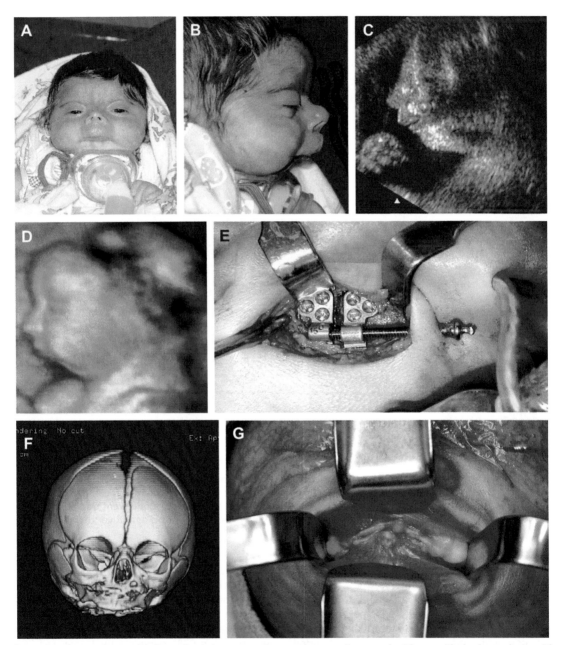

Fig. 7. (*A–E*) A newborn with Cornelia de Lange syndrome who was diagnosed with mandibular hypoplasia with ultrasound techniques as a fetus. She underwent an ex utero intrapartum treatment procedure with a tracheostomy performed using maternal circulation for a brief period of time to establish an airway. The typical mandibular hypoplasia of this disorder is evident on the lateral view. (*F* and *G*) Mandibular hypoplasia is evident in this patient with a physical impediment to growth of the mandible. This child has congenitally fused maxilla and mandible, which will prevent the mandible from functioning and may contribute to hypoplasia over time.

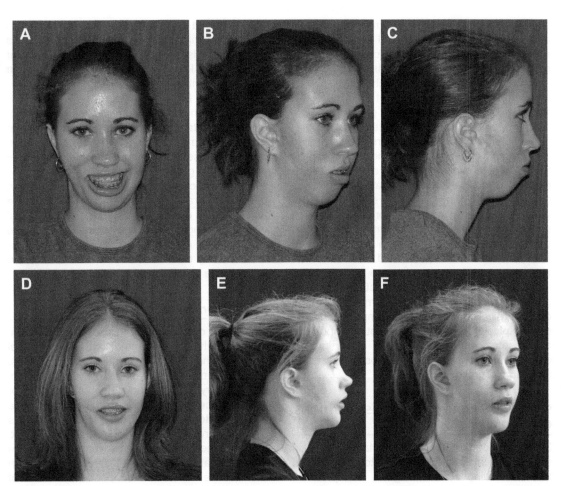

Fig. 8. (*A–C*) A teenager with craniofacial microsomia who was born with a Tessier #7 right lateral commissure cleft. The cleft was repaired in infancy by another surgeon, but she retains the right-sided hypoplasia seen with this disorder. (*D–F*) A Le Fort I osteotomy, bilateral sagittal split osteotomies, and a genioplasty provide improved facial balance and occlusion in the postoperative views. (*From* Fonseca RJ, Marciani RD, Turvey TA. Oral and maxillofacial surgery. 2nd edition. Saunders; 2009. Figure 43-8, p. 857; with permission.)

intervention for severe deformities may include either growth modification devices or early osteotomies with or without distraction osteogenesis.

CLINICAL EVALUATION OF CRANIOFACIAL GROWTH

There is considerable individual variation in the growth of the craniofacial skeleton, and many methods have been developed to assess the individual growth of patients considered for surgical treatment of a craniofacial deformity. The evaluation of the craniofacial skeleton can be performed by several simple methods based on both expected norms and concepts of growth and development. There are considerable data on the growth of the facial skeleton in patients without significant deformity or growth discrepancy.[15,16,31,33,34]

Individual measurements can be made and compared with existing age-matched control data to gain some information about the extent of the deformity. In comparison, there is a limited amount of data available on the various anomalies, and therefore only generalizations can be made with respect to the differences observed with the abnormal relationships.

Hand-wrist plain films have been used for many years to assess skeletal growth and to predict the maturation point of the craniofacial skeleton.[35] The same process can be performed by analyzing the maturation of the cervical spine, and the predictive value of the cervical spine analysis has been purported to be similar to the hand-wrist technique.[36]

One of the best methods to ascertain an individual's craniofacial growth is to evaluate serial cephalometric radiographs. Minimal or no change in velocity of the maxillofacial growth during adolescence is a good indicator of skeletal maturation. Cephalometric radiographs from the same machine using the same technique can be compared 6 or 12 months apart to evaluate for any significant change indicating growth.[16,37]

Anthropometric measurements can be performed on individuals with calipers and correlated with normative data sets.[20–23] These data can be helpful in determining either the amount of treatment to be undertaken or in evaluating the success of treatment.[37] Posnick and others[3,4,38] have evaluated individual types of deformities and the success of various surgical treatments using this type of approach, in addition to data generated from measurements performed on computed tomography (CT) scans. Although the measurements on CT are generally not practical for clinical practice, they are helpful in outcome assessment of the surgical correction.[3,4,38] Computer-assisted surgery planning software allows superimposition of expected normative data or mirror-imaged data, which may be helpful in grossly evaluating comparative growth.

SURGICAL MANAGEMENT CONSIDERATIONS
Cranio-Orbital Dysmorphology

Dysmorphology of the craniofacial skeleton is seen in patients with craniosynostosis of various types, including coronal, sagittal, metopic, and the various combinations of multiple-suture craniosynostosis. Craniosynostosis is an excellent example of the balance that is required when considering early treatment of a dysmorphology.

By definition, craniosynostosis is the early fusion of 1 or multiple sutures of the cranial vault, which causes both a telltale dysmorphology and a concern that the intracranial volume is less than the amount required for the rapidly developing brain. This mismatch can cause issues with brain growth, optic nerve function, and overall neurologic development. For this reason, expansion of the cranial vault is considered for some children with this disorder to both increase the volume available to the brain for growth and improve the dysmorphology caused by the restriction of cranial vault growth in the affected area.

The importance of brain growth requires that the surgeon consider the treatment of craniosynostosis before the ultimate maturity of the skull, but very early treatment is associated with marked relapse and the need for reoperation. For this reason, most surgeons tend to surgically dismantle the cranial vault before 1 year of age but after some growth has occurred; typically,

this is beyond the 6-month time period. In cases in which multiple sutures are involved, the need for treatment is more urgent, and earlier treatment is considered knowing that additional cranial vault expansions will likely be required.

The need for revision surgery is higher in patients who have undergone very early treatment of cranio-orbital dysmorphology. The concept that early surgery may unlock growth has not proven to be sound based on the current understanding of craniofacial growth. However, delaying the surgical correction significantly may have adverse effects on brain development and optic nerve function. The exact timing remains controversial because no predictable and repeatable measure of either brain growth velocity or intracranial pressure is easily obtainable to allow the clinician to better judge the timing of surgical expansion.

Mandibular Hypoplasia

Mandibular deficiency, with class II malocclusion, is one of the most common patterns of facial deformity and presents in a variety of expressions. When the mandible is particularly hypoplastic, early surgery in this group is often considered for airway concerns, such as obstructive sleep apnea or tracheostomy dependence. Contrasting results have been reported in the literature pertaining to the outcome of mandibular advancement before skeletal maturation.[7,10–12,38] Direct comparison between these studies is not possible because of the heterogeneity of several factors: variation in age, number of patients, presence of associated craniofacial deformities, and osteotomy and fixation techniques. Huang and colleagues[12] reviewed the outcomes of mandibular advancement in 22 growing children and found a variation of response, which appeared to be influenced by the amount of advancement. In those who underwent advancement of 10 mm or more, significant condylar remodeling and/or resorption was shown, with remodeling in the posterior symphyseal region also observed in some cases. These patients had significant relapse that continued over several years after the operation. In contrast, the group that underwent advancements of 9 mm or less showed a milder degree of relapse. No significant mandibular growth occurred after 11 years of age, and the mandible returned to its preoperative growth direction within 2 years following surgery. The patient sample was mixed with the inclusion of 4 patients with recognized craniofacial syndromes and 2 with juvenile rheumatoid arthritis. These associated features are significant confounding factors when attempting to analyze the outcomes.

In contrast, several investigators have reported favorable results following early mandibular advancement.[7,10,11,38] A study by Schendel and colleagues[10] examined the results of sagittal split mandibular advancement, with nonrigid fixation, in 12 growing patients. They showed minimal skeletal relapse and the maintenance of harmonious growth between the mandible and maxilla. In a group of 12 patients, Snow and colleagues[38] showed postoperative mandibular growth in the vertical dimension following sagittal split advancement in 11 of the patients. Vertical maxillary growth was found in several cases, and a concurrent vertical lengthening of the ramus was observed, which resulted in the maintenance of the chin position in the horizontal plane and harmonious facial balance. In addition, the occlusion was maintained, in a class I relationship, over a 5-year period after surgery in the 12 cases.

The risk factors for true relapse in following mandibular advancement seem to be similar to those seen in the skeletally mature patients. Although the number of patients in the studies in growing children is limited, they seem to indicate that preexisting condylar pathologic conditions, high mandibular plane angles, and mandibular advancements of greater than 10 mm are potential factors for significant relapse and concur with the findings from adult studies.[39–42]

Since the development of mandibular distraction osteogenesis techniques, there have been numerous reports of mandibular lengthening in the growing child for treatment of facial deformity or obstructive sleep apnea. There are some short-term follow-up reports on growth and development following the distraction procedure; however, there are no convincing, published, long-term prospective studies examining subsequent facial growth patterns and outcomes through to skeletal maturation.[43,44] It is not possible to extrapolate the early results and attempt to draw conclusions about long-term outcomes. A study by Hopper and colleagues[45] retrospectively assessed mandibular stability in 7 cases following advancement with an external distraction appliance at 12 months after the operation. During the consolidation phase, relapse of the mandible was shown with variable amounts of change. Cephalometric analysis revealed clockwise rotation of the mandible with relapse of advancement and posterior movement of the pogonion. The amount of mandibular relapse during the consolidation phase was shown to be greater than that between the postconsolidation phase and the subsequent 12-month follow-up in some cases. They found an average relapse of 22% during the consolidation phase (range 4%–41%), and, from the period following

the end of the consolidation phase to a 12-month follow-up, there was an additional mean relapse of 28% (range 7%–58%). This degree of relapse forces the question of what benefit is gained from early osteotomy in this patient population. Long-term, longitudinal studies are needed to further evaluate the success of these procedures during the growth phase.

Surgery in the small child or infant is potentially challenging for several reasons. The performance of sagittal split osteotomies in the growing child can be technically challenging because of the small amount of cancellous bone and increased pliability of the bone, in conjunction with the presence of second molar and impacted third molar teeth. There is a paucity of literature describing the complications that are seen after early osteotomy with or without the use of distraction osteogenesis. Complications include traumatic injury to tooth buds, nerve injury, malunion, nonunion, trismus, ankylosis of the temporomandibular joint, and intraoral and extraoral scarring. For many patients, the hoped-for advantages are outweighed by the number of complications seen. As with most complicated procedures in surgery, patient selection is paramount (**Fig. 9**).

Despite these concerns, early advancement of the mandible can have several advantages for patients who are approaching skeletal maturity and have significant deformity. For this population, the benefit is potentially significant (see **Fig. 7**). Even very small children with serious functional concerns (ie, severe obstructive sleep apnea) may benefit from early advancement of the facial structures despite knowing that revision surgery is likely or even certain.

Mandibular Hyperplasia

For skeletally mature patients who undergo the surgical treatment of mandibular prognathism, long-term stability remains a problem, and the nature of the relapse seems to be multifactorial. It is recognized that postpubertal mandibular growth is common, and it is unpredictable in individual patients. The positioning of the proximal segments following mandibular setback and seating of the condyle can be technically difficult, resulting in subsequent forward movement of the mandible after surgery. These factors combine to make the treatment of mandibular prognathism during growth challenging, with difficulty in predicting the final position of the mandible. The risk of relapse of this procedure in the growing child is significant. Because it is not possible to predict the amount of future mandibular growth and accommodate that growth with surgical overcorrection at the time of

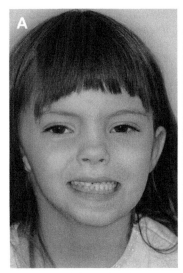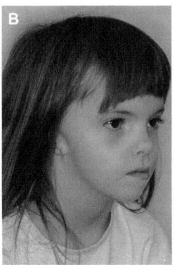

Fig. 9. (*A* and *B*) A child born with hemifacial microsomia at age 6 years who was distracted by another surgeon at an earlier age to improve symmetry and occlusion. The previous asymmetry has recurred, and relapse is evident with crossbites and three-dimensional hypoplasia on the affected side. Early surgery can be helpful in many cases for psychosocial or functional reasons, but may require revision osteotomies and additional procedures that may have a higher degree of complexity in the secondary phase. In this case, the distraction procedure offered little functional or aesthetic benefit. A more definitive treatment could be performed at skeletal maturity without incurring iatrogenic growth restriction. (*From* Fonseca RJ, Marciani RD, Turvey TA. Oral and maxillofacial surgery. 2nd edition. Saunders; 2009. Figure 43-9. p. 859; with permission.)

the setback, the procedure does not guarantee a successful outcome. For similar reasons in the growing child, orthopedic treatment with functional appliances of skeletal class III patients with mandibular excess and/or vertical excess are poor candidates for growth modification.[46] Buschang and colleagues[47] showed a worsening of the horizontal relationship between the anterior nasal spine and pogonion positions during adolescence as a result of the differential growth movements of the mandible. It was usual for the anterior-posterior relationship to worsen by greater than 4 mm during adolescence. These results concur with the findings of Harris and colleagues,[48] who also observed a progressive worsening of dental relationships in class III cases.

There is a paucity of literature on the effect of surgical mandibular setback in the growing child because the procedure is rarely undertaken before skeletal maturity. Wolford and colleagues[49,50] have some experience with the early management of this deformity. They performed bilateral high condylectomies with articular disk repositioning, either simultaneously with mandibular setback or as a staged procedure, with condylectomies followed by orthognathic surgery for the management of condylar hyperplasia. The concept of this combined approach is to remove the active growth center and therefore retard further

mandibular growth potential. They reported stable long-term outcomes, with predictable results of the mandibular position, in 25 patients managed with concomitant high condylectomy and mandibular reduction, with a mean age of 16.7 years and range of 13 to 24 years. There are few published reports examining this combined approach for comparison. In general, the procedure of high condylectomy has been reserved for severe cases of condylar hyperplasia during growth, with the treatment of the skeletal malocclusion performed after puberty and following the stabilization of the condylar growth pattern (**Figs. 10** and **11**).

Maxillary Hypoplasia

In the adult patient, the Le Fort I maxillary advancement has been shown to be a stable procedure, and, in patients undergoing large maxillary advancements, the stability has been found to be improved by the use of interpositional grafting and rigid fixation.[2,13,51] In the consideration of performing maxillary advancement before the completion of growth, it is imperative to assess the nature of the associated skeletal class III malocclusion, which may be a consequence of isolated maxillary hypoplasia, mandibular hyperplasia, or a combination of both. As previously discussed, mandibular growth commonly occurs

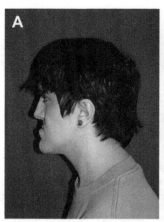 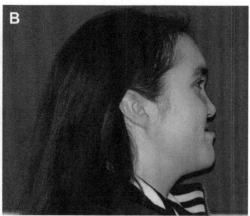

Fig. 10. Varying degrees of maxillary hypoplasia associated with unilateral cleft lip and palate. (*A*) This patient exhibits a degree of mandibular hypertrophy and maxillary hypoplasia. (*B*) This patient displays a similar degree of discrepancy, but a greater degree of maxillary hypoplasia without the severe mandibular hypertrophy. (*From* Fonseca RJ, Marciani RD, Turvey TA. Oral and maxillofacial surgery. 2nd edition. Saunders; 2009. Figure 43-10, p. 859; with permission.)

through puberty and can influence the outcome of a surgical result leading to a degree of relapse of the class III malocclusion. If the maxillary deficiency is the underlying cause of the class III malocclusion, it may be possible to overcorrect the maxillary position at the time of advancement; however, the planning of the amount of overcorrection is an empirical decision by the clinician because there are no predictive guidelines for growth potential. In the presence of mandibular hyperplasia, the surgical correction of the skeletal deformity in the maxilla and/or mandible before the completion of growth can be undertaken with the proviso that a second surgical procedure may be required in the future to compensate for any significant malocclusion.[14]

In patients with a cleft lip and palate or other craniofacial anomalies associated with significant maxillary hypoplasia, there are potential indications for undertaking maxillary advancement during growth. In patients with skeletal class III discrepancies of greater than 15 mm, there may be consideration for performing 2-stage surgical procedures: (1) maxillary advancement during growth to reduce the degree of deformity and improve facial aesthetics, followed by (2) definitive orthognathic surgery at skeletal maturity. Treatment of these large skeletal discrepancies as a single-jaw procedure is associated with significant relapse and may be detrimental to facial balance and aesthetics.[13] Undertaking these large movements even as an early single-stage maxillary and mandibular procedure may still show significant relapse.[13,14,52,53] The first-stage procedure of maxillary advancement can be performed

either by conventional advancement osteotomy or by the technique of distraction osteogenesis, although in some cases distraction osteogenesis may permit larger advancements to be performed.[52,53]

Whether conventional orthognathic or distraction techniques are used for midfacial or maxillary advancement, the underlying restriction of maxillary growth remains unchanged. Disproportionate maxillary growth in relation to the mandible following staged advancement will continue (see **Fig. 6**). The control of the vector of movement and the maintenance of proportionate bilateral movement in distraction osteogenesis is technically more difficult. The best occlusal and aesthetic postgrowth outcomes are obtained by experienced orthognathic surgeons using standard techniques of advancement. There have been several reported complications using the technique of distraction, especially if there is inadequate mobilization of the maxilla at the time of surgery, which may result in the unfavorable propagation of forces in the midfacial complex, causing unusual fractures and difficulty with vector control.[54–56]

The maxillary hypoplasia present in craniofacial dysostosis cases, such as Apert and Crouzon syndromes, is often severe and occurs concomitantly with fronto-orbital hypoplasia and exophthalmus. The treatment of the position of the fronto-orbital complex is usually undertaken between the ages of 5 and 7 years, when approximately 85% of orbital and zygomatic growth has been completed.[20–22,37] The surgical technique undertaken is based on the amount of movement

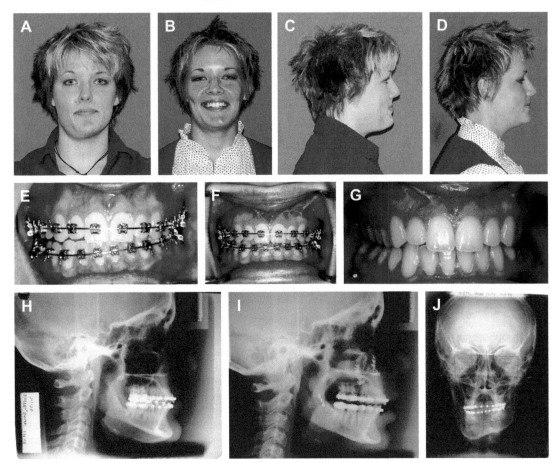

Fig. 11. (*A–M*) A 19 year-old woman with hemimandibular hypertrophy that is now stable based on sequential radiographic reviews and a quiescent bone scan. Preoperative views show the significant degree of three-dimensional asymmetry caused by the growth disturbance. Postoperative views show the balanced facial thirds and optimized occlusion.

desired at levels of both the frontal bone and orbital complex, and differential movement may be required. The fronto-orbital advancement can be achieved by a monobloc procedure or by a staged approach with frontal advancement followed by Le Fort III advancement. The surgery at this stage is undertaken to treat the fronto-orbital complex position and is not based on the occlusion. The Le Fort III advancement can also be performed by conventional osteotomy or distraction osteogenesis techniques (see **Fig. 5**).[57,58] At the completion of skeletal growth, the patient usually requires definitive orthognathic surgery for management of the malocclusion, which is typically a class III pattern with or without an anterior open bite.

There are several technical considerations that are important to consider when performing midface osteotomies in the growing patient. The positioning of the second and third molars and the canines are of importance in patients undergoing early maxillary osteotomies. Performance of the osteotomy cut with the provision of sufficient space above the apices of the permanent dentition is critical. These teeth may still be unerupted or partially erupted. Failing to provide sufficient space at the osteotomy may result in potentially adverse outcomes for the tooth, such as ankylosis, impairment of root growth, or devitalization. Due consideration for the location of the tooth roots is also imperative during the placement of plates and screws.

Vertical Maxillary Excess

Vertical maxillary excess (VME) has a well-recognized pattern of facial growth and characteristics. There is characteristic elongation of the maxilla vertically and differential lengthening of the maxilla, which result in the development of

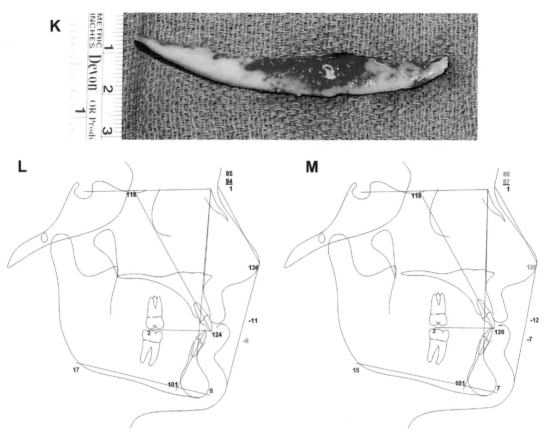

Fig. 11. (*continued*)

an anterior open bite in some patients. The VME influences the position of the mandible, with the clockwise rotation of the mandible posterior and inferior, and results in an increase in the mandibular plane angle and increased lower facial height. Early animal experiments indicated a beneficial response to maxillary impaction during growth, with a 50% to 70% reduction in vertical growth after surgery.[59] However, these experiments were performed in animals with a normal maxillary position without the underlying predisposition for the development of VME. In a report by Freihofer[7] in 1977, 3 growing patients who underwent maxillary impaction for correction of anterior open bite deformities showed marked relapse with continued downward movement of the maxillary molars with growth. Subsequent studies have concurred with the findings of the Freihofer[7] study and contrasted with the results of the animal investigations. Mojdehi and colleagues[60] examined the outcome of maxillary impaction in VME in a series of 15 growing patients, with a mean age of 12.8 years, and found that maxillary repositioning did not change the vertical growth pattern of the maxilla. The growth was neither normalized nor retarded by early surgical impaction of the maxilla. In addition, they found that there was evidence of adaptive changes in the mandible with postoperative mandibular and condylar remodeling and repositioning. Washburn and colleagues[8] reviewed the subsequent growth of the maxilla in 16 patients following maxillary impaction undertaken between 10 and 16 years of age. In the group of patients with bimaxillary protrusion before surgery, counterclockwise mandibular rotation with growth of the mandible downward and forward was observed, with a mild degree of increase in the height of the lower face.

Continued vertical growth of the maxilla can be anticipated despite early maxillary impaction, and this vertical growth rate is similar to that observed preoperatively, resulting in relapse and recurrence of the VME. The additional feature of differential maxillary or mandibular growth and the development of an anterior open bite tendency further complicate the potential for undertaking surgery before skeletal maturation (**Fig. 12**).

If the patient would benefit from early surgical intervention for psychosocial reasons, adequate warnings regarding the propensity for relapse

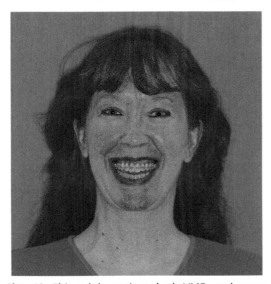

Fig. 12. This adult patient had VME and some mandibular hypoplasia young in life, but developed a late growth phase open bite in her teen years as a result of disproportionate growth of the posterior maxilla. She reports not having an open bite in the younger years of her childhood. She has a long history of obstructive nasal breathing, tonsil hypertrophy, and loud snoring.

and the necessity for an additional surgical procedure at the completion of growth are required. To reduce the chance of development of an open bite after surgery, it is advisable to maximize the overbite with orthodontic mechanics before surgery rather than compensating for the open bite with orthodontic extrusion of anterior teeth.

SUMMARY

The purpose of craniomaxillofacial surgery is to improve function, occlusion, craniofacial balance, and aesthetics. Accurate diagnosis, assessment, and careful treatment planning are essential in achieving a successful outcome, and an understanding of the pattern of facial growth is integral in this process.[14,61] Patients with craniofacial congenital dysmorphologies, posttraumatic asymmetries, or disturbances of facial balance from radiation may have functional and/or aesthetic issues that require treatment. Understanding the complexities of growth in the skull and face is a key component to appropriate treatment planning for these disorders.

The psychological implications of dentofacial deformity are important to consider and have been investigated in several studies.[13,62,63] Psychological parameters, such as self-confidence, self-esteem, insecurity, and identification with body image, are intrinsically related to patients' perception of their facial appearance. A self-perception of an abnormal facial appearance may affect an individual's psychosocial development and interactions, especially during adolescence, which may have important longer-term ramifications. Although a single definitive operation performed at skeletal maturity is preferable for patients who have a significant deformity, psychological implications may present a compelling reason to consider early surgery.

The decision to proceed with surgery before the completion of growth is complex and should not be made lightly. Comprehensive understanding of the development of the facial skeleton is critical in this decision process. Patients and their families must be fully apprised of all the implications and involved in the decision process. When early surgery is considered, the risk of relapse following surgery during growth necessitating a further surgical procedure at maturity should be discussed in detail with the patient and family. In some cases, a 2-stage surgical approach may be part of the overall treatment plan. There are several patients who benefit from early surgical intervention before maturation, and careful diagnosis and treatment planning and full consultation with the patient and family are vital when considering craniomaxillofacial surgery in the growing patient.

REFERENCES

1. Proffit WR, White RP, Sarver DM. Contemporary treatment of dentofacial deformity. Philadelphia: Mosby; 2003.
2. Proffit WR, Turvey TA, Phillips C. Orthognathic surgery: a hierarchy of stability. Int J Adult Orthodon Orthognath Surg 1996;11:191–204.
3. Waitzman AA, Posnick JC, Armstrong DC, et al. Craniofacial skeletal measurements based on computed tomography: I. Accuracy and reproducibility. Cleft Palate Craniofac J 1992;29:112.
4. Waitzman AA, Posnick JC, Armstrong DC, et al. Craniofacial skeletal measurements based on computed tomography: II. Normal values and growth trends. Cleft Palate Craniofac J 1992;29:118.
5. Precious DS, Jensen GM, McFadden LR. Correction of dentofacial deformities in children and adolescent patients. Int J Oral Surg 1985;14:399.
6. Precious DS, McFadden LR, Fitch SJ. Orthognathic surgery for children. Analysis of 88 consecutive cases. Int J Oral Surg 1985;14:466.
7. Freihofer HP. Results of osteotomies of the facial skeleton in adolescence. J Maxillofac Surg 1977;5:267.
8. Washburn MC, Schendel SA, Epker BN. Superior repositioning of the maxilla during growth. J Oral Maxillofac Surg 1982;40:142.

9. Vig KW, Turvey TA. Surgical correction of vertical maxillary excess during adolescence. Int J Adult Orthodon Orthognath Surg 1989;4:110.

10. Schendel SA, Wolford LM, Epker BN. Mandibular deficiency syndrome. III. Surgical advancement of the deficient mandible in growing children. Treatment results in twelve patients. Oral Surg 1978;45:364.

11. Wolford LM, Schendel SA, Epker BN. Surgical-orthodontic correction of mandibular deficiency in growing children. Long term treatment results. J Maxillofac Surg 1979;7:61.

12. Huang CS, Ross RB. Surgical advancement of the retrognathic mandible in growing children. Am J Orthod 1982;82:89.

13. Posnick JC, Tompson B. Cleft orthognathic surgery: complications and long-term results. Plast Reconstr Surg 1995;96:255.

14. Turvey TA, Simmons K. Orthognathic surgery before the completion of growth. Oral Maxillofac Surg Clin North Am 1994;6:121.

15. Scott JH. The analysis of facial growth from fetal life to adulthood. Angle Orthod 1963;33:11–113.

16. Riola ML, Moyers RE, McNamara JA Jr, et al. An atlas of craniofacial growth: cephalometric standards from the University School Growth Study. Ann Arbor (MI): University of Michigan Center for Human Growth and Development; 1974.

17. Moss M. The functional matrix hypothesis revisited. I. The role of mechanotransduction. Am J Orthod Dentofacial Orthop 1997;112:1.

18. Enlow DH, Hans M. Essentials of facial growth. Philadelphia: WB Saunders; 1996.

19. Enlow DH, Kuroda T, Lewis A. The morphological and morphogenic basis for craniofacial form and pattern. Angle Orthod 1971;41:3.

20. Farkas LG, Posnick JC, Hreczko TM. Anthropometric growth study of the head. Cleft Palate Craniofac J 1992;29:306.

21. Farkas LG. Anthropometry of the head and face in medicine. New York: Elsevier; 1981.

22. Farkas LG, Posnick JC. Growth and development of regional units in the head and face based on anthropometric measurements. Cleft Palate Craniofac J 1992;29:301.

23. Farkas LG, Posnick JC, Hreczko T. Growth patterns of the face: a morphometric study. Cleft Palate Craniofac J 1992;29:303.

24. Gorski JL, Estrada L, Hu C, et al. Skeletal-specific expression of FGD1 during bone formation and skeletal defects in faciogenital dysplasia. Dev Dyn 2000;218:573–86.

25. Mooney MP, Losken HW, Siegel MI, et al. Development of a strain of rabbits with congenital simple, nonsyndromic coronal suture synostosis. Part 2: somatic and craniofacial growth patterns. Cleft Palate Craniofac J 1994;31:8.

26. Putz DA, Smith TD, Burrows AM, et al. Cranial base changes following coronal suturectomy in craniosynostotic rabbits. Orthod Craniofac Res 2002;5:90–103.

27. Kjaer I, Keeling JW, Fischer-Hansen B. The prenatal human cranium-normal and pathologic development. Hoboken (NJ): Blackwell Science; 1999.

28. Aizenbud D, Morrill LR, Schendel SA. Midfacial trauma and facial growth: a longitudinal case study of monozygotic twins. Am J Orthod Dentofacial Orthop 2010;138:641.

29. Grymer LF, Bosch C. The nasal septum and the development of the midface. A longitudinal study of a pair of monozygotic twins. Rhinology 1997;35:6.

30. Precious DS, Delaire J, Hoffman CD. The effects of nasomaxillary injury on future facial growth. Oral Surg Oral Med Oral Pathol 1988;66:525.

31. Scott JH. The analysis of facial growth. I. The anteroposterior and vertical dimensions. Am J Orthod 1958;44:507.

32. Dostálová S, Sonka K, Smahel Z, et al. Cephalometric assessment of cranial abnormalities in patients with acromegaly. J Craniomaxillofac Surg 2003;31:80.

33. Posnick JC, Farkas LG. The application of anthropometric surface measurements in craniomaxillofacial surgery. In: Farkas LG, editor. Anthropometry of the head and face. 2nd edition. New York: Raven Press; 1994.

34. Posnick JC, Lin KY, Chen P, et al. Sagittal synostosis: quantitative assessment of presenting deformity and surgical results based on CT scans. Plast Reconstr Surg 1993;92:1015.

35. Grave KC, Brown T. Skeletal ossification and the adolescent growth spurt. Am J Orthod 1977;71:406–20.

36. Franchi L, Baccetti T, McNamara JA. Mandibular growth as related to cervical vertebral maturation. Am J Orthod Dentofacial Orthop 2000;118:335–40.

37. Hajnis K, Hajnisova M. Determination of the time for the corrective operations of the face according to the dynamics of its growth. Anthropos 1967;19:123.

38. Snow MD, Turvey TA, Walker D, et al. Surgical mandibular advancement in adolescents post surgical growth related to stability. Int J Adult Orthodon Orthognath Surg 1991;6:143.

39. DeClercq CA, Neyt LF, Mommaerts MY, et al. Condylar resorption in orthognathic surgery: a retrospective study. Int J Adult Orthodon Orthognath Surg 1994;9:233.

40. Arnett GW, Milam SB, Gottesman L. Progressive mandibular retrusion - idiopathic condylar resorption. Part I. Am J Orthod Dentofacial Orthop 1996;110:8.

41. Crawford JG, Stoelinga PJ, Blijdorp PA, et al. Stability after reoperation for progressive condylar resorption after orthognathic surgery: report of seven cases. J Oral Maxillofac Surg 1994;52:460.

42. Morabarak KA, Espeland L, Krogstad O, et al. Mandibular advancement in high angle and low angle class II patients: different long term skeletal responses. Am J Orthod Dentofacial Orthop 2001; 119:368.

43. Swennen G, Schliephake H, Dempf R, et al. Craniofacial distraction osteogenesis: a review of the literature: part I: clinical studies. Int J Oral Maxillofac Surg 2001;30:89.

44. Swennen G, Dempf R, Schliephake H. Craniofacial distraction osteogenesis: a review of the literature: part II. Experimental studies. Int J Oral Maxillofac Surg 2002;31:123.

45. Hopper RA, Itug AT, Grayson BH, et al. Cephalometric analysis of the consolidation phase following bilateral pediatric mandibular distraction. Cleft Palate Craniofac J 2003;40:233.

46. Kluemper GT, Spalding PM. Realities of craniofacial growth modification. Atlas Oral Maxillofac Surg Clin North Am 2001;9:23.

47. Buschang PH, Martins J. Childhood and adolescent changes of skeletal relationships. Angle Orthod 1998;68:199.

48. Harris EF, Behrents RG. The intrinsic stability of class I molar relationships: a longitudinal of untreated cases. Am J Orthod Dentofacial Orthop 1988;94:63.

49. Wolford LM, Mehra P, Reiche-Fischel O, et al. Efficacy of high condylectomy for management of condylar hyperplasia. Am J Orthod Dentofacial Orthop 2002;121:136.

50. Wolford LM, Karras SC, Mehra P. Considerations for orthognathic surgery during growth. Part 1. Mandibular deformities. Am J Orthod Dentofacial Orthop 2001;119:95.

51. Bishara SE, Chu GW. Comparisons of postsurgical stability of the Le Fort I impaction and maxillary advancements. Am J Orthod Dentofacial Orthop 1992;102:335.

52. Costello BJ, Ruiz RL. The role of distraction osteogenesis in orthognathic surgery of the cleft patient. Selected Readings in Oral and Maxillofacial Surgery 2001;10:1–27.

53. Posnick JC, Ruiz RL. Discussion of: management of secondary orofacial cleft deformities. In: Goldwyn RM, Cohen MN, editors. The unfavorable result in plastic surgery: avoidance and treatment. 3rd edition. Philadelphia: Lippincott Williams & Wilkins; 2000. p. 349. Chapter 23.

54. Cohen SR, Rutrick RE, Burstein FD. Distraction osteogenesis of the human craniofacial skeleton: initial experience with a new distraction system. J Craniofac Surg 1995;6:368.

55. Cohen SR, Burstein FD, Stewart MB, et al. Maxillary-midface distraction in children with cleft lip and palate: a preliminary report. Plast Reconstr Surg 1997;99:1421.

56. Lo LJ, Hung KF, Chen YR. Blindness as a complication of LeFort I osteotomy for maxillary disimpaction. Plast Reconstr Surg 2002;109:688–98.

57. Holmes AD, Wright GW, Meara JG, et al. Le Fort III internal distraction in syndromic synostosis. J Craniofac Surg 2002;13:262.

58. Polley JW, Figueroa AA, Charbel FT, et al. Monoblock craniomaxillofacial distraction osteogenesis in a newborn with severe craniofacial synostosis: a preliminary report. J Craniofac Surg 1995;6:421.

59. Nanda R, Bouayad O, Topazian RG. Facial growth subsequent to Le Fort I osteotomies in adolescent monkeys. J Oral Maxillofac Surg 1987;45:123.

60. Mojdehi M, Buschang PH, English JD, et al. Postsurgical growth changes in the mandible of adolescents with vertical maxillary excess growth pattern. Am J Orthod Dentofacial Orthop 2001;119:106.

61. Wolford LM, Karras SC, Mehra P. Considerations for orthognathic surgery during growth. Part 2. Maxillary deformities. Am J Orthod Dentofacial Orthognath Surg 2001;119:102.

62. Bertolini F, Russo V, Sansebastiano G. Pre- and postsurgical psychoemotional aspects of orthognathic surgery. Int J Adult Orthodon Orthognath Surg 2000;15:16.

63. Gerzanic L, Jagsch R, Watzke IM. Psychologic implications of orthognathic surgery in patients with skeletal class II or class III malocclusion. Int J Adult Orthodon Orthognath Surg 2002;17:75.

Ear and Nose Reconstruction in Children

Edward I. Lee, MD, Amy S. Xue, BS, Larry H. Hollier Jr, MD,
Samuel Stal, MD*

KEYWORDS

• Ear • Nose • Reconstruction • Pediatric • Children

KEY POINTS

- Pediatric ear and nasal deformities, congenital and acquired, are common.
- One must weigh the benefits of reconstruction on form and function versus risks of growth disturbance and donor site morbidity.
- A number of local flap options are available for traumatic ear deformities depending on the location and size of injury. In larger defects, using congenital auricular reconstruction techniques may give better results.
- The paramedian forehead flap is very useful for nasal reconstruction because local flap options are generally limited in this patient population. The goal of reconstruction is to preserve airway while re-establishing nasal lining, structural framework, and external skin envelop.

INTRODUCTION

The ear and the nose are two prominent appendages of the face that are crucial to overall facial aesthetics. As such, auricular and nasal deformities can have significant social ramifications; therefore, proper repair of these deformities is critically important to a child's well-being. Moreover, the benefits of reconstruction in the pediatric population must be weighed against added concerns about potential growth restriction on the ear and the nose with any manipulation. This article reviews various methods of auricular and nasal reconstruction and discusses some of the technical pearls for improved outcome. A complete discourse on treatment of total ear and nasal reconstruction is beyond the scope of this article. Attention is focused primarily on partial to subtotal defects.

EAR RECONSTRUCTION

The structure of the human ear is composed of three primary complexes: (1) the helix-antihelix, (2) the concha, and (3) the lobule (**Fig. 1**). Moreover, the ear is a composite construct of skin, soft tissue, and cartilage of various shape and thickness depending on the location. A more detailed anatomic description along with embryology, neurovascular, and aesthetic considerations can be found elsewhere in literature.[1]

Critical to any discussion about pediatric ear reconstruction is the issue of auricular growth. Although ear width continues to increase until age 10, it is well established that 85% of ear development is attained by 3 years of age.[2] For congenital defects, this issue is compounded by a certain degree of growth arrest attributable to the underlying pathophysiology. For congenital and traumatic defects, the goal of reconstruction should

The authors have nothing to disclose.
Division of Plastic Surgery, Baylor College of Medicine, 6701 Fannin, CC 610.00, Houston, TX 77030, USA
* Corresponding author.
E-mail address: sstal@bcm.edu

Oral Maxillofacial Surg Clin N Am 24 (2012) 397–416
doi:10.1016/j.coms.2012.04.004
1042-3699/12/$ – see front matter © 2012 Elsevier Inc. All rights reserved.

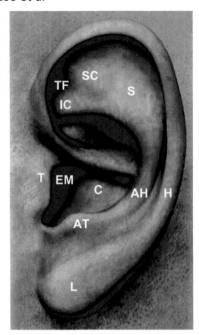

Fig. 1. External ear anatomy. AH, antihelix; AT, antitragus; C, concha; EM, external auditory meatus; H, helix; IC, inferior crus; L, lobule; S, scapha; SC, superior crus; T, tragus; TF, triangular fossa.

be to achieve symmetry with the contralateral side. For practical purposes, the ear is fully developed at 6 years of age.[3]

ACQUIRED AURICULAR DEFORMITIES

There are several principles to keep in mind for traumatic injuries to the ear and the nose. First, rule out other more serious injuries, such as skull base fractures, hearing loss, and facial nerve injury. Second, thoroughly examine the area and remove traumatic debris with only minimal debridement because aggressive removal of tissue can lead to untoward distortion of structures.[4] Third, close primarily where feasible without suturing through the cartilage. If immediate closure is not feasible, then clean, debride, and perform frequent dressing changes with topical antibiotics and nonadherent dressing to avoid desiccation before definitive reconstruction.

When evaluating the ear for reconstruction the ear is divided into five zones following the subunit principle: (1) helical rim, (2) superior third of auricle, (3) middle third of auricle, (4) lower third of auricle, and (5) lobule (Fig. 2). Auricular defects can be of partial thickness or full thickness and may involve the underlying cartilaginous framework. Therefore, identifying the location in these five zones and ascertaining the depth of injury during clinical evaluation is critical in formulating the appropriate reconstructive plan.

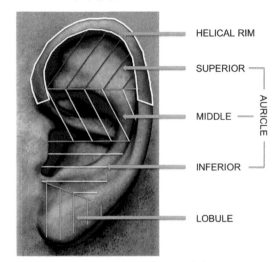

Fig. 2. Five reconstructive subunits of the ear.

In partial-thickness wounds, regardless of the location, the presence of perichondrium dictates the treatment so it is important to establish its presence or absence. When underlying perichondrium is present, partial skin avulsions can be reattached or a skin graft can be taken from the postauricular region to resurface the wound. When perichondrium is absent, then wedge excision should be considered to close the wound if the defect is less than 1.5 cm. Larger defects can be covered with any of the many variations of preauricular or postauricular flaps. Lastly, small avulsed ear pieces that are clean can be reattached as composite grafts within 6 hours.[5]

Helical Rim Defects

For full-thickness helical rim defects, the size of the defect drives the treatment approach. Where the defect is less than 2 cm, a contralateral composite graft or an ipsilateral chondrocutaneous rotation flap can be used. The chondrocutaneous flap, as described by Antia and Buch, is a versatile flap that can be advanced superiorly, inferiorly, or in both directions and requires only one stage without damaging the donor site (Fig. 3).[6] Where the defect is larger than 2 cm, superiorly based preauricular or postauricular flaps with or without cartilage grafts can be used. For larger defects, the Davis conchal transposition flap, which transposes the chondrocutaneous conchal surface on a skin pedicle to fill a marginal defect, is also an option, but a skin graft is needed to close the donor site.[7]

Another useful flap, first described by Dieffenbach, is the posterior auricular skin flap (Fig. 4), which is elevated the same width as the defect

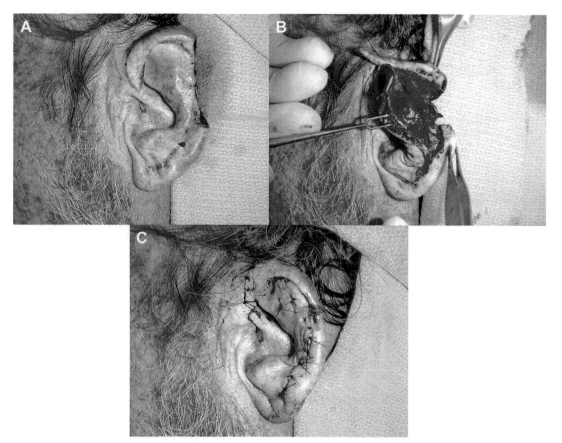

Fig. 3. Antia-Buch chondrocutaneous flap. (*A*) Preoperative markings. (*B*) Flap elevation. (*C*) Postoperative result.

up to the hairline.[6,8] Cartilage, if needed, can be taken from the ipsilateral or contralateral ear. It is important to reduce tension on the closure by temporarily suturing the conchal cartilage down to the mastoid. The flap pedicle can be divided at 3 weeks and donor defect skin grafted.

Many other reconstructive options, including tubed-pedicle flaps and tunneled techniques, have also been described but these techniques, by and large, are difficult to perform and to obtain consistent results.[9–11]

Superior Defects

In the superior third of the ear, like helical rim defects, the size of the defect also drives the reconstructive technique. Defects less than 2 cm can be reconstructed with various methods of auricular reduction. To this end, Tanzer excision patterns are useful to optimize wound closure while maximizing the amount of soft tissue available (**Fig. 5**).[12] Defects larger than 2 cm in this region without cartilaginous involvement can be resurfaced with preauricular flaps alone. Large composite defects may require a costal cartilage

graft along with either a skin flap or graft for coverage. Chondrocutaneous composite flaps, such as the Ortichochea conchal rotational flap (**Fig. 6**), provide another option for full-thickness defects.[13]

Middle and Lower Defects

Auricular reduction is useful for small defects in the middle and lower third of the ear. However, defects larger than 2 cm require a more complex reconstructive option, such as a contralateral composite graft with posterior auricular skin flap or chondrocutaneous flap.

Lobular Defects

Lobular defects are generally closed primarily because there is ample amount of soft tissue without need for cartilaginous support. However, cleft earlobe from traumatic earring avulsion requires special attention. A wedge excision can be performed but the wound edges must be everted or z-plasty performed to prevent notching. If the patient plans on wearing earrings, then a local

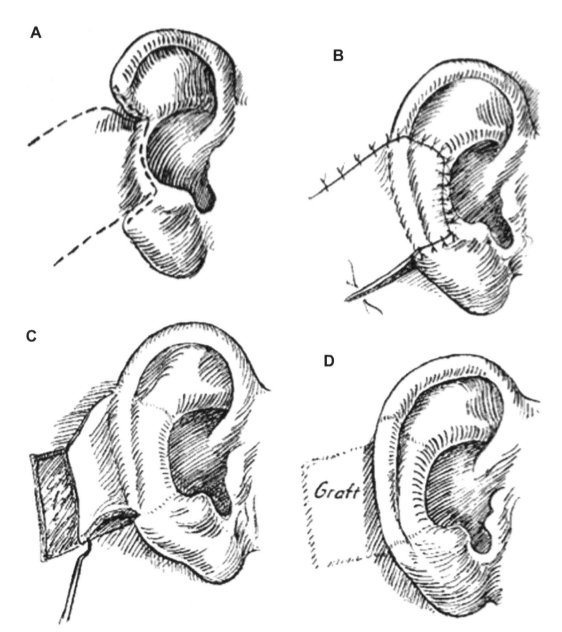

Fig. 4. Diffenbach flap. (*A*) Defect and outline of flap. (*B*) Flap advanced over the defect. (*C*) Flap divided at second stage. (*D*) Flap folded around posteromedial aspect of the ear and donor side skin grafted. (*From* Brent B. Reconstruction of the auricle. In: McCarthy JG, editor. Plastic surgery, vol. 3. Philadelphia: WB Saunders; 1990. p. 2094–152; with permission.)

flap can be rolled to create a tract with epidermal lining or the defect can be closed around a suture as a stent for future earring use.[14]

Total and Subtotal Defects

With larger defects, local options become limited. Moreover, many surgeons believe that reconstruction with local tissue rearrangement gives rise to imperfect outcomes. Consequently, many have abandoned the use of local tissue in favor of using principles of congenital auricular reconstruction to repair partial and total acquired deformities.[15–17] Some centers are performing two-stage Nagata technique (**Fig. 7**) for traumatic partial ear amputations.[16] Ali and colleagues[15] modified the Nagata technique into a single-stage procedure to treat patients with acquired segmental auricular

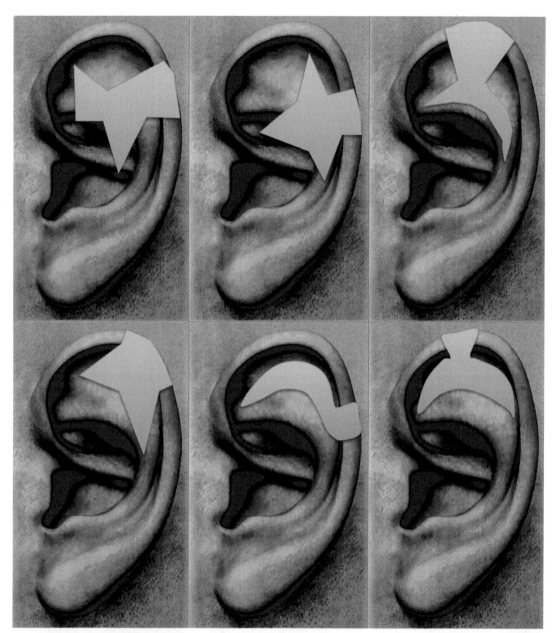

Fig. 5. Tanzer excision patterns for auricular reduction. (*Adapted from* Tanzer RC. Deformities of the auricle. In: Converse JM, editor. Reconstructive plastic surgery. 2nd edition. Philadelphia: WB Saunders; 1977. p. 1671–719; with permission.)

defects. They report a low complication rate and high satisfaction rate in 20 patients with the use of costal cartilage, temporoparietal fascial flap, and split-thickness skin graft.

For total auricular avulsion, an attempt at replantation can be made; however, the lack of reliable veins, need for lengthy procedure with long hospital stays, frequent complications, and need for leeching for venous congestion with subsequent blood transfusion handicaps the efficacy of this technique.[18] Some argue that the results of ear replantation are seldom rewarding and that it is better to discard the amputated segment, allow rapid primary healing, and perform formal elective ear reconstruction with costal cartilage.[19]

In the case of a total traumatic defect where immediate reconstruction is not a viable strategy, banking the auricular cartilage for future reconstruction has

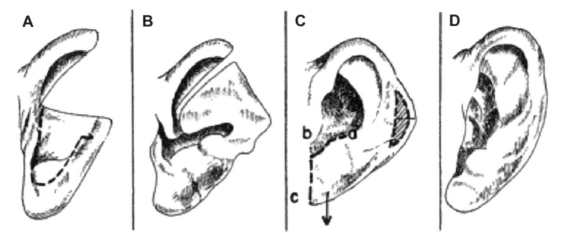

Fig. 6. Orticochea composite chondrocutaneous rotation flap. (*A, B*) First stage. A compound flap based on lateral helical rim is created containing whole concha and carrying the external-anterior skin, cartilage, and retroauricular skin. The concha donor site is covered with skin graft. (*C, D*) Second stage. Helix and lobule are adjusted to match the opposite normal side. (*From* Orticochea M. Reconstruction of partial losses of the auricle. Plast Reconstr Surg 1970;46:403–5; with permission.)

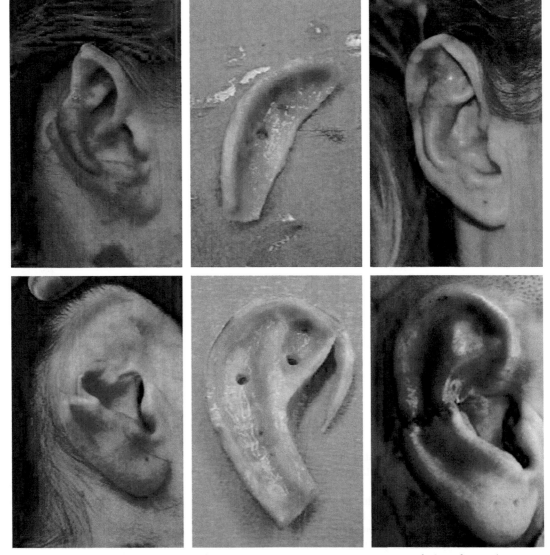

Fig. 7. Reconstruction of traumatic partial ear amputation using two-stage Nagata technique for total ear reconstruction. (*Top*) Upper pole defect. (*Bottom*) Superior half defect. (*From* Pearl RA, Sabbagh W. Reconstruction following traumatic partial amputation of the ear. Plast Reconstr Surg 2011;127:621–9; with permission.)

been described.[20] The banking of cartilage is based on the "pocket principle" and several modifications have been used to improve outcomes, including dermabrading and fenestrating the amputated segment.[21] However, banking remains an unreliable, ineffective method because it often causes cartilage to go through significant warping.[16,17] Furthermore, a salvage procedure with costal cartilage is often needed in auricular amputations of this degree. Also, because the skin flap has already been elevated in creating the retroauricular pocket, the soft tissue coverage and reconstruction becomes more difficult.[17]

Burn Injuries and Keloids

Auricular burns and frostbite occur with relative frequency in the pediatric population. Typically, auricular burns are managed topically with mafenide acetate cream to prevent desiccation and infection. Compressive dressings should not be used because they may compromise vascularity to the injured tissues. Conservative debridement of eschar after demarcation should be performed and the defect reconstructed according to the depth and location of defect. A patient commonly needs prophylactic antibiotic coverage because *Pseudomonas* infection regularly causes suppurative eschar in this type of injury.[22] Frostbite wounds are managed with rapid rewarming using warm, saline-soaked dressings. Tetanus prophylaxis is

recommended and the use of systemic prostaglandin inhibitors (ie, ibuprofen) or topical thromboxane inhibitors (ie, aloe vera) has been advocated to limit thrombosis and tissue loss.[5]

The earlobe is the most common site of keloid formation because of an association with ear piercing, which occurs with relative frequency in the pediatric population. Treatment modalities for keloid scars in this region run the gamut from simple excision to corticosteroid injection, radiation therapy, and silicone dressings. Proper treatment usually requires serial treatment using multiple modalities. Unfortunately, regardless of the treatment technique, there is a very high recurrence rate ranging from 19% to 100%.[23]

Postoperative Care

Postoperative care is equally as important as the reconstruction itself with auricular injuries. A postoperative hematoma or seroma can cause permanent warping of cartilage, known as "cauliflower deformity," which is difficult to repair. The use of bolster dressings and a careful follow-up in these patients is helpful in preventing unwanted complications (**Fig. 8**).[24]

CONGENITAL AURICULAR DEFORMITIES

Congenital ear deformities can be divided into three broad categories: (1) complete absence, (2) hypoplasia, and (3) hyperplasia. Complete auricular

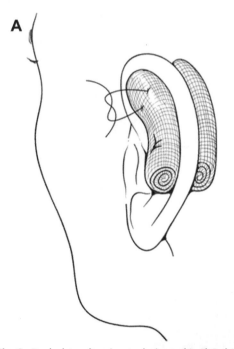
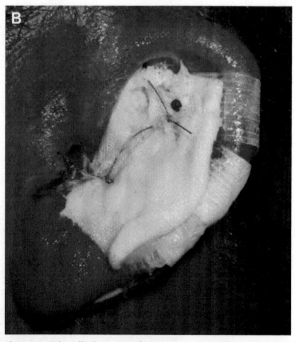

Fig. 8. Ear bolster dressing technique. (*A, B*) Bolster the ear with rolled up Xeroform gauze (Covidien, Mansfield, MA, USA) sutured in place with through and through 2-0/3-0 nylon or Prolene (Ethicon, Somerville, NJ, USA).

reconstruction for total and subtotal auricular deformities and otoplasty for prominent ears are beyond the scope of this article. Instead, addressed next are varying degrees of microtia and auricular malformations.

Clinical variations of microtia materialize from stunted development during 6 to 8 weeks of gestation.[25] The severity of the deformity diminishes the later in gestational age the malformation occurs. A detailed history and physical examination is important because auricular malformations are associated with many syndromic abnormalities, including Goldenhar syndrome, Treacher Collins syndrome, and cleft lip and palate. Isolated microtia is considered the mildest form of hemifacial microsomia.[26]

The degree of the external auricular defect does not correlate with the functionality of the middle ear; therefore, a complete radiographic and audiologic evaluation is needed to fully assess any damage to the middle ear.[27] The need for otologic surgery must be taken into consideration when planning for ear reconstruction, because most surgeons recommend auricular reconstruction before middle ear surgery.

The age of the child is important in determining the timing of reconstruction. For example, in larger defects requiring cartilaginous support, the costal cartilage is rarely of sufficient size until 5 to 6 years of age.[28] Because most children start school at this age, any physical abnormality has obvious psychosocial implications. Therefore, most surgeons recommend reconstruction to be performed during this time. Other factors that also affect the timing of surgery include the maturity of a child, recognition of the deformity of the child, the rate of the ear growth, and the elasticity of the cartilage.[29]

Some minor to moderate microtia deformities are amenable to the use of local tissue, including local flaps, composite grafts, and skin and cartilage grafts. The subunit principle described for trauma reconstruction can also be applied as a tool in determining the surgical method to be used in the reconstruction of these types of deformities. Furthermore, incisions must be carefully placed to maintain perfusion to surrounding tissue in the event that total ear reconstruction is needed as a salvage procedure. Often, a malformed cartilaginous remnant must be removed and replaced with cartilage grafts for optimal results.

Lastly, osseointegrated implants are a valuable reconstructive option that can be used to support a prosthetic ear in extreme microtia or anotia. In certain patients, these implants have shown

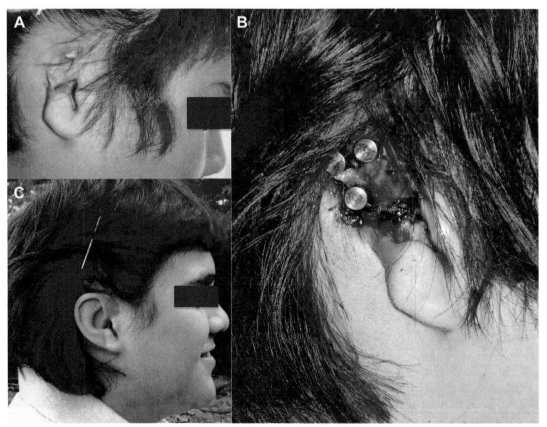

Fig. 9. Osseointegrated implant. (*A*) Preoperative defect. (*B*) Osseointegrated implant. (*C*) Postoperative result.

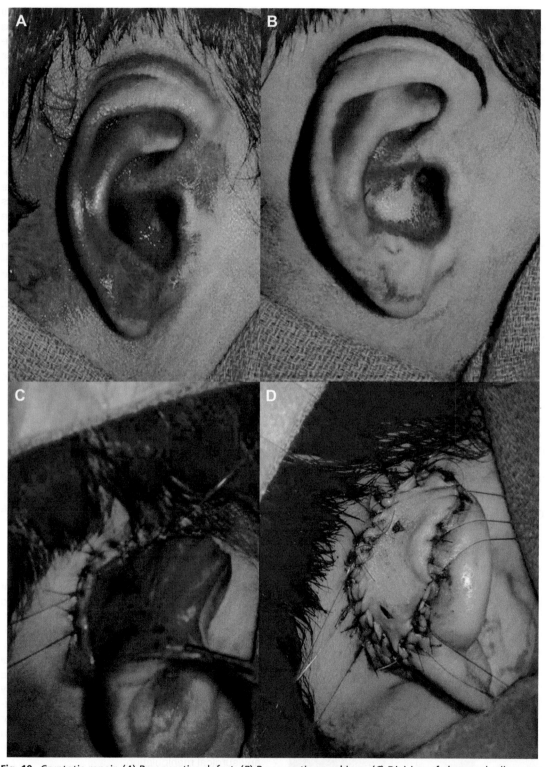

Fig. 10. Cryptotia repair. (*A*) Preoperative defect. (*B*) Preoperative markings. (*C*) Division of abnormal adherence. (*D*) Application of skin graft.

positive long-term results with high patient satisfaction and can be easily combined with hearing aids (**Fig. 9**).[30,31] However, the prosthesis is costly and they generally need to be replaced every 5 years from wear and tear and from the child's growth. Moreover, upkeep and maintenance of the implants is necessary and tedious to prevent peri-implantitis, infection, and loss of the implants.

Cryptotia

Cryptotia, known as "hidden ear," occurs as a result of abnormal adherence of the ear to temporal skin resulting in absent superior auriculocephalic sulcus. This condition is associated with various degrees of cartilage malformation. Splinting to slowly mold and elevate the cryptotic ear away from the postauricular surface may be attempted initially but definitive treatment involves division of the adherent skin and placement of a split-thickness skin graft to create a sulcus (**Fig. 10**).[32]

Stahl Ear

The defining features of Stahl ear, also known as Spock ear, are the presence of a third crus, flat helix, and malformed scaphoid fossa (**Fig. 11**). The deformity can be corrected by splinting in neonates while the cartilage is still soft and malleable. There are several surgical options that have been described, including z-plasty, cartilage reversal, and wedge excision of the third crus with helical advancement.[33]

Constricted Ear

Constricted ear is a continuum of deformities involving the upper third of auricular cartilage that ranges from slight lidding to virtual microtia

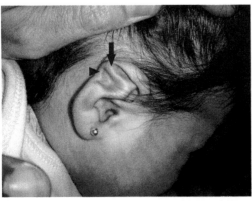

Fig. 11. Stahl ear. Defining characteristics include a third crus (*arrow*) and poorly formed helical rim (*arrowhead*).

(**Fig. 12**). Although there are several colloquial terms for this deformity, including lop, canoe, and cup ear, lidded helix, and cockle shell, all involve some permutation of the following four features: (1) lidding caused by deficient fossa triangularis, scapha, and superior crus; (2) protrusion caused by a flattened antihelix and helical rim with a deepened conchal fossa; (3) low ear position with or without hooding; and (4) decreased ear size.[29]

Constricture can be divided into mild, moderate, and severe deformities. Most mild deformities resolve spontaneously. Splinting can be useful for milder cases early on but most deformities require surgical correction. In mild cases, surgical efforts are concentrated on improving helical definition and height because native cartilage frequently maintains near-normal auricular infrastructure. Local skin and subcutaneous tissue reshaping produces excellent results. The surgical approach to moderate ear constricture is varied and debatable. The literature describes many different techniques but most surgeons conclude that regardless of the technique, successful reconstruction hinges on proper expansion of the skin envelope, reshaping the cartilage, and prevention of helical collapse.[29] Moderate to more severe deformities often require complete autologous reconstruction with costal cartilage (**Fig. 13**). Adequate soft tissue coverage must be available when planning for extensive cartilage fabrication. As such, the combination of an autologous cartilaginous framework in conjunction with an expanded skin graft is a reliable, effective means of recreating auricular form.[34] In addition, a mastoid hitch may be useful to tether the easily malleable neohelix to a more structurally sound mastoid fascia after substantial cartilage manipulation.

NASAL RECONSTRUCTION

The nose is perhaps the single most prominent aesthetic feature of the face. The same structured anatomic characteristics that give it such importance in appearance also contribute to its corporeal vulnerability. Moreover, external deformities, congenital or acquired, can cause significant nasal airway obstruction, which is a challenge for infants who are obligate nasal breathers. Therefore, any attempt at nasal reconstruction must simultaneously account for the functional and aesthetic component of nasal deformity with the caveat that it is possible to exacerbate the problem with any surgical manipulation.

Development

During embryologic development, the face is formed by five facial prominences: frontonasal

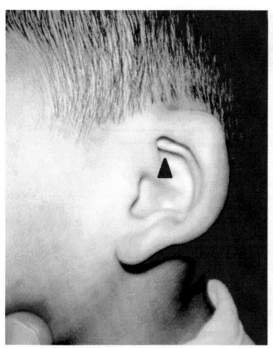 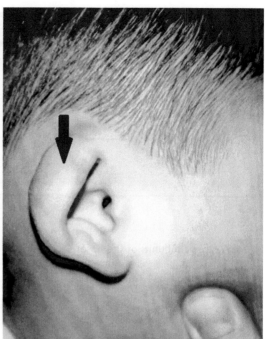

Fig. 12. Constricted ear. Lidding (*arrow*) results from deficiency in the fossa triangularis, scapha, and superior crus. The antihelix is typically flat leading to protrusion of the upper third of the ear (*arrowhead*).

prominence, two maxillary prominences, and two mandibular prominences. The nose forms from the frontonasal prominence through neural crest migration during the third to tenth weeks of gestation.[35] These cells ultimately differentiate into the medial and lateral nasal processes. The two lateral nasal processes develop into the external walls of the nose: the nasal bones, upper lateral cartilages, ala, and the lateral crus of the lower lateral cartilage.[36] The two medial nasal processes fuse to form the nasal septum and the medial crus of the lower lateral cartilage. The medial processes also interact with the maxillary prominence to create the midface. Facial clefts result from disruptions to the fusion of these processes.

The growth of the midface is contingent on the normal growth of the cartilaginous nasal septum. The sphenodorsal zone of the septum coordinates

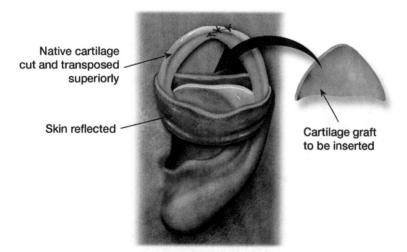

Native cartilage
cut and transposed
superiorly

Skin reflected

Cartilage graft
to be inserted

Fig. 13. Correction of a constricted ear with a moderate deformity using the double-banner technique.

408

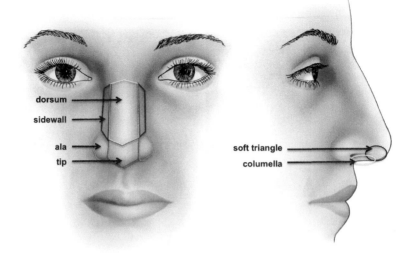

Fig. 14. Aesthetic subunits of the nose.

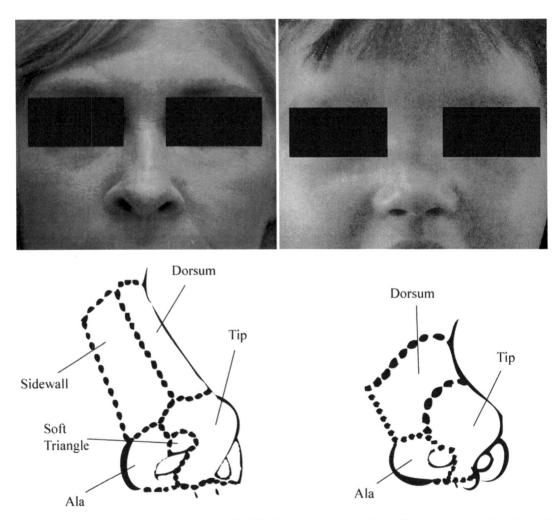

Fig. 15. An infant nose versus an adult nose. Modified subunit approach for pediatric nasal reconstruction (left, adult; right, child). Only three convex subunits are used: tip, dorsum, and ala. (*From* Giugliano C, Andrades PR, Benitez S. Nasal reconstruction with a forehead flap in children younger than 10 years of age. Plast Reconstr Surg 2004;114:316–25; with permission.)

the development of the nasal dorsum, and the sagittal growth of the basal rim guides the forward outgrowth of the premaxilla.[37] Complete loss of the septum arrests the growth of the nose and the maxilla. Therefore, surgeons should always avoid harvesting grafts from a developing septum.

In a growing child, the nose follows a particular growth pattern. Nasal bridge length increases the fastest between 4 and 5 years of age for boys and 6 and 7 years of age for girls.[38] Girls finish nasal growth at the age of 12, whereas boys continue to grow in length.[39,40]

Critical to any discussion about nasal reconstruction in the pediatric population are issues regarding nasal growth and timing of surgery. Because the septum is a major growth center of the face, any significant septal trauma, including iatrogenic, can adversely affect midfacial development. In addition, any manipulation of the nasal anatomy and resultant scarring of the nasal structures can have significant adverse consequences to nasal form and function. Furthermore, the smaller surface area of the nose and lack of potential donor sites of adequate size in children means local flap options are limited. Although most surgeons agree that the optimal time for extensive nasal reconstruction is during adolescence when most nasal growth has occurred, reconstruction may be performed earlier because of psychosocial factors and despite possible reoperation at a later age.[41] Moreover, satisfactory results can be obtained with careful planning and execution.

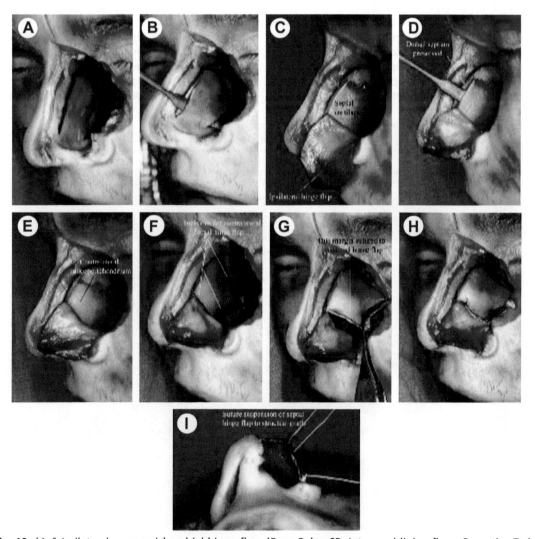

Fig. 16. (*A–I*) Ipsilateral mucoperichondrial hinge flap. (*From* Baker SR. Intranasal lining flaps. Operative Techniques in Otolaryngology 2011;22:72–83; with permission.)

Anatomy

First, it is important to understand the complex nasal anatomy, which can be simplified to the "Rule of 3s." The nose can be divided into three layers: (1) the external skin envelope, (2) skeletal-cartilaginous framework, and (3) internal nasal lining. The nose can be divided into three vaults based on the underlying skeletal structure (proximal, middle, and distal). Lastly, the external nose can be divided into aesthetic subunits. Modified from Burget and Menick's subunit principle, the adult nose is divided into nine subunits: unpaired dorsum, tip, and columella and paired sidewall, ala, and soft triangle (**Fig. 14**).[42] However, unlike the ear, which has fully developed subunits from birth, the nose goes through significant development and change throughout life. Some of the subunits, depending on the age of the child, can hardly be observed in early childhood. The pediatric nose has a bulbous tip and no distinctive side walls. The nasal apertures are typically rounder. As such, Giugliano and colleagues[43] advocate using a modified approach to the subunit principle in the pediatric population to include just 3 subunits: (1) tip, (2) dorsum, and (3) ala (**Fig. 15**).

Principles of Nasal Reconstruction

Whether managing a traumatic or congenital deformity, a proper defect analysis is critical to optimize outcomes. The "Rule of 3's" can be used to simplify defect analysis because any assessment of the defect must address the location (upper, middle, or lower third), the depth (skin and soft tissue, skeletal framework or lining), and the dimensions of defect (aesthetic subunits and absolute size). The goal of reconstruction is to preserve airway patency while optimizing nasal aesthetics through replacement of like tissues and re-establishment of distinct nasal layers.

Patients can be divided into three broad categories: (1) young children who have indistinct nasal subunits, (2) mid-aged children who have developing subunits, and (3) older children who have completed nasal growth and have fully developed subunits. In infants and toddlers, it may be prudent to attempt primary closure if at all possible to minimize further distortion of adjacent structures. Revision is inevitable in this population as the child grows, but the importance of minimizing distortion of adjacent structures and significant scarring cannot be overemphasized. Older children who

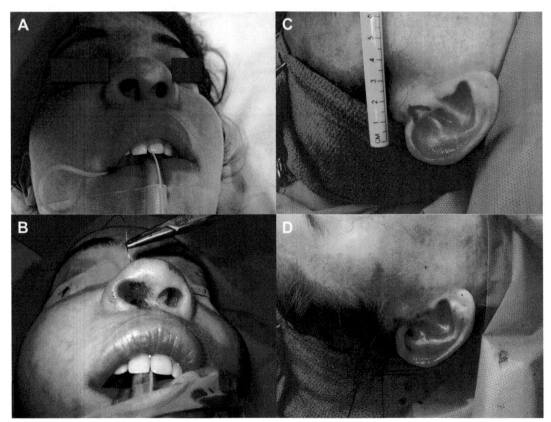

Fig. 17. Reconstruction of soft triangle defect with auricular composite graft. (*A*) Preoperative defect. (*B*) Postoperative result. (*C*) Donor site markings. (*D*) Closure of donor defect.

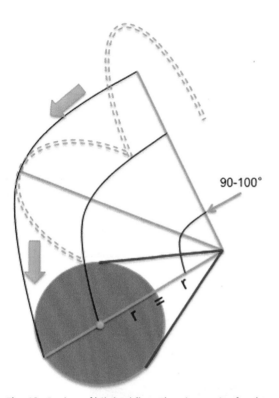

modality of treatment should be determined on a case-by-case basis. The following discussion is more pertinent to treatment of nasal deformities in older children but the principles discussed can be applied to the entire pediatric population.

Regardless of the age of the patient, significant contraction or distortion of the external nose can cause external valve collapse and stenosis, which are troublesome functional problems. Whether it be congenital or acquired, it is imperative to release all deforming forces on the nose and recreate the defect. In doing so, it is likely that the defect will require replacement of the nasal lining, structural framework, and skin.

Nasal Lining

Defects that involve the nasal lining are often overlooked. In the experience of the authors and others, a proper re-establishment of the nasal lining is critical to maintain long-term durability of any repair. Several options exist for lining replacement but septal mucoperichondrium (**Fig. 16**) remains the workhorse flap for small to moderate sized defects at any age.[44] As a rule, septal procedures should be minimized until 12 to 13 years old to prevent growth arrest of the midface. Turnover flaps or skin grafts can also be used in smaller defects.[45,46] Larger defects often require a free tissue transfer for lining replacement in a staged manner, most often with free radial forearm fasciocutaneous flap.

Structural Framework

As for reconstruction of the structural framework, the use of septal cartilage should be avoided in the pediatric population. Instead, auricular cartilage should be used for small defects and those

Fig. 18. Design of bilobed flap. The pivot point for the flap is set at one radius length from the edge of the defect. First lobe is measured to be the same size as the defect, whereas second lobe is smaller to allow donor site closure. Allow no more than 50 degrees of rotation for each lobe and undermine widely just above the perichondrium and periosteum.

have completed growth should be treated as adults from a reconstructive standpoint. The difficulty lies in treating those patients in the intermediate category and the decision to treat and the

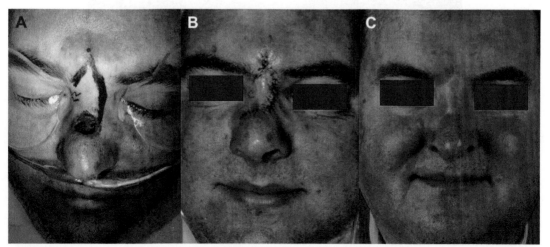

Fig. 19. Dorsal nasal flap. (*A*) Preoperative defect and marking. (*B*) Immediate postoperative result. (*C*) One-year postoperative result.

involving the ala, whereas costal cartilage can be used for larger defects. Costal cartilage is generally taken from the sixth or seventh rib.[45]

Skin and Soft Tissue

External defects can be addressed after the lining and framework have been re-established. Partial-thickness or small defects less than 1 cm, especially those located in concave regions, such as the medial canthal region, nasal sidewall-facial junction, and alar-facial sulcus, often heal with favorable aesthetic results by secondary intention.[47] Moreover, wound contracture that occurs with secondary intention can be used to reduce the size of defect for locoregional closure of

a wound that would have otherwise required a more complex option.

Skin Grafts and Composite Grafts

There are anatomic and subjective considerations for use of skin grafts versus local flaps in smaller defects. Full-thickness skin grafts taken from the preauricular, postauricular, and supraclavicular regions work well in defects that are less than 1 cm, in partial-thickness defects, and in those involving the thin skin of the upper two-thirds of the nose. However, skin grafts can be used in larger, deeper defects depending on patient preference, underlying case considerations, and as a temporary coverage for eventual flap reconstruction.

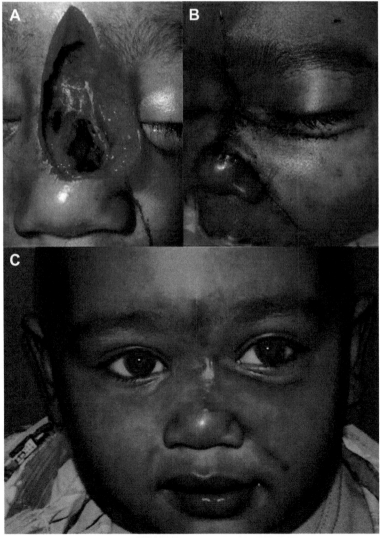

Fig. 20. Cheek advancement flap. (*A*) Intraoperative nasal defect in a child after an extensive ablative procedure. (*B*) Immediate postoperative result. (*C*) Six-month postoperative result.

Small full-thickness defects (<1.5 cm) of the nasal ala and tip can be repaired with auricular chondrocutaneous composite grafts to supply the lining, skeletal framework, and external skin. Grafts can be taken from the root of the helix or conchal bowl depending on the reconstructive need. The auricular composite graft is also an excellent option for defects in the soft triangle or columella (**Fig. 17**). It is imperative to obliterate the dead space between graft and flap with a bolster suture in larger defects because graft viability can be an issue.[48] Lastly, the auricular composite graft can be an option in patients who wish to avoid reconstruction using a forehead flap or free tissue transfer, which are associated with larger donor site morbidities.[49]

Local Flaps

Several local flaps exist and a complete description of each of these flaps is beyond the scope of this article. There are four local flaps worth mentioning: (1) bilobed flap; (2) dorsal nasal (Rieger) flap; (3) cheek advancement flap; and (4) nasolabial flap.

Bilobed flap
This is an excellent option for defects up to 1.5 cm in the thicker-skinned, lower third of the nose (**Fig. 18**). It is a double transposition flap with two flaps having a common base and no more than 50 degrees of rotation for each lobe.[50] The diameter of the first lobe is equal to that of the defect, whereas the diameter of the second lobe is smaller to allow easier donor site closure. Generally, a laterally based flap is designed for defects of the tip of the nose, whereas a medially based flap is used for lobular defects.

Dorsal nasal (Rieger) flap
This flap is based on the angular artery whereby the entire skin of the nasal dorsum can be rotated and advanced caudally to cover lobular defects up to 2 cm (**Fig. 19**).[51] The disadvantage of this flap is the creation of a large scar that does not follow skinfolds or wrinkles; careful planning of incisions along aesthetic subunits can mitigate this issue. The superior incision can be placed across the root of the nose to be concealed in the radix crease.[52] This flap should only be used in patients who have completed nasal growth because the distortion and scarring created by this method can cause significant growth restriction and disturbance.

Cheek advancement flap
This robust flap can replace nasal sidewall defects up to 2.5 cm (**Fig. 20**). Paranasal and cheek areas can be advanced with primary closure of the donor

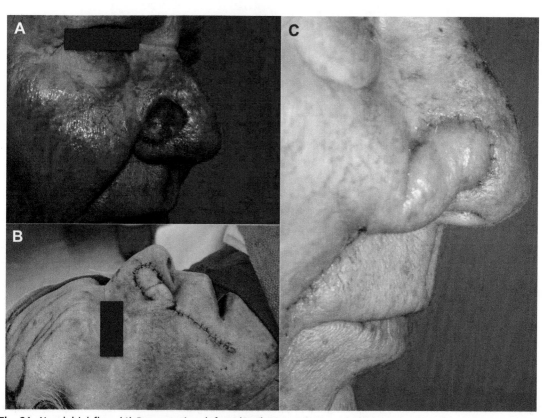

Fig. 21. Nasolabial flap. (*A*) Preoperative defect. (*B, C*) Postoperative results.

site but the flap must be anchored to the nasal-facial junction to prevent long-term distortion in larger advancements.[48]

Nasolabial flap
Defects of the nasal sidewall, ala, and tip (if superiorly based) and defects of the nasal floor and columella (if inferiorly based) can be reconstructed with nasolabial flaps based on the angular artery (**Fig. 21**). It can be designed as a transposition flap in a single stage or interpolated flap in multiple stages, especially if cartilage graft is needed for support.[53]

By and large, the use of local flaps is limited in the pediatric population because of a smaller donor surface area, tight and inelastic skin envelope, and greater degree of nasal distortion caused by tension on the closure. Therefore, the paramedian

forehead flap is the preferred local flap in this patient population.

Paramedian forehead flap
The forehead flap is reliable with good donor site morbidity and has the capacity to grow as the patient grows.[45] Moreover, no other loco-regional flap furnishes the benefit of a more sweeping coverage of defects involving multiple nasal subunits or nasal tip and accomplishes the acceptable aesthetic and functional results (**Fig. 22**).

The paramedian forehead flap is centered over the supratrochlear artery, which is located reliably between 1.7 and 2.2 cm from midline with a Doppler probe.[54] The flap is designed vertically along the path of the supratrochlear artery but can be designed obliquely to gain additional length. Where additional length is desirable, the

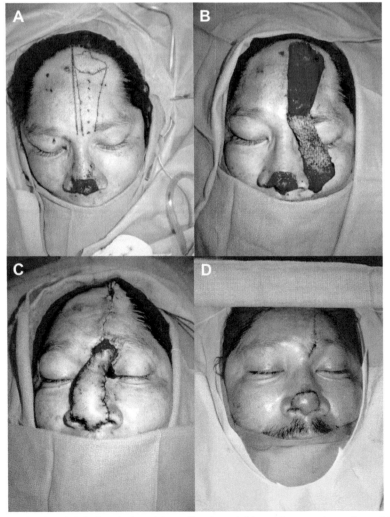

Fig. 22. Paramedian forehead. (*A*) Flap design. (*B*) Application of skin graft on undersurface of flap. (*C*) Completion of first stage. (*D*) After division and inset of flap 3 weeks later.

flap can be extended into the hair-bearing scalp or pre-expanded with placement of a subgaleal tissue expander.

The flap is elevated just above the loose areolar tissue over the frontal bone and the pedicle width should be no more than 1.5 cm because a wider pedicle may obstruct venous return after making the necessary 180-degree pivot for inset.[45] Some surgeons choose to cover the undersurface of the pedicle with a split-thickness skin graft.[45] At 3-week intervals, the second- and third-stage procedures can be done to divide the flap, further thin the distal flap, and revise the tip and donor site.

SUMMARY

Pediatric ear and nasal deformities, congenital and acquired, are common. One must weigh the benefits of reconstruction on form and function versus risks of growth disturbance and donor site morbidity. It is important to understand the anatomy and know the technical principles to optimize outcome. With careful planning and execution, ear and nasal reconstruction in children can be predictable and rewarding.

REFERENCES

1. Beahm EK, Walton RL. Auricular reconstruction for microtia. Part I. Anatomy, embryology, and clinical evaluation. Plast Reconstr Surg 2002;109(7):2473–82.

2. Adamson JE, Horton CE, Crawford HH. The growth patterns of the external ear. Plast Reconstr Surg 1965;36:466–70.

3. Farkas LG. Anthropometry of normal and anomalous ears. Clin Plast Surg 1978;5:401–12.

4. Hackney FL. Plastic surgery of the ear. In: Selected readings in plastic surgery, vol. 9, number 16. Dallas (TX): Selected Readings in Plastic Surgery, Inc.; 2001. p. 1–26.

5. Bullocks JM, Hsu PW, Izaddoost SA, et al. Plastic surgery emergencies: principles and techniques. New York: Thieme; 2008. p. 29–53.

6. Ottat MR. Partial reconstruction of the external ear after a trauma: simple and efficient techniques. Braz J Otorhinolaryngol 2010;76(1):7–13.

7. Donelan MB. Conchal transposition flap for postburn ear deformities. Plast Reconstr Surg 1989;83:641–54.

8. Dieffenbach JF. Die operative chirrurgie. Leipzig (Germany): Brockhaus; 1845.

9. Converse JM. Reconstruction of the auricle. Part I. Plast Reconstr Surg 1958;22:150–63.

10. Preaux J. Un procede simple de reconstruction de la partie inferieure du pavilion de l'oreille. Ann Chir Plast 1971;16(3):60–2.

11. Brent B. The acquired auricular deformity: a systemic approach to its analysis and reconstruction. Plast Reconstr Surg 1977;59:475–85.

12. Tanzer RC. Congenital deformities (of the auricle). In: Converse JM, editor. Reconstructive plastic surgery, vol. 3. 2nd edition. Philadelphia: WB Saunders; 1977. p. 1671–719.

13. Orticochea M. Reconstruction of partial losses of the auricle. Plast Reconstr Surg 1970;46:403–5.

14. Pardue AM. Repair of torn earlobe with preservation of the perforation for an earring. Plast Reconstr Surg 1973;51:472–3.

15. Ali SN, Khan MA, Farid M, et al. Reconstruction of segmental acquired auricular defects. J Craniofac Surg 2010;21:561–4.

16. Pearl RA, Sabbagh W. Reconstruction following traumatic partial amputation of the ear. Plast Reconstr Surg 2011;127:621–62.

17. Steffen A, Katzbach R, Klaiber S. A comparison of ear reattachment methods: a review of 25 years since Pennington. Plast Reconstr Surg 2006;118: 1358–64.

18. O'Toole G, Bhatti K, Masood S. Replantation of an avulsed ear, using a single arterial anastomosis. J Plast Reconstr Aesthet Surg 2008;61:326–9.

19. Gault D. Post traumatic ear reconstruction. J Plast Reconstr Aesthet Surg 2008;61:S5–12.

20. Pribaz JJ, Crespo LD, Orgill DP, et al. Ear replantation without microsurgery. Plast Reconstr Surg 1997;99(7):1868–72.

21. Mladick RA. Salvage of the ear in acute trauma. Clin Plast Surg 1978;5:427–35.

22. Ray E, Wu T, Mobin SS, et al. Review of options for burned ear reconstruction. J Craniofac Surg 2010; 21:1165–9.

23. Ogawa R. The most current algorithms for the treatment and prevention of hypertrophic scars and keloids. Plast Reconstr Surg 2010;125:557–68.

24. Giffin CS. Wrestler's ear: pathophysiology and treatment. Ann Plast Surg 1992;28:131–9.

25. Melnick M, Myrianthopoulos NC. External ear malformations: epidemiology, genetics and natural history. Birth Defects Orig Artic Ser 1979;15:i–ix, 1–140.

26. Bennum RD. Microtia: a microform of hemifacial microsomia. Plast Reconstr Surg 1985;76:859–65.

27. Schuknecht NF. Reconstructive procedures for congenital aural atresia. Arch Otolaryngol 1975; 101:170–2.

28. Brent B. The correction of microtia with autogenous cartilage grafts. I. The classic deformity. Plast Reconstr Surg 1980;66:1–12.

29. Janz BA, Cole P, Hollier LH, et al. Treatment of prominent and constricted ear anomalies. Plast Reconstr Surg 2009;124(Suppl 1):27e–37e.

30. Hamming KK, Lund TW, Lander TA, et al. Complications and satisfaction with pediatric osseointegrated

external ear prosthesis. Laryngoscope 2009;119: 1270–3.

31. Grandstrom G, Berstrom K, Odersjo M, et al. Osseointegrated implants in children: experience from our first 100 patients. Otolaryngol Head Neck Surg 2001;125:85–92.

32. Hirose T, Tomono T, Matsuo K, et al. Cryptotia: our classification and treatment. Br J Plast Surg 1985; 38:352–60.

33. Nakajima T, Yoshimura Y, Kami T. Surgical and conservative repair of Stahl's ear. Aesthetic Plast Surg 1984;8:101–7.

34. Hu XG, Zhuang HX, Yang QH, et al. Subtotal ear reconstruction for correction of type 3 constricted ears. Aesthetic Plast Surg 2006;30:455–9.

35. Losee JE, Kirschner RE, Whitaker LA, et al. Congenital nasal anomalies: a classification scheme. Plastic Reconstr Surg 2004;113:676–89.

36. Skevas A, Tsoulias T, Papadopoulos N, et al. Proboscis lateralis, a rare malformation. Rhinology 1990;28:285–9.

37. Verwoerd CD, Verwoerd-Verhoef HL. Rhinosurgery in children: basic concepts. Facial Plast Surg 2007;23: 219–30.

38. Sforza C, Grandi G, De Menezes M, et al. Age- and sex-related changes in the normal human external nose. Forensic Sci Int 2011;204:205.e1–9.

39. Genecov JS, Sinclair PM, Dechow PC. Development of the nose and soft tissue profile. Angle Orthod 1990;60:191–8.

40. Ferrario VF, Sforza C, Poggio CE, et al. Three-dimensional study of growth and development of the nose. Cleft Palate Craniofac J 1997;34:309–17.

41. Pittet B, Montandon D. Nasal reconstruction in children: a review of 29 patients. J Craniofac Surg 1998;9:522–8.

42. Burget GC, Menick FJ. The subunit principle in nasal reconstruction. Plast Reconstr Surg 1985;76: 239–47.

43. Giugliano C, Andrades PR, Benitez S. Nasal reconstruction with a forehead flap in children younger than 10 years of age. Plast Reconstr Surg 2004; 114:316–25.

44. Burget GC, Menick FJ. Nasal support and lining: the marriage of beauty and blood supply. Plast Reconstr Surg 1989;84:189–202.

45. Burget GC. Preliminary review of pediatric nasal reconstruction with detailed report of one case. Plast Reconstr Surg 2009;124(3):907–18.

46. Menick FJ. A 10-year experience in nasal reconstruction with the three-stage forehead flap. Plast Reconstr Surg 2002;109(6):1839–55.

47. Van der Eerden PA, Lohuis PJ, Hart AA, et al. Secondary intention healing after excision of nonmelanoma skin cancer of the head and neck: statistical evaluation of prognostic values of wound characteristics and final cosmetic results. Plast Reconstr Surg 2008;122(6):1747–55.

48. Chang JS, Becker SS, Park SS. Nasal reconstruction: the state of the art. Plast Reconstr Surg 2004; 12(4):336–43.

49. Rapley JH, Lawrence WT, Witt PD. Composite grafting and hyperbaric oxygen therapy in pediatric nasal tip reconstruction after avulsive dog-bite injury. Ann Plast Surg 2001;46:434–8.

50. Zitelli JA. The bilobed flap for nasal reconstruction. Arch Dermatol 1989;125:957–9.

51. Rieger RA. A local flap for repair of the nasal tip. Plast Reconstr Surg 1967;40:147–9.

52. Rohrich RJ, Barton FE, Hollier L. Nasal reconstruction. In: Aston SJ, Beasley RW, Thorne CH, editors. Grabb & Smith's plastic surgery. 5th edition. Philadelphia: Lippincott; 1997. p. 513–28.

53. Jin HR, Jeong WJ. Reconstruction of nasal cutaneous defects. Auris Nasus Larynx 2009;36:560–6.

54. Asaria J, Pepper JP, Baker SR. Key issues in nasal reconstruction. Curr Opin Otolaryngol Head Neck Surg 2010;18:278–82.

Craniofacial and Orbital Dermoids in Children

Brent A. Golden, DDS, MD[a,b],*,
Michael S. Jaskolka, MD, DDS[a,c],
Ramon L. Ruiz, DMD, MD[d,e,f]

KEYWORDS

- Dermoid - Pediatric - Craniofacial

KEY POINTS

- Dermoid lesions in the craniofacial and orbital region comprise a spectrum of pathologic conditions that range from extraorbital extracranial cysts to complex sinus tracts extending intracranially.
- The goals of surgical treatment include complete excision to obtain the proper histopathologic diagnosis, prevent recurrence, and for select lesions, prevent neurologic complications.
- Cranio-orbital lesions in the midline pose a higher risk for penetration of the facial skeleton with coincident neurologic involvement requiring special attention.
- Simple lesions are amenable to direct excision. Deeper lesions may require a coordinated surgical approach between a neurosurgeon and craniofacial surgeon after characterization by radiographic imaging.

INTRODUCTION

Dermoid lesions of the craniofacial region comprise a spectrum of pathologic conditions that range from simple localized cysts to complex lesions with fistula formation and intracranial extension. When encountered in children, they are commonly considered to be congenital in nature and to arise from active ectodermal cell rests that are trapped in an abnormal position.[1]

When considering all dermoids, 7% arise in the head and neck,[2] and more than half will be diagnosed before 6 years of age.[3] Additionally, when including orbital rim lesions, numerous reports in children identify the dermoid cyst as the most commonly encountered orbital lesion.[4–6]

Congenital dermoids in the head and neck are classified as periorbital, nasal, submental, and midventral/middorsal neck.[1] More focused approaches to the craniofacial region have highlighted nasoglabellar, orbital, and frontotemporal occurrences.[7,8] Within these craniofacial groups, pathologic conditions as varied as epidermal inclusion cysts, encephaloceles, gliomas, eosinophilic granulomas, lipomas, neurofibromas, and

The authors have nothing to disclose.
[a] Department of Oral and Maxillofacial Surgery, University of North Carolina Chapel Hill, CB 7450, 101 Manning Drive, Chapel Hill, NC 27599, USA; [b] Department of Pediatrics, University of North Carolina Chapel Hill, 260 MacNider Building, CB 7220, UNC School of Medicine, Chapel Hill, NC 27599, USA; [c] First Appalachian Craniofacial Deformities Specialists Cleft Center, Charleston Area Medical Center, Women and Children's Hospital, 830 Pennsylvania Avenue, Suite 302, Charleston, WV 25302, USA; [d] Pediatric Craniomaxillofacial Surgery, Arnold Palmer Hospital for Children, 83 West Columbia Street, Orlando, FL 32806, USA; [e] Department of Children's Surgery, Arnold Palmer Hospital for Children, Orlando, FL, USA; [f] University of Central Florida College of Medicine, Orlando, FL, USA
* Corresponding author. Department of Oral and Maxillofacial Surgery, University of North Carolina, CB 7450, 101 Manning Drive, Chapel Hill, NC 27599.
E-mail address: brent.golden@gmail.com

Oral Maxillofacial Surg Clin N Am 24 (2012) 417–425
doi:10.1016/j.coms.2012.04.006
1042-3699/12/$ – see front matter © 2012 Published by Elsevier Inc.

hemangiomas may overlap with respect to clinical presentation.

Often the simple dermoid cyst remains asymptomatic but when neglected may exhibit a slowly progressive nature resulting in pain, hard or soft tissue distortion, functional impairment, or drainage with or without infection. The more rarely encountered dermal sinus tract also harbors the notable potential for morbid neurologic complications including tumor formation, meningitis, or brain abscess if improperly managed.[9]

The goals of surgical treatment include complete excision to obtain proper histopathologic diagnosis, prevent recurrence, and for select lesions, prevent neurologic complications. Given the congenital nature of these lesions, their relative frequency, and the range of pathologic conditions that must be differentiated, the pediatric craniomaxillofacial surgeon must be familiar with their presentation and management.

HISTOPATHOLOGY

Dermoid cysts are cystic neoplasms that demonstrate ectodermal and mesodermal features. This is in contrast to epidermal inclusion cysts, which only include ectodermal elements, or teratomas, which have ectodermal, mesodermal, and endodermal components. More precisely, dermoid cysts are lesions with a stratified squamous epithelial lining in a fibrous connective tissue that includes skin adnexa, such as hair follicles, sebaceous glands, or sweat glands (**Fig. 1**). The lumen often contains keratin or sebaceous material produced by these components.[3] The cyst is usually subcutaneous and is often adherent to the periosteum overlying a craniofacial suture.

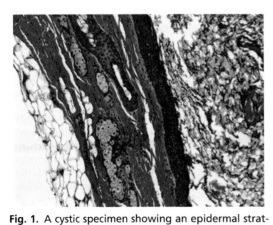

Fig. 1. A cystic specimen showing an epidermal stratified squamous epithelium with intraluminal keratin and a connective tissue wall containing sebaceous glands and hair follicle (hematoxylin-eosin, original magnification ×100).

ORIGINS

Dermoid cysts may be congenital in origin or, more rarely, acquired.[2,7,8] The congenital dermoid in the craniofacial region most often is thought to be of an inclusion type whereby epithelial remnants are sequestered abnormally to a deeper location.[1,8] In contrast, the teratoma type of congenital dermoid is primarily found in the ovaries or testes and is derived from displaced cells in the blastomere.[1]

Focusing on congenital inclusion dermoids, the embryologic origin stems from the activation of ectodermal cells dislocated secondary to nondisjunction from deeper neuroectodermal elements during the migration and maturation of these primordial tissues.[10] The general pattern of distribution of these lesions along the lines of embryologic fusion supports this hypothesis.[1]

This disturbance may result in the formation of a simple cyst or a continuous tract with extension to a dural or even intradural location. These dermal inclusion tracts show a greater propensity for the neural axis closure line, most commonly at the lumbosacral region and posterior cranial fossa in the midline.[11] The fronto-nasal region is less commonly implicated but is also notable for penetrating dermal sinus formation.[11]

CLASSIFICATION

Although most congenital inclusion dermoids in the craniofacial region are thought to develop through a common mechanism, the differential diagnosis and the risk of involvement of deeper structures varies based on anatomic location. Because of this, the classification of craniofacial space occupying lesions in the pediatric patient by site can help guide diagnostic testing and treatment decisions. Craniofacial midline lesions clearly pose a higher risk for neurologic involvement and deserve special attention. Additionally, the management of scalp and calvarial lesions must be considered separately from orbitomaxillofacial lesions based on the range of pathologic conditions that can be encountered. Useful anatomic groupings that have evolved are nasofrontoethmoidal, frontotemporal, orbital, and calvarial lesions.[7,8]

The characterization of the risk of involvement of structures deep to the craniofacial skeleton is also required to develop a proper treatment plan. Simple dermoids have a clearly intact skeletal barrier between the lesion and deeper structures (eg, dura or orbit). Complex lesions will demonstrate features of a tract or cyst that penetrate or are likely to penetrate underlying bone or cartilage. Importantly, diagnostic imaging will not always provide a definitive picture of depth but can serve to provide information that may suggest extension or penetration. Surgical exploration is required to fully define a lesion's relationship to the surrounding structures. It follows that within each anatomic location, lesions may be subclassified as simple or complex relative to their risk of extension into deeper structures.

EVALUATION AND TREATMENT
Frontotemporal and Orbital Lesions

The dermoid cyst is the most common locally palpable periorbital lesion in children with more than half of all craniofacial dermoids found in this area.[1,6,12,13] The superotemporal quadrant associated with the zygomaticofrontal suture is the site most frequently involved.[12,13]

Brow cysts in the frontotemporal region with easily palpable borders and no skin involvement are generally considered uncomplicated. The treatment must consider a differential diagnosis that includes epidermal inclusion cyst, lipoma, neurofibroma, benign adnexal tumor, or teratoma.[8] If the depth of involvement or character is unclear, ultrasound evaluation has been shown to be diagnostic in the craniofacial region for dermoids (**Fig. 2**).[1]

Although some reports suggest imaging and then observation without excision may allow for some of these simple cysts to spontaneously involute,[14,15] the definitive treatment remains excision. The excision is most often performed through a lateral brow or upper-lid blepharoplasty approach.[4,8] (**Fig. 3**) The deep surface of the dermoid lesion is often adherent at the suture, and the inclusion of the periosteum with the cyst is recommended to facilitate delivery. Every effort should be made to deliver the lesion unruptured to decrease the risk of incomplete removal and subsequent recurrence as well as to limit the

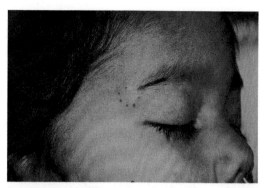

Fig. 3. Markings of a brow approach to a lateral orbital dermoid cyst.

inflammatory response associated with the spillage of the cyst contents into the surrounding tissues.

Endoscopic techniques have been used to hide the access scar in the hairline; however, limitations include longer operating time and difficulty recontouring any potential soft tissue depressions caused by lesion removal.[16] The direct approaches remain simple, rapid, and cosmetic. Excision is expected to be curative when the lesion is completely removed.

Frontotemporal and orbital lesions harbor the potential for complex features with orbital or even transcranial involvement. In fact, Sathananthan and colleagues[17] reported a high incidence of radiographic extension into or through bone around the orbit despite limited clinical indications of such. Concern for deeper involvement may come from a lesion that has borders difficult to palpate, is immobile and firmly adherent to the underlying facial skeleton, exhibits a draining fistula, or results in proptosis. When clinical features or ultrasound evaluation suggest deeper involvement, fine-cut axial and coronal orbital computed tomography (CT) greatly improves the diagnostic yield and is mandatory for surgical planning (**Fig. 4**).

Orbital lesions may exist as bilobed dumbbell lesions with intraorbital and extraorbital components connected through the medial or lateral orbital wall.[18] The goal remains complete excision, which may require incision of the orbital septum with intraorbital exploration. Another approach involves posterior subperiosteal dissection into the orbit followed by incision of the periosteum to deliver the cyst.[12] For larger or posterior lesions, a lateral orbitotomy may be necessary for access and complete cyst removal.[4] Orbital dermoids may also be of conjunctival origin.[18] These occur more commonly in a superonasal orientation, and excision can be performed through either a conjunctival or cutaneous lid approach.[4]

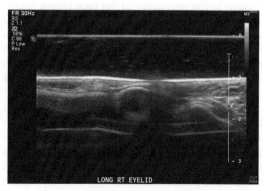

LONG RT EYELID

Fig. 2. Ultrasound image of simple dermoid cyst.

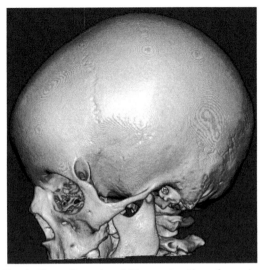

Fig. 4. Three-dimensional CT reconstruction of complex lateral orbital dermoid cyst.

Craniofacial dermal sinuses with deep extension in the frontotemporal region occurring away from the midline are extremely rare, with less than a dozen cases reported previously.[7,19] When a frontotemporal lesion demonstrates CT evidence of transcranial extension, magnetic resonance imaging (MRI) is useful to further characterize the relationship to the dura. Combined neurosurgical and craniofacial approach via a coronal flap and craniotomy may be necessary to provide wide exposure to allow for safe excision and prevent neurologic sequela. Depending on the depth of invasion, a portion of the dura may be excised, which requires primary repair or a patch. Given the rarity of reported cases, the surgical approach needs to be tailored to the clinical presentation (**Fig. 5**).

Frontonasoethmoidal Lesions

Frontonasoethmoidal dermoid cysts compose approximately 10% of head and neck dermoid lesions.[2,9,11,13] They belong to the category of midline nasal masses that occur in approximately 1 in 20,000 live births and includes dermoids, gliomas, and encephaloceles.[20,21] Most reports describe few instances of concurrent congenital anomalies, but Wardinsky and colleagues[22] report other pathologic findings in more than 40% of their sample. Most are not considered to have a familial predisposition, although occasional reports of familial occurrence do exist in the literature.[21]

Understanding the range and pattern of frontonasoethmoidal masses requires particular attention to the local embryology. Embryologic descriptions largely arise from 2 theories of tissue origin: one cranial and the other cutaneous.[21,23]

Although simple cysts may come from a cutaneous source, the cranial origin more adequately explains the spectrum of frontonasoethmoidal pathologic conditions.

Grunwald[24] is credited with the initial description of the embryologic development of cranial dermoid pathologic conditions in 1910. Brunner and Harned[25] and Pratt[26] further elaborated on the frontonasal origin and development of midline masses. According to their descriptions, intramembranous formation of the nasal bones and cranial vault progresses from discontinuous sites leaving transitory intervening spaces (**Fig. 6**). The anterior and posterior fontanelles that persist in the early infant skull are well-known examples of this developmental process.

Two lesser-discussed spaces are of particular relevance for frontonasal development: the fonticulus nasofrontalis and the prenasal space. The anatomic space between the developing nasal and frontal bones is known as the fonticulus nasofrontalis (**Fig. 7**). The transitory prenasal space extends from the anterior cranial base to the nasal tip lying just deep to the nasal bones and just above the cartilaginous nasal capsule that forms its deep surface.

It is proposed that during development, chords of dural diverticula temporarily extend into these embryologic spaces. Normally, when the fonticulus nasofrontalis closes to form the frontonasal suture, there is regression of these dural projections with resultant obliteration of all communication between the dura and overlying skin. In the developing nose, the dural diverticulum that extends into the prenasal space regresses into the anterior cranial base and is encircled with bone leaving only the foramen cecum (see **Fig. 7**).

Rarely, chords of cells may adhere to the surface ectoderm in either of these spaces resulting in the inclusion of abnormal cells along embryologic lines. As with other midline locations, these two frontonasal spaces seem to have an increased tendency for inclusion tract formation relative to the remainder of the face where superficial dermoid cysts are more common. Consistent with these embryologic routes, most frontonasal tracts that exhibit intracranial extension will travel beneath the nasal bones to penetrate the foramen cecum or, less commonly, may directly traverse the frontonasal junction.

Not only may skin elements be drawn deeper but also neural elements may be drawn superficially resulting in glioma or encephalocele formation. Any child with a midline or paramidline lesion in the frontonasal region should undergo CT or MRI evaluation to identify and distinguish between these pathologic entities.

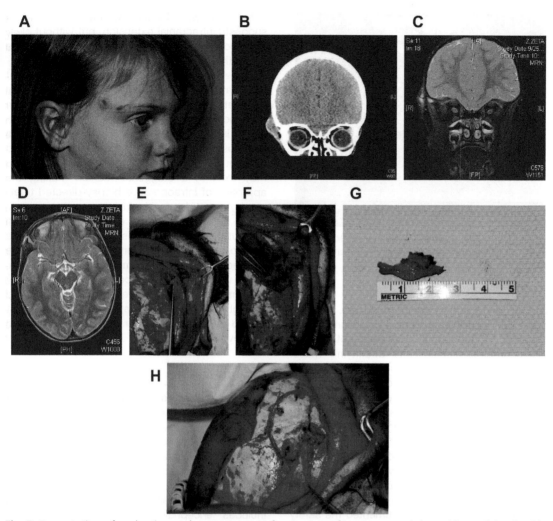

Fig. 5. Presentation of evaluation and management of a recurrent frontotemporal dermoid cyst. (*A*) A healthy 4-year-old girl presented for evaluation and treatment of a right frontotemporal draining fistula associated with pain and intermittent swelling. Before presentation, she had undergone 2 attempts at local removal through direct and lateral brow incisions without any preoperative imaging. A dermoid cyst was diagnosed by histopathologic examination. (*B*) CT imaging demonstrating a space-occupying lesion of the right temporal region associated with a full-thickness calvarial defect lateral to the orbit. (*C, D*) MRI confirmed intracranial extension of a soft tissue tract that extended to the dura. (*E*) Combined neurosurgical and craniomaxillofacial treatment consisted of dissection of the cutaneous remnants and fistulous tract, a coronal flap for access to the pterional region, full-thickness bone flap for dural exposure, and excision of the lesion and tract to the level of the dura (*F, G*). The bone flap was replaced using biodegradable bone plates and screws for reconstruction (*H*). Final histopathology demonstrated a dermoid cyst with associated tract.

Frontonasal lesions with transcranial extension will have significant implications for surgical planning and intervention. The literature variably reports the incidence of intracranial extension ranging from less than 5%[23] up to 40%.[9,13,21,27] Nevertheless, the potential for intracranial extension necessitates a methodical approach to the diagnosis and management for all complex dermoids.

A cutaneous nasal sinus opening may occur anywhere from glabella to the columella but is most commonly found on the lower third of the nose.[21] A tract may have a short blind course or continue deep to the midline with variable presence of an underlying cyst (**Fig. 8**). Although intra-axial extension has been reported, with transcranial involvement the tracts most commonly extend up to the dura or the anterior falx and remain extra-axial.[28] CT scans may identify a frank tract but can also demonstrate indirect features of deep involvement, such as a bifid

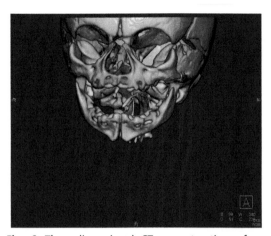

Fig. 6. Three-dimensional CT reconstruction of an infant skull demonstrates the patency of sutures and fontanelles at birth.

septum, an enlarged foramen cecum, or bifid crista galli.[9,21] When a dermal inclusion tract is identified, MRI is helpful in delineating its course and characterization of any underlying mass. Prompt diagnosis and treatment decreases the chance of morbidity associated with infection.

If an intracranial pathologic condition is identified or patients are at a high risk for involvement, a combined intracranial-extracranial approach is recommended. Nasal skin incisions are used to isolate the identified tract. A coronal flap is then elevated and followed by a low frontal craniotomy for access. Complete excision is followed by any necessary reconstruction with autogenous bone. Posnick and colleagues[28] documented the safety of performing this as a single-stage surgical treatment when intracranial involvement is encountered.

The treatment of lesions with a sinus tract that suggests intracranial extension, but without clear CT evidence, may proceed by excision of the lesion through a transnasal approach. An intraoperative biopsy of the terminal fibrous chord at the cranial base is recommended to confirm complete excision.[8,21,27] If a tract or cystic lesion is found at the proximal extent, a formal craniotomy is advocated for access and treatment as previously described.[8,21,27] Even so, Posnick and colleagues[28] note that dural or epidural elements may exist in a staggered fashion making the approach of intraoperative biopsy-directed treatment more at risk for recurrence.

The surgical treatment of the dermoid lesion without intracranial extension is also complete excision. Lesions with skin involvement may be excised through a direct midline nasal approach, which will heal with an acceptable scar (**Fig. 9**).[28] Lesions without skin involvement may be removed through an open nasal approach. Every effort should be made to deliver the lesion unruptured as previously noted.

Calvarial Lesions

Calvarial dermoids deserve special attention because of the wide diagnostic differential and may initially present to a range of providers, including neurosurgeons, maxillofacial surgeons, pediatric surgeons, otolaryngologists, or plastic surgeons who commonly see a variety of scalp lesions.

The differential diagnosis of a scalp mass in a child includes encephalocele, meningioma, calcified cephalohematoma, eosinophilic granuloma, malignant tumor, hemangioma, sinus pericranii, fibrous

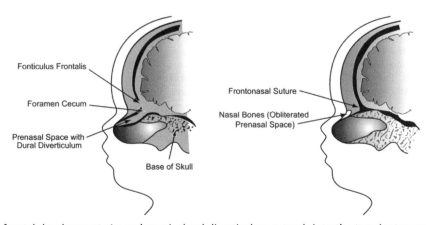

Fig. 7. Nasofrontal development. An embryonic dural diverticulum extends into the transient prenasal space via the foramen cecum. Then the dural diverticulum completely regresses back into the cranium. Finally, the prenasal space and fonticulus frontalis close. (*From* Baxter DJ, Shroff MM. Developmental maxillofacial anomalies. Semin Ultrasound CT MR 2011;32(6):555–68; with permission.)

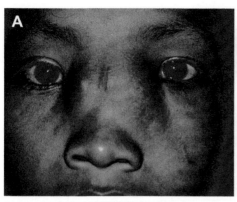
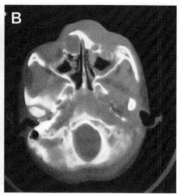

Fig. 8. (*A*) Clinical presentation of a frontonasal lesion with coincident hypertelorism. (*B*) CT examination demonstrates features of extension into the intracranial compartment.

dysplasia, osteoma, or posttraumatic tumor.[29,30] When grouped by age, Martinez-Lage and colleagues[29] found that children aged up to 1 year were predisposed to encephaloceles and cephalo-hematomas; children aged from 1 to 7 years were predisposed to cysts, posttraumatic masses, and eosinophilic granulomas; and those aged from 8 to 18 years were predisposed to fibrous dysplasia, osteoma, and eosinophilic granuloma.

Lesions located in the cranial vault region should be stratified by those that are located in the midline and those that are not. Midline dermoid lesions have a particular propensity for transcranial involvement with dermoid cysts commonly presenting over the anterior fontanelle and dermal sinus tracts at the occipital squama.[10,19]

The most common location for a calvarial dermoid cyst is over the anterior fontanelle in the bregmatic region.[10] These cysts lie between the pericranium and galea. The initial evaluation and diagnosis may be undertaken with plain skull radiographs, but CT imaging provides detailed information required for surgical planning. It is important in these cases to rule out encephalocele or meningocele. The treatment of cysts that extend to the dura without intervening calvarium remains excision with inclusion of the deep periosteal layer. Transcranial dermoid cysts in the bregmatic region can usually be dissected off the dura and rarely involve the underlying sagittal sinus (**Fig. 10**).[10]

Dermal inclusion tracts of the calvarium are considered a type of craniospinal dysraphism and are most frequently found in the suboccipital midline.[31] Intracranial dermoid sinus cysts are rare and compose only 0.1% to 0.7% of all intracranial tumors[32] but may be seen more frequently in patients with Klippel-Feil syndrome, Dandy-Walker malformation, or agenesis of the corpus callosum.[31] Any dorsal midline dimpling or subcutaneous mass should be approached with great care. Fistulography should be avoided secondary to the concern for seeding bacterial contamination or rupturing the cyst itself.[33] Radiographic workup should include CT or MRI studies. MRI evaluation will most often show intrinsic hyperintense T1 signal and absent central contrast enhancement for intracranial dermoids.[34]

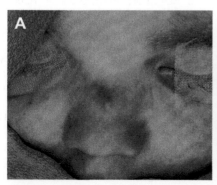
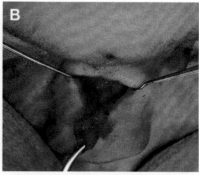

Fig. 9. (*A*) Nasal cutaneous fistula secondary to a dermoid pathologic condition. (*B*) Direct midline nasal approach for lesion excision.

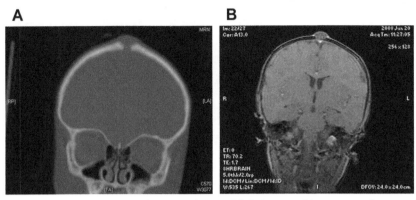

Fig. 10. (*A*) CT image of dermoid cyst over the sagittal sinus. (*B*) CT image with contrast of a second dermoid cyst over the sagittal sinus.

Compared with frontonasoethmoidal dermoids, which are more often extradural, lesions found in a more cephalad position dorsally are more frequently intradural.[35] The treatment may include the need for a posterior fossa craniotomy for complete excision. Given the risk of intracranial involvement at this location, the surgical evaluation and treatment of these lesions should be executed under the direction of a neurosurgeon.

An intradiploic cyst can be found at any location in the cranial vault. They should be removed by full-thickness craniectomy and immediate split-thickness calvarial reconstruction with a neurosurgeon and craniofacial surgeon.[36] An intrabony lesion may actually be a persistent remnant from a previous attempt at removal by simple excision. Any dermoid over a suture or prior area of boney fusion has this potential. Long-term clinical follow-up is not unreasonable with periodic imaging.

The surgical treatment of simple nonmidline scalp lesions with an intact underlying calvarium can proceed by complete excision, most often through a direct approach. Again, every effort should be made to deliver the lesion unruptured, which often necessitates incorporation of the periosteum.

SUMMARY

Dermoid cysts are congenital lesions that arise most commonly from nondisjunction of the surface ectoderm from deeper neuroectodermal structures. Because of this, they tend to be found along planes of embryonic closure. Classification by site is helpful for diagnostic planning and surgical treatment. A distinction can be made between frontotemporal, orbital, frontoethmoidal, and calvarial lesions. Additionally, the risk of extension into deeper tissues must be determined before surgical intervention. Simple lesions are amenable to direct excision. Deeper lesions often require a coordinated surgical approach between a neurosurgeon and craniofacial surgeon after thorough radiographic imaging. Follow-up through the developmental years is recommended for complex dermoid lesions.

REFERENCES

1. McAvoy JM, Zuckerbraun L. Dermoid cysts of the head and neck in children. Arch Otolaryngol 1976; 102:529–31.
2. New GB, Erich JB. Dermoid cysts of the head and neck. Surg Gynecol Obstet 1937;65:48–55.
3. Luna MA, Pfaltz M. Cysts of the neck. In: Gnepp, editor. Diagnostic surgical pathology of the head and neck. Philadelphia: WB Saunders; 2001. p. 664.
4. Shields J, Shields C. Orbital cysts of childhood – classification, clinical features and management. Surv Ophthalmol 2004;49(3):281–99.
5. Pollard ZF, Harley RD, Calhoun J. Dermoid cysts in children. Pediatrics 1976;57:379–82.
6. Brownstein MH, Helwig EB. Subcutaneous dermoid cysts. Arch Dermatol 1973;107:237–9.
7. Lacey M, Gear AJ, Lee A. Temporal dermoids: three cases and a modified treatment algorithm. Ann Plast Surg 2003;51:103–9.
8. Bartlett SP, Lin KY, Grossman R, et al. The surgical management of orbitofacial dermoids in the pediatric patient. Plast Reconstr Surg 1993;91(7): 1208–15.
9. Posnick JC, Costello BJ. Dermoid cysts, gliomas, and encephaloceles: evaluation and treatment. Atlas Oral Maxillofac Surg Clin North Am 2002;10: 85–99.
10. Pannell BW, Hendrick EB, Hoffman HJ, et al. Dermoid cysts of the anterior fontanelle. Neurosurgery 1982;10:317–22.
11. Soto-Ares G, Vinchon M, Delmaire C, et al. Report of eight cases of occipital dermal sinus: an update, and MRI findings. Neuropediatrics 2001; 32(3):153–8.

12. Shields JA, Kaden IH, Eagle RC, et al. Orbital dermoids cysts: clinicopathologic correlations, classification and management. Ophthal Plast Reconstr Surg 1997;4:265–76.

13. Pryor SG, Lewis JE, Weaver AL, et al. Pediatric dermoids cysts of the head and neck. Otolaryngol Head Neck Surg 2005;132:938–42.

14. Riebel T, David S, Thomale UW. Calvarial dermoids and epidermoids in infants and children: sonographic spectrum and follow-up. Childs Nerv Syst 2008;24:1327–32.

15. Holthusen W, Lassrich MA, Steiner C. Epidermoids and dermoids of the calvarian bones in early childhood: their behavior in the growing skull. Pediatr Radiol 1983;13:189–94.

16. Lee S, Persing JA. Refinement in technique for pediatric dermoid cyst excision: technical note. Plast Reconstr Surg 2008;122(4):1059–61.

17. Sathananthan N, Moseley IF, Rose GE, et al. The frequency and clinical significance of bone involvement in outer canthus dermoids cysts. Br J Ophthalmol 1993;77:789–94.

18. Emerick G, Shields CL, Shields JA, et al. Chewing-induced visual impairment from a dumbbell dermoid cyst. Ophthal Plast Reconstr Surg 1997;13(1):57–61.

19. Mack WJ, Ghatan S. Congenital pterional dermal sinus in an 18 month old child: case report. Neurosurgery 2007;61:e661.

20. Hughes GB, Sharpino G, Hunt W, et al. Management of the congenital midline nasal mass: a review. Head Neck Surg 1980;2:222–33.

21. Sessions RB. Nasal dermal sinuses – new concepts and explanations. Laryngoscope 1982;92(Suppl 29): 1–28.

22. Wardinsky TD, Pagon RA, Kropp RJ, et al. Nasal dermoid sinus cysts: associations with intracranial extension and multiple malformations. Cleft Palate Craniofac J 1991;28:87.

23. Bradley PJ. The complex nasal dermoid. Head Neck Surg 1983;5:469–73.

24. Grunwald L. Beitrage zur Kenntnis Kongenitaler Geschwulste und Missbildungen an Ohr und Nase. Ztsch f Ohrenhik 1910;60:270 [in German].

25. Brunner H, Harned JW. Dermoid cysts of the nose. Arch Otolaryngol 1942;36:86–94.

26. Pratt LW. Midline cysts of the nasal dorsum: embryologic origin and treatment. Laryngoscope 1965;75: 968–80.

27. Pensler JM, Bauer BS, Naidich TP. Craniofacial dermoids. Plast Reconstr Surg 1988;82:953–8.

28. Posnick JC, Bortoluzzi P, Armstrong DC, et al. Intracranial nasal dermoid sinus cysts: computed tomographic scan findings and surgical results. Plast Reconstr Surg 1994;93(4):745–54.

29. Martinez-Lage JF, Capel A, Costa TR, et al. The child with a mass on its head: diagnostic and surgical strategies. Childs Nerv Syst 1992;8:247–52.

30. Martinez-Lage JF. Choux M, Di Rocco C, Hockley AD, et al. editor. In: Dermoid cysts and other mass lesions over the anterior fontanelle. Pediatric neurosurgery. London: Churchill Livingston; 1999. p. 109.

31. Douvoyiannis M, Goldman DL, Abbott IR, et al. Posterior fossa dermoid cyst with sinus tract and meningitis in a toddler. Pediatr Neurol 2008;39(1):63–6.

32. Caldarelli M, Massimi L, Kondageski C, et al. Intracranial midline dermoid and epidermoid cysts in children. J Neurosurg 2004;100(Suppl 5):473–80.

33. Tekkok I, Baeesa S, Higgins MJ, et al. Abscedation of posterior fossa dermoid cysts. Childs Nerv Syst 1996;12:318–22.

34. Baxter DJ, Schroff MM. Developmental maxillofacial anomalies. Semin Ultrasound CT MR 2011;32:555–68.

35. Mann GS, Gupta A, Cochrane DD, et al. Occipital dermoid cyst associated with dermal sinus and cerebellar abscesses. Can J Neurol Sci 2009;36: 487–90.

36. Jimenez DF, Barone CM. Encephaloceles, meningoceles, and dermal sinuses. In: Albright, editor. Operative techniques in pediatric neurosurgery. New York: Thieme; 2001. p. 37–50.

Craniofacial Fibrous Dysplasia

Pat Ricalde, DDS, MD[a],*, Kelly R. Magliocca, DDS, MPH[b],
Janice S. Lee, DDS, MD[c]

KEYWORDS

- Fibrous dysplasia • Bone tumor • Monostotic • Polyostotic • Fibrous

KEY POINTS

- Craniofacial fibrous dysplasia is a genetic disorder resulting in slow growing lesions composed of immature bony and fibrous tissues that replace normal bone.
- Ninety percent of lesions in craniofacial fibrous dysplasia are present before the age of five.
- There is much unknown about the natural history of fibrous dysplasia.
- Surgery is the mainstay of treatment in fibrous dysplasia, but the technique, timing and in some instances, indications, remain controversial.

INTRODUCTION

Fibrous dysplasia (FD) is a nonheritable, genetic disorder characterized by the replacement of normal bone by immature, haphazardly distributed bony and fibrous tissues. The cause of this disorder is a gene mutation that prevents the differentiation of cells within the osteoblastic lineage. Despite these important advances in the understanding of FD, this disorder remains enigmatic, with many unanswered questions concerning its epidemiology, natural history, and management.

CLASSIFICATION

Monostotic and polyostotic forms of FD have classically been described, with the monostotic form representing about 70% of all patients.[1] Most investigators consider the disease process to be monostotic even if contiguous bones are affected as long there is only 1 disease focus, as is the case in gnathic and craniofacial FD.[2] A large European multicenter clinicopathologic study of FD determined that, of those patients with monostotic disease, the most common site of involvement was the femur.[3] Other common sites of involvement included the ribs and the craniofacial skeleton.[3,4] The incidence of craniofacial involvement in FD has been reported as 10% to 25% in the monostotic form and at least 50% to as high as 90% in polyostotic FD.[2,5] Polyostotic FD is characterized by multiple foci involving several bones. The lesions more commonly affect 1 side of the body, but can be found on both.[3] Various associated disorders are noted in the spectrum of polyostotic FD (PFD), including Jaffe- Lichtenstein syndrome (JLS), McCune-Albright syndrome (MAS), and Mazabraud syndrome. JLS is characterized by PFD and pigmented café-au-lait skin lesions, whereas MAS has the additional features of hyperfunctioning endocrinopathies. In children, the most commonly encountered endocrinopathy in MAS is precocious puberty, predominantly in girls.[6] In adults, hyperthyroidism, acromegaly, and renal phosphate wasting are the most common endocrine complications of MAS.[7,8] Mazabraud syndrome is defined by the association of FD and intramuscular myxomas.[7]

PATHOGENESIS/NATURAL HISTORY

The pathologic basis for FD is a postzygotic (ie, it occurs after fertilization in somatic cells) mutation in the GNAS-1 gene located on chromosome 20,

[a] St Joseph's Craniofacial Center, 4200 North Armenia Avenue, Suite 3, Tampa, FL 33607, USA; [b] Department of Pathology and Laboratory Medicine, 1364 Clifton Road, Atlanta, GA 30322, USA; [c] Department of Oral & Maxillofacial Surgery, UCSF, 521 Parnassus Avenue C522, San Francisco, CA 94143-0440, USA
* Corresponding author.
E-mail address: pricalde@tampabay.rr.com

Oral Maxillofacial Surg Clin N Am 24 (2012) 427–441
doi:10.1016/j.coms.2012.05.004

which results in the formation of excess 3′,5′-cyclic adenosine monophosphate (cAMP) in mutated cells. The increase in cAMP is thought to prevent the differentiation of cells within the osteoblastic lineage.[7] The mutation occurs in the 201 position, which is usually occupied by an arginine (R201) but, in FD, is replaced by either a cysteine (R201C), a histidine (R201H), or a guanine (R201G).[9,10] The GNAS-1 mutation and subsequent cAMP excess impairs the ability of cells in the osteoblastic lineage to fully differentiate. The condition of cAMP excess contributes to the overexpression of interleukin (IL)-6 by mutated osteoblastic cells, which in turn activates surrounding osteoclasts, permitting these bony lesions to expand.[7] The accepted explanation for the variability in the severity and extent of the disease is related to the stage at which the postzygotic mutation occurred. Severe disease is associated with an early mutational event such that all 3 germ cell layers are affected with a more widespread distribution of mutant cells, as seen in MAS.[7,9,11] A mutational event occurring later in development is thought to result in a limited distribution of the mutant cells and the resulting phenotype is less severe, as seen in monostotic FD.[7] This hypothesis also provides a biologic basis for the observation that monostotic FD does not convert to polyostotic disease over time.

The natural history of FD is difficult to predict, but a study of 109 patients over 32 years at the National Institutes of Health found that, in the craniofacial region, 90% of craniofacial lesions were present by 3.4 years. In the extremities, 90% were present by 13.7 years, and, in the axial skeleton, 90% were present by 15.5 years.[12] The activity of lesions seems to decrease after puberty; however, there are several reported cases that FD remains or becomes active well into adulthood.[1,13]

Craniofacial FD (CFD) is typically a slow-growing lesion that is often identified incidentally with routine imaging, particularly for monostotic disease, or when gradual swelling and facial asymmetry become noticeable. The behavior of the lesion may change if associated with other rapidly growing lesions such as an aneurysmal bone cyst, or in the setting of poorly controlled endocrinopathies, especially growth hormone (GH) excess.[5,14–18] In such cases, referral to the appropriate craniofacial specialist and/or endocrinologist is recommended.

DIAGNOSIS

The diagnosis of FD should be based on the clinical history and physical, radiographic, and histopathologic findings.[19] In those cases in which the location, age of patient, or other factors make it difficult to obtain a satisfactory biopsy (especially in polyostotic FD or MAS), the radiographic and clinical findings may be sufficient to provide a high probability of the diagnosis. A broad differential diagnosis may exist for monostotic FD that is influenced by the age of the patient and the variability in the radiographic appearance. In these circumstances, a bone biopsy may be prudent to confirm the diagnosis of FD.[19] The risks of the procedure should be carefully weighed against the benefits, and an informed decision reached as to whether a biopsy is warranted. Should a biopsy be performed, it is imperative for the pathologist to have the imaging studies for review in order to differentiate the lesion from others that have similar histopathologic features. The differential diagnosis of FD is largely determined by the age of presentation, the clinical extent, and severity (**Table 1**).

Plain radiography, computed tomography (CT), magnetic resonance imaging (MRI), and bone scintigraphy are all modalities that have been used in the evaluation of FD. In general, the radiographic appearance can be variable because it is influenced by the proportion of mineralized tissue and fibrous tissue in the lesion. This variability results in a range of appearances from the classically described ground-glass appearance with ill-defined borders, to a mixed radiolucent-opaque lesion, to one that is primarily radiolucent (**Figs. 1 and 2**).[7,20]

Plain Radiography

A panoramic radiograph is a simple, inexpensive modality that has its greatest usefulness for those lesions occurring in the jaws (**Fig. 3**). The classic radiographic findings include ground-glass trabeculation with loss of the lamina dura.[20,21] One study suggested that superior displacement of the mandibular canal in the setting of a fibro-osseous lesion may be unique to FD.[21] The cortex of the mandible is often described as thinned or indistinct.[20]

CT Scan

CT without contrast is the best technique for showing the radiographic characteristics and extent of disease. The radiographic bone involvement on a CT scan has been characterized as ground-glass, sclerotic, pagetoid, and cystic,[2] some of which are clearly seen in **Fig. 1**. One study suggested that, regardless of the dominant radiographic pattern, there is at least some component of the classic ground-glass bone pattern that can be detected on CT.[4] In a recent study, it was suggested that the variation of radiographic

Table 1
Differential diagnosis of gnathic FD in children

	Fibrous Dysplasia	SOD	ROD	Cherubism	JAOF	Jv Chronic Osteo	Renal OD
Inheritance	Nonhereditary	Nonhereditary	Nonhereditary	Autosomal dominant	Nonhereditary	Nonhereditary	Nonhereditary
Chromosome	20q13	–	–	4p16	Few cases studied	–	–
Cause	Postzygotic mutation	UK	UK	SH3BP2	UK	Infectious? UK	Chronic renal fail
Age	Usually childhood	Childhood	Childhood	Childhood	Usually childhood	Childhood	Any
Site	Maxilla > mandible	Maxilla	Maxilla	Mandible > maxilla	Maxilla > mandible	Mandible	Any
Multifocal disease	– in monostotic + in polyostotic	–	Rarely	+	–	Usually –	Possible
Plain Radiography of lesion	Classic: Ground-glass Other patterns: Cystic Pagetoid	Vertically oriented trabecular pattern of bone; coarse trabeculae	Ghost teeth	Multilocular radiolucencies in posterior mandible > maxilla	Mixed opaque and radiolucent or predominantly opaque	Periosteal new-bone reaction Ground-glass or cotton wool	Ground-glass Loss of lamina dura
Histopathology	BFOL	Mosaic woven and lamellar bone Many osteocytes	Abnormal enamel and dentinal morphology	Giant cells in a fibrous proliferation	BFOL, 2 variants: Psammomatoid Trabeculae	BFOL Inflammation +/–	BFOL, occasional giant cells
Increased laboratory values	+/– GH +/– ALP	–	–	–	–	+/– ESR	ALP
Extragnathic features	+/– CALMS	+/– Hypertrichosis	–	Possible if associated with other syndromes (Ramon, Noonan)	None	+ if syndrome associated (SAPHO)	Patient on dialysis
Alveolar ridge expansion	+	+	+/– may be soft tissue in origin (ie, gingival tissue)	+	+ if gnathic disease	+	+
Orodental features	Tooth rotation Oligodontia Tooth displacement[31,33]	Hypodontia within diseased site, usually premolars Local gingival hyperplasia	Hypodontia Delayed eruption Malformed teeth Local gingival hyperplasia	Unerupted teeth Delayed eruption Displaced teeth[31]	–	–	Displaced teeth

Abbreviations: ALP, alkaline phosphatase; BFOL, benign fibro-osseous lesion; CALMS, café-au-lait macules; ESR, erythrocyte sedimentation rate; JAOF, juvenile active ossifying fibroma[49]; Jv Chronic Osteo, juvenile mandibular chronic osteomyelitis[50,51] (encompasses diffuse sclerosing osteomyelitis, sclerosing osteomyelitis); Renal OD, renal osteodystrophy[55]; ROD, regional odontodysplasia[54]; SAPHO, synovitis, acne, pustulosis, hyperostosis, osteitis; SOD, segmental odontodysplasia[31,53]; UK, unknown.

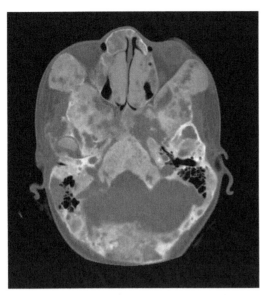

Fig. 1. Axial CT image showing extensive FD in MAS.

appearance of FD depends on the age of the patient.[22] Within the first decade of life, the lesions most often appear as homogeneous, radiodense lesions on CT. As these patients enter the second decade of life, the lesions progress to a mixed radiodense/radiolucent appearance that stabilizes in adulthood but does not necessarily return to a ground-glass appearance (**Fig. 4** show this progression).

It is important to differentiate the natural progression of these lesions from the development of a secondary disorder, such as an aneurysmal bone cyst, which has been reported and may be associated with rapid swelling, vision changes, and hearing loss, in which case an updated CT should be obtained to rule out intralesional hemorrhage and compression. The head and neck, maxilla, orbit, frontal bones, and cranial base are commonly affected by FD.[5,23] In the craniofacial region where overlap of anatomic structures limits the usefulness of plain radiography, CT is particularly helpful to show lesion extent and cortical thinning (**Fig. 4**). FD abutting or compressing vital structures such as the orbit, optic nerve (**Fig. 5**), epitympanum, and external auditory canal may result in neuropathy, obstruction, and functional compromise.[5,7,24]

Scintigraphy

It is important to consider performing radionuclide bone scintigraphy or a skeletal survey at the initial presentation and when there is a history of fractures or endocrinopathies, in order to map the sites of the disease and survey for polyostotic involvement. Increased uptake in FD lesions is expected, but this uptake may become less intense as the lesion matures over time.[19] Increased tissue activity is nonspecific and cannot be distinguished from the uptake seen in malignancy, which has been reported in FD.[25,26] The specific diagnosis of CFD may be suggested by bone scintigraphy, particularly in cases involving the sphenoid wing or other associated facial bones as a result of the distinctive pattern of uptake, which has been described as resembling a pirate wearing an eyepatch.[4]

MRI

Gadolinium-enhanced MRI is helpful in defining a lesion suspected to have undergone malignant transformation in the setting of FD. It is useful in the detection of irregular or focal contrast enhancement and these features may indicate malignant change within the dysplastic lesion.[27]

Histopathology

Three distinct histologic patterns of FD have been described: the classic Chinese-character form, the pagetoid type, and the hypercellular type (**Fig. 6**).[7,10] Some have speculated that the different microscopic patterns may be site specific, whereas others have suggested that the differences are correlated with mechanical stress.[28] A description of the differences between these histologic patterns is beyond the scope of this article and does not affect patient prognosis. The overall impression of classic FD histopathology is

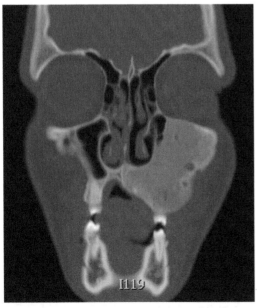

Fig. 2. Coronal CT image of FD involving the left zygomatic-maxillary region.

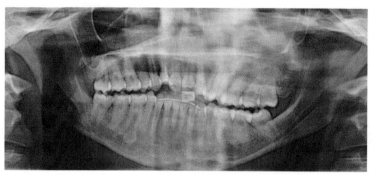

Fig. 3. Panorex radiograph showing monostotic FD in the posterior left maxilla.

the presence of immature, non–stress-oriented, bony trabeculae enmeshed in a fibrous stroma of variable cellularity. The extensive proliferation of fibrous tissue is produced by the mutated cells of the osteoblastic lineage.[7] The stromal cells tend to be plump and slightly spindled but do not show cytologic atypia, and variation in cellularity probably depends on the phase of the disease.[19] Enmeshed in the fibrous stroma are thin, often curved, disconnected osseous trabeculae of woven bone with a characteristic absence of significant osteoblastic rimming (**Fig. 6**B).[29] Because these trabeculae often fail to undergo remodeling, they seldom possess cement lines.[9] Collagen fibers may emerge perpendicular to the bone surface along the bony trabeculae.[9,30] Of surgical interest is the finding of multiple dilated vascular channels along the lesional bone trabeculae and interspersed in the stroma, which may result in brisk bleeding during surgery.[3,9]

In the gnathic and craniofacial bones, there are at least 3 differences in histopathology compared with FD in other bony sites. First, it is unusual to find cartilaginous differentiation in FD of the jaw or craniofacial bones, unless the patient has a history of a fracture. Although pathologic fracture of the long bones is common in severe cases of FD, it is uncommon in gnathic or CFD. Second, in contrast with FD of long bones, the bony trabeculae in gnathic or CFD may acquire a lamellar configuration, rather than being strictly composed of woven bone.[31] Third, it is possible to detect some evidence of osteoblastic rimming in CFD. These histologic differences do not affect prognosis, but may confound a pathologist, leading to delay or even misclassification in the diagnosis.

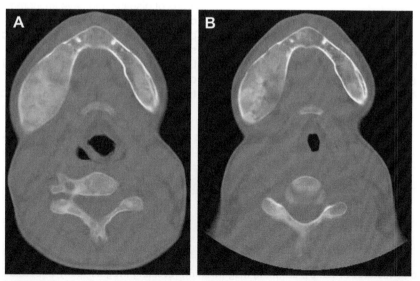

Fig. 4. CT axial images showing transformation of FD lesions. (*A*) The mandible of a 15-year old boy with FD. (*B*) Same patient 2 years later. The FD changes from a ground-glass appearance to a more mixed radiodense/radiolucent lesion.

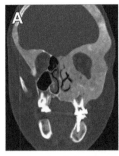
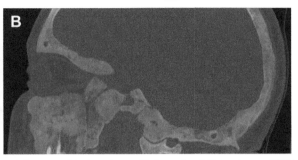

Fig. 5. CT image of PFD of skull base and fronto-orbital region with loss of orbital volume. (*A*) Coronal image showing changes in orbital volume, obliteration of the paranasal sinuses, and skeletal expansion. (*B*) Sagittal image showing narrowing and lengthening of the optic tract.

Genetic Testing

Through genetic amplification techniques such as polymerase chain reaction, it is now possible to test for the genetic mutation in peripheral blood samples and paraffin-embedded tissues, but the probability of detection may be proportional to the number of mutated cells and the severity of the disease.[9,32] Detection of the activating GNAS mutation is useful to confirm a diagnosis in those cases in which there is diagnostic uncertainty surrounding the microscopic features.[7,9] However, testing is not routine, and ideally requires samples that are either fresh or have not been subject to the routine harsh decalcification procedures. Furthermore, testing may not be easily available, which makes anticipating costs and coverage by insurance providers unpredictable.

PROGNOSIS

The prognosis of FD is influenced by the clinical presentation and extent of the disease. Estimating prognosis can be difficult in FD and, in some cases, takes time to assess, but it is an important step in establishing an individualized plan of treatment. Monostotic lesions tend to enlarge in proportion to skeletal growth and, in general, the prognosis is good. Lesions are characteristically firm and expansile and, depending on their location, symptoms manifest because of compression and mass effect. Lesions surrounding foramina may show some sensory disturbances or pain. Lesions adjacent to the sinuses can grow into and completely obliterate the sinus resulting in congestion, headaches, and/or hyposmia.

In the jaws, dental shifting and malocclusion may be noted.[33] Lesions involving the bones of the orbit are of particular interest and are discussed later. Most sites of FD become quiescent after cessation of skeletal growth, but some continue to enlarge after skeletal maturity and well into adulthood, with progressive deformity.[1]

Prognosis in PFD is best considered as proportional to the extent of disease. The lesions in MAS, especially in the context of uncontrolled endocrinopathies, develop into larger and more persistent areas of disease and have an increased frequency of complications.[9,18] By adolescence, many patients with widespread PFD and MAS have severe deformities and functional impairment. Laboratory evaluation of biochemical markers of bone turnover, such as serum osteocalcin, total and bone-specific alkaline phosphatase,

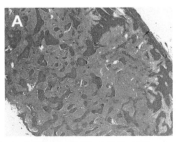
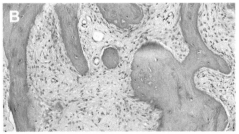

Fig. 6. Histologic features of FD. (*A*) Scanning magnification revealing irregular bony trabeculae embedded in a fibrous stroma. Numerous small blood vessels present within the stroma (hematoxylin and eosin [H&E], original magnification ×20). (*B*) Trabeculae of woven bone with minimal to no osteoblastic rimming, fibrous and vascular stroma (H&E, original magnification ×200).

and C-terminal type I collagen cross-links have been advocated as a means of following activity and progression of disease. These markers are expected to decrease with medical therapy for FD.[7]

MANAGEMENT

Successful clinical management begins with an accurate diagnosis, careful documentation, interdisciplinary consultation (where appropriate), and thorough radiographic assessment. Estimating prognosis can be difficult in FD and, in some cases, takes time to assess, but is an important step in establishing an individualized plan of treatment. Patients and caregivers should understand that there is no cure for this disorder. A monostotic lesion is occasionally resectable; however, most treatment plans are variable, staged, and depend on the behavior of the lesions; long-term follow-up is paramount. Most lesions in the craniofacial structures deemed suitable for surgery are managed by debulking procedures. Depending on location, this can be accomplished by staged, serial shaving; more aggressive debulking maneuvers; or resection, contouring, and reconstruction. **Fig. 7** shows an adult patient with a large FD lesion in the right mandible. After orthodontic preparation, he underwent a combined orthognathic surgery and debulking of the tumor.

Depending on the site of involvement, patients with CFD may benefit from the services of various subspecialists, and consideration should be given for follow-up through an interdisciplinary craniofacial team. In cases of orbital bone involvement, thorough ophthalmologic testing including a visual field assessment, color vision, visual acuity, and funduscopic examination by a neuro-ophthalmologist is necessary.[5] Otolaryngologic and audiological assessments are necessary if there is temporal bone involvement.[1] Patients with skull base involvement may also benefit from an evaluation by a neurologist and neurosurgeon. PFD may be associated with endocrine and metabolic abnormalities that require early diagnosis and appropriate treatment.[9] Psychosocial well-being during the developmental years is vital, therefore children with a chronic and deforming disorder should receive pediatric psychological evaluation and prompt intervention if necessary.

Serial clinical observation may be indicated in patients in whom the lesions do not seem to progress, cause deformity, or functional impairment.[34] Vigilant interval follow-up and radiographic assessment in an asymptomatic individual depend on the site(s) of bone involvement and the age of the patient. Those lesions involving the orbit, skull base, and temporal bone in children need

particular vigilance and scrutiny that can only take place through an interdisciplinary effort.

Medical Therapy

No medical treatment is available to cure or definitively halt the progression of FD. As stated earlier, one of the effects of excess cAMP is the overexpression of IL-6 by abnormal osteoblasts. This overexpression leads to osteoclastic bone resorption, which is the rationale for treating patients with antiresorptive agents such as bisphosphonates (BP).[19] Medical management has had a greater role in noncraniofacial FD, in which fractures and chronic pain are more common. There has been mixed success in craniofacial FD for pain reduction and to reduce the rate of growth of the lesion.[35] With the increased risk of BP-related osteonecrosis, the unclear efficacy in the management of FD, and the unknown long-term effects of BP treatment in children, further studies are necessary before these medications can be recommended.

Surgical Intervention

Surgery is the mainstay of treatment in FD, but the technique, timing, and, in some instances, indications remain controversial. In many cases, particularly in the jaws, the dysplastic bone can be successfully contoured by conservative surgical measures to approximate facial symmetry and/or relieve symptoms, without attempting complete resection (**Fig. 7**). Surgical treatment performed at a young age may require revision surgery sooner than in cases performed on a postpubescent patient. This relative disadvantage is offset by the improvement in quality of life or relief of existing symptoms achieved through early surgical intervention. There is always some risk of regrowth, even when conservative therapy is performed after puberty.[36] Kusano and colleagues[37] noted that, in their long-term follow-up of 11 patients with FD, growth of monostotic FD arrested in adolescence, but PFD was less predictable.

In some anatomic locations, a shave procedure is technically challenging to accomplish, but the use of a surgical navigation system may assist in overcoming some of this difficulty.[36] Other cases may require complete surgical excision and immediate reconstruction of the defect, such as those with an amenable monostotic lesion or those with a particularly aggressive lesion.[38,39] Deciding between a procedure designed to contour versus an excisional surgery is influenced by the anatomic location of the disease, type of FD, rate of tumor growth and behavior of the lesion, nature of the

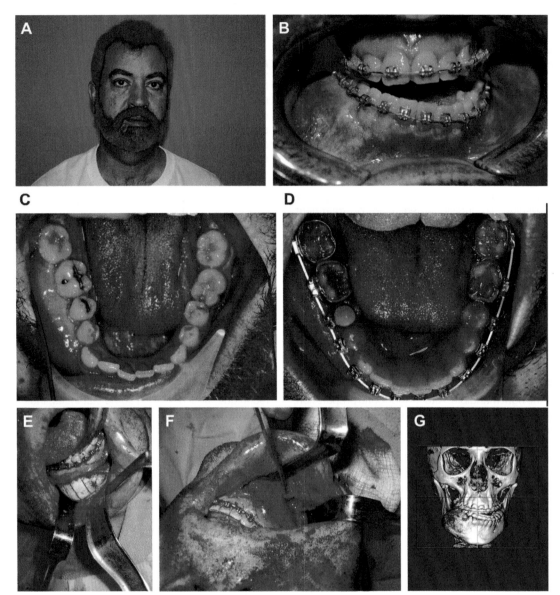

Fig. 7. (*A, B*) Patient with FD right mandible, facial asymmetry, and severe malocclusion. (*C*) Before and (*D*) after orthodontic level and alignment of mandibular arch. (*E*) Picket-fence–type osteotomies in preparation for debulking. (*F*) Surgery complete with preservation of nerve. (*G, I*) Preoperative CT scans. (*H, J*) Postoperative CT scans (Parts *C* and *D Courtesy of* Dr Sharon Durrett).

symptomatic disturbance (aesthetic, functional, neurosensory), an assessment of the potential for reactivation or regrowth, consideration of the patient's age and expectations, and the surgeon's preference. The indications for surgery include:

- Restoration of facial contour and aesthetics. Procedures to restore aesthetics can be accomplished at most ages; however, in younger patients, the risk of regrowth is greater than in older patients. Orthognathic

surgery with or without contouring may be indicated in patients with facial deformity or a malocclusion with normal healing.[40] Most studies recommend waiting until patients are beyond puberty, skeletally mature, and the lesions are quiescent before contouring and jaw surgery.[38] In preparation for correction of malocclusion and asymmetry, presurgical orthodontic treatment can be undertaken without concern for increased activation of the disease state while plans

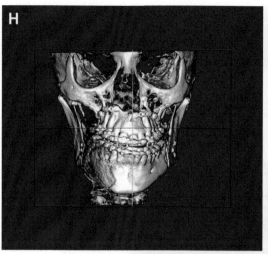

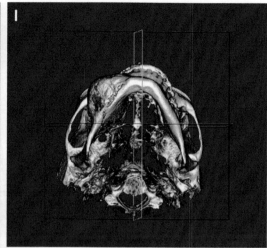

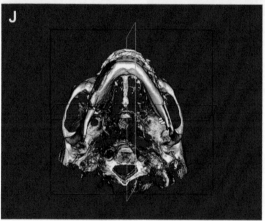

Fig. 7. (*continued*)

are underway for orthognathic surgical correction at the cessation of growth. **Fig. 8** show preoperative and postoperative orthognathic management.[33]

- Control of secondary disorder. Benign lesions (mucocoele,[41] aneurysmal bone cyst[42]) and malignancy (usually sarcomas[43]) have the potential to develop in the primary lesion, and may contribute to rapid growth, symptoms, and complications. Many secondary benign entities (eg, sinus and lacrimal obstruction, nasal stenosis) require surgical treatment. Malignant entities require management through a pediatric cancer center. The treatment in these situations is dictated by the secondary disorder.
- Removal of aggressive lesions. Lesions showing aggressive, accelerated behavior or those lesions associated with significant growth potential, particularly in the setting of endocrinopathies (as seen in MAS, and

GH excess) are surgical candidates. There must be concomitant control and management of the underlying endocrinopathy.[2,18] Complete excision is desirable, but may not be possible.

- Restoration or preservation of function. FD is benign and natural progression occurs slowly. Adaptation of vital structures typically takes place and patients, particularly young children, do not often complain of symptoms. However, there are instances in which symptoms develop such as visual changes, conductive or sensorineural hearing loss, numbness, and pain.[1,18,44] In such cases, surgical intervention, usually decompression of canal or nerve foramina, may be necessary but the risks associated with treatment must be reviewed. However, there is a dearth of studies reviewing the success of such procedures and the long-term sequelae.

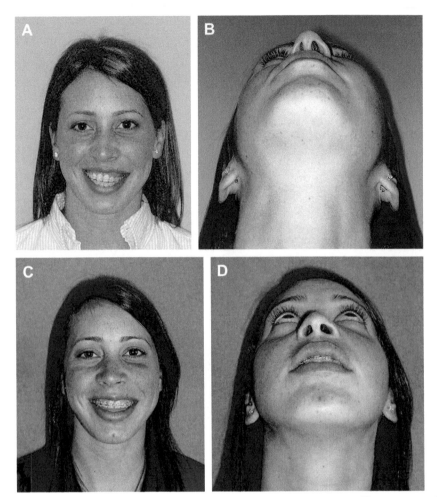

Fig. 8. Surgical treatment of a patient with facial asymmetry and left zygomatic-maxillary FD treated by orthognathic surgery. (*A, B*) Preoperative views of left-sided FD. (*C, D*) Same patient 2 months after Le Fort I maxillary osteotomy.

LONG-TERM CONSIDERATIONS

- Evaluation of serum values such as alkaline phosphatase (ALP) and GH (if there is a history of GH excess) may be useful in select cases
- Interval radiographic assessment may be used to monitor residual FD and survey for the development of secondary disorders or malignant transformation
- Open communication between all members of the patient's care team is encouraged to avoid duplication of laboratory and imaging evaluation
- The patient and family members should have a good understanding of signs and symptoms that warrant immediate evaluation
- Regular and periodic clinical assessment by the surgical team and relevant consultant services is recommended

- General mental, physical, and social well-being need to be considered as an important aspect of FD management, and referral for specialty services should be made in those cases in which deficiencies are noted.

Dental Considerations

Patients with FD involving the maxilla and mandible are more likely to have malocclusion, and have a higher caries rate. It seems that they are able to undergo routine dental interventions without event, including orthodontics.[33] Orthognathic surgery has been successful in the management of facial asymmetry in these patients (refer to **Figs. 7** and **8**).

Akintoye and colleagues[33] examined 32 patients with CFD. Twenty-three patients had PFD/MAS and 9 had monostotic disease. In this study,

28% of the patients had a dental anomaly within FD bone. The most common anomalies included tooth rotation, oligodontia, displacement, enamel hypoplasia, enamel hypomineralization, taurodontism, retained deciduous teeth, and attrition. There was no correlation between endocrine dysfunction and tooth anomalies. The patients who had received routine dental care did not report any complications or exacerbation of their lesions after dental restorations, orthodontic therapy, or oral surgical procedures such as tooth extractions, odontoma removal, maxillary cyst removal, or biopsy of the jaws. Among the 10 patients who received orthodontic therapy, the duration of treatment was longer (2–4 years in duration) than in conventional cases, with unsatisfactory results because of persistent growth and relapse.

For patients with missing teeth, dental endosseous implants may be considered. In a recent case report, a 32-year old woman with MAS and quiescent FD lesions underwent successful integration and loading of long dental implants (>15 mm) in the maxilla and mandible. The dental implants remained functional after 5 years.[45] The literature is limited, and it is unclear whether there is an increased risk of implant failure or risk of osteomyelitis in the setting of a failed implant. For these reasons, long-term follow-up and further studies are needed to direct implant care in this population.

Orbital Considerations

The optimal management of FD in the region of the optic nerve remains controversial. The status of the optic nerve when associated with FD may be considered in 3 categories: no evidence of neuropathy, subtle and gradual optic neuropathy, and acute neuropathy with rapid visual changes or vision loss. Because of the lack of large cohort studies and long-term follow-up, particularly for the scenario of gradual optic neuropathy, guidelines in managing FD around the optic nerve are limited. The following synopsis is a review of some of the current literature and the potential mechanisms that are thought to contribute to the development of optic neuropathy.[46–48]

- No evidence of optic neuropathy. Although prophylactic decompression (unroofing) has been considered for a completely encased optic nerve that is asymptomatic, studies have shown that optic neuropathy and vision loss are not necessarily the natural progression in encased optic nerves, and close observation may be an acceptable treatment. The presence of a narrowed optic canal is not necessarily associated with visual loss.[5,18] Even with complete encasement of the optic nerve by FD, most patients (88% in Cutler and colleagues'[18] study of 87 patients) have no evidence of optic neuropathy and those who have some degree of neuropathy cannot be definitively explained by encasement by FD (**Fig. 9**). No relationship between patient age and the degree of involvement of the bony optic canal has been established, suggesting that optic canal encasement is not simply an inevitable consequence of increasing age.

- Subtle and gradual optic neuropathy. The presence of GH excess has been associated with an increase in the relative risk (RR) for complete encasement (RR = 4.1) and optic neuropathy (RR = 3.8).[18] GH excess occurs in approximately 20% of patients with MAS[49] and MAS itself is thought to be under recognized.[49,50] GH excess may not be clinically evident early in the course of MAS, but is a potentially treatable disease at this early asymptomatic stage.[50] An increased GH level is correlated with an increase in head circumference, or macrocephaly. Either compression or traction on the optic nerve that accompanies bony expansion of the skull may be the mechanism of gradual vision loss in some patients.[14,18] Early evaluation of GH excess is essential, with the assumption that control of GH excess may prevent long-term craniofacial morbidity.[51] Optic neuropathy is difficult to evaluate and follow

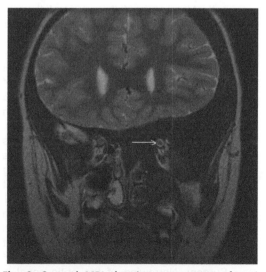

Fig. 9. Coronal MRI showing encasement of optic canal with FD and preservation of the canal contents, including the optic nerve (*arrow*).

because the changes may be gradual and subtle, without evidence of papilledema or visual compromise.

In those few cases with demonstrated progressive visual compromise, some surgeons have advocated an attempt at decompression via endoscopic techniques.[52–54]

- Acute visual changes. In cases of acute visual loss, secondary disorders arising within the lesions of FD, such as an aneurysmal bone cyst and/or mucocele, are usually the cause of the visual disturbance, and not the presence of the FD lesion alone.[5,14,42] The mechanism of acute vision loss is thought to be intralesional hemorrhage (associated with aneurysmal bone cyst) and compression of the optic nerve.[18,51,54] These pathologic entities develop unpredictably and can result in acute visual loss in a short period of time, therefore patients with known cystic development near the optic canal or with increased GH require vigilance, as outlined earlier.[2] Surgical decompression and medical control of intracanal (cranial) pressure with acetazolamide may be indicated in acute vision loss. The risk factors for the development of secondary disorders are unknown.

General recommendations for lesions involving optic canal

- Clinical and laboratory evaluation. Once optic canal encasement is diagnosed, patients must be followed carefully with a regular and detailed assessment of their visual acuity, color vision, visual fields, and fundus examination by a neuro-ophthalmologist.[5,55–61] Serum levels of GH and ALP may be an additional source of information.[38,49,51] Patients with increased levels of GH should be evaluated by an endocrinologist and managed aggressively.
- Imaging. Detailed visual field assessments performed by an ophthalmologist are more sensitive than CT imaging in detecting gradual visual deterioration. Nonetheless, it remains critical to survey patients with CT scanning at established intervals, and an acute change in vision should prompt an immediate imaging evaluation to rule out the development of secondary disorders.[42]
- Surgery. Narrowing of the optic canal is not necessarily associated with visual changes, so decompression in the absence

of subjective and objective manifestations of optic neuropathy cannot be recommended (ie, from imaging alone).[39,51] Immediate surgical decompression can be considered for patients with acute visual loss (or within 1 week of sudden visual loss),[1] in the presence of objective signs of optic neuropathy and deteriorating vision.[1,55] A multidisciplinary approach is important, especially in patients with subtle neuropathic changes with unclear prognosis. The team may include a craniofacial surgeon, skull base surgeon, neurosurgeon, and neuro-ophthalmologist. Reviewing surgical outcomes in the literature is a challenge given the heterogeneity of the patient population and their associated characteristics. Outcomes and reporting can be influenced by the surgical technique, experience of the surgeon, the original indication for the decompression (type and degree of visual deficit, presence of secondary disorders), and variability in interpretation of the imaging and laboratory results. Surgery can range from endoscopic decompression of 1 or more orbital walls to a complete fronto-orbital craniotomy for resection, or possibly recontouring (debulking) and reconstruction of certain affected units.[52–55]

In summary, the overall status of the patient, including an assessment of the laboratory values and clinical findings mentioned earlier, must be taken into consideration when discussing surgical intervention. Future studies documenting the risks, benefits, and outcomes of surgery in the setting of optic nerve decompression will be important in shaping surgical management algorithms.

Malignant Transformation

The rate of malignant transformation in FD has been estimated to range between 0.5% and 4%. The craniofacial region is reported as the most common site of involvement, followed by the femur, tibia, and pelvis.[43] Changes in the clinical presentation suggesting malignant transformation include a rapid increase in the size of the site of FD, a new onset of pain or tenderness, sensory changes, and changes in imaging characteristics. Radiotherapy was historically used for attempted treatment of FD but was shown to be highly associated with malignant transformation and has since been abandoned.[19] Osteosarcoma is the most commonly reported malignancy, followed by various other sarcomas.[43]

SUMMARY

Despite recent advances in the understanding of the natural history and molecular abnormalities, many questions remain surrounding the progression and management of FD. In the absence of comorbidities such as GH excess or secondary disorders, the expected behavior of CFD is slow growing and without functional consequence. In order to optimize patient care, understanding of the pathophysiologic mechanisms contributing to the various phenotypes of this condition, as well as the predictors of the different behaviors of FD lesions, must be improved. The importance of long-term follow-up of patients with CFD cannot be overstated because spontaneous recovery is unlikely, and the course of disease can be unpredictable.

REFERENCES

1. Ricalde P, Horswell BB. Craniofacial fibrous dysplasia of the fronto-orbital region: a case series and literature review. J Oral Maxillofac Surg 2001; 59:157–67 [discussion: 167–8].

2. Rahman AM, Madge SN, Billing K, et al. Craniofacial fibrous dysplasia: clinical characteristics and long-term outcomes. Eye (Lond) 2009;23:2175–81.

3. Ippolito E, Bray EW, Corsi A, et al. Natural history and treatment of fibrous dysplasia of bone: a multi-center clinicopathologic study promoted by the European Pediatric Orthopaedic Society. J Pediatr Orthop B 2003;12:155–77.

4. Lisle DA, Monsour PA, Maskiell CD. Imaging of craniofacial fibrous dysplasia. J Med Imaging Radiat Oncol 2008;52:325–32.

5. Lee JS, FitzGibbon E, Butman JA, et al. Normal vision despite narrowing of the optic canal in fibrous dysplasia. N Engl J Med 2002;347:1670–6.

6. Feller L, Wood NH, Khammissa RA, et al. The nature of fibrous dysplasia. Head Face Med 2009;5:22.

7. Chapurlat RD, Orcel P. Fibrous dysplasia of bone and McCune-Albright syndrome. Best Pract Res Clin Rheumatol 2008;22:55–69.

8. Collins MT, Chebli C, Jones J, et al. Renal phosphate wasting in fibrous dysplasia of bone is part of a generalized renal tubular dysfunction similar to that seen in tumor-induced osteomalacia. J Bone Miner Res 2001;16:806–13.

9. DiCaprio MR, Enneking WF. Fibrous dysplasia. Pathophysiology, evaluation, and treatment. J Bone Joint Surg Am 2005;87:1848–64.

10. Riminucci M, Liu B, Corsi A, et al. The histopathology of fibrous dysplasia of bone in patients with activating mutations of the Gs alpha gene: site-specific patterns and recurrent histological hallmarks. J Pathol 1999;187:249–58.

11. Bianco P, Riminucci M, Majolagbe A, et al. Mutations of the GNAS1 gene, stromal cell dysfunction, and osteomalacic changes in non-McCune-Albright fibrous dysplasia of bone. J Bone Miner Res 2000; 15:120–8.

12. Hart ES, Kelly MH, Brillante B, et al. Onset, progression, and plateau of skeletal lesions in fibrous dysplasia and the relationship to functional outcome. J Bone Miner Res 2007;22:1468–74.

13. Barontini F, Maurri S, Sita D. Peripheral ophthalmoplegia as the only sign of late-onset fibrous dysplasia of the skull. J Clin Neuroophthalmol 1986;6:109–12.

14. Michael CB, Lee AG, Patrinely JR, et al. Visual loss associated with fibrous dysplasia of the anterior skull base. Case report and review of the literature. J Neurosurg 2000;92:350–4.

15. Diah E, Morris DE, Lo LJ, et al. Cyst degeneration in craniofacial fibrous dysplasia: clinical presentation and management. J Neurosurg 2007;107:504–8.

16. Sadeghi SM, Hosseini SN. Spontaneous conversion of fibrous dysplasia into osteosarcoma. J Craniofac Surg 2011;22:959–61.

17. Reis C, Genden EM, Bederson JB, et al. A rare spontaneous osteosarcoma of the calvarium in a patient with long-standing fibrous dysplasia: CT and MR findings. Br J Radiol 2008;81:e31–4.

18. Cutler CM, Lee JS, Butman JA, et al. Long-term outcome of optic nerve encasement and optic nerve decompression in patients with fibrous dysplasia: risk factors for blindness and safety of observation. Neurosurgery 2006;59:1011–7 [discussion: 1017–8].

19. Chapurlat RD, Meunier PJ. Fibrous dysplasia of bone. Baillieres Best Pract Res Clin Rheumatol 2000;14:385–98.

20. MacDonald-Jankowski D. Fibrous dysplasia: a systematic review. Dentomaxillofac Radiol 2009; 38:196–215.

21. Petrikowski CG, Pharoah MJ, Lee L, et al. Radiographic differentiation of osteogenic sarcoma, osteomyelitis, and fibrous dysplasia of the jaws. Oral Surg Oral Med Oral Pathol Oral Radiol Endod 1995;80:744–50.

22. Lee JS, Butman JA, Collins MT, et al. Radiographic appearance of craniofacial fibrous dysplasia is dependent on age. J Oral Maxillofac Surg 2002; 60(Suppl):88–91.

23. Chen YR, Wong FH, Hsueh C, et al. Computed tomography characteristics of non-syndromic craniofacial fibrous dysplasia. Chang Gung Med J 2002;25:1–8.

24. Megerian CA, Sofferman RA, McKenna MJ, et al. Fibrous dysplasia of the temporal bone: ten new cases demonstrating the spectrum of otologic sequelae. Am J Otol 1995;16:408–19.

25. Stegger L, Juergens KU, Kliesch S, et al. Unexpected finding of elevated glucose uptake in fibrous

dysplasia mimicking malignancy: contradicting metabolism and morphology in combined PET/CT. Eur Radiol 2007;17:1784–6.

26. Basu S, Baghel NS, Puri A, et al. 18 F-FDG avid lesion due to coexistent fibrous dysplasia in a child of embryonal rhabdomyosarcoma: source of false positive FDG-PET. J Cancer Res Ther 2010;6:92–4.

27. Cappabianca S, Colella G, Russo A, et al. Maxillofacial fibrous dysplasia: personal experience with gadoliniumenhanced magnetic resonance imaging. Radiol Med 2008;113:1198–210.

28. Maki M, Saitoh K, Horiuchi H, et al. Comparative study of fibrous dysplasia and osteofibrous dysplasia: histopathological, immunohistochemical, argyrophilic nucleolar organizer region and DNA ploidy analysis. Pathol Int 2001;51:603–11.

29. Shidham VB, Chavan A, Rao RN, et al. Fatty metamorphosis and other patterns in fibrous dysplasia. BMC Musculoskelet Disord 2003;4:20.

30. Pollandt K, Engels C, Kaiser E, et al. Gsalpha gene mutations in monostotic fibrous dysplasia of bone and fibrous dysplasia-like low-grade central osteosarcoma. Virchows Arch 2001;439:170–5.

31. Eversole R, Su L, ElMofty S. Benign fibro-osseous lesions of the craniofacial complex. A review. Head Neck Pathol 2008;2:177–202.

32. Dumitrescu CE, Collins MT. McCune-Albright syndrome. Orphanet J Rare Dis 2008;3:12.

33. Akintoye SO, Lee JS, Feimster T, et al. Dental characteristics of fibrous dysplasia and McCune-Albright syndrome. Oral Surg Oral Med Oral Pathol Oral Radiol Endod 2003;96:275–82.

34. Fernandez E, Colavita N, Moschini M, et al. "Fibrous dysplasia" of the skull with complete unilateral cranial nerve involvement. Case report. J Neurosurg 1980;52:404–6.

35. Chao K, Katznelson L. Use of high-dose oral bisphosphonate therapy for symptomatic fibrous dysplasia of the skull. J Neurosurg 2008;109:889–92.

36. Nowinski D, Messo E, Hedlund A, et al. Computer-navigated contouring of craniofacial fibrous dysplasia involving the orbit. J Craniofac Surg 2011;22:469–72.

37. Kusano T, Hirabayashi S, Eguchi T, et al. Treatment strategies for fibrous dysplasia. J Craniofac Surg 2009;20:768–70.

38. Park BY, Cheon YW, Kim YO, et al. Prognosis for craniofacial fibrous dysplasia after incomplete resection: age and serum alkaline phosphatase. Int J Oral Maxillofac Surg 2010;39:221–6.

39. Valentini V, Cassoni A, Marianetti TM, et al. Craniomaxillofacial fibrous dysplasia: conservative treatment or radical surgery? A retrospective study on 68 patients. Plast Reconstr Surg 2009;123:653–60.

40. Yeow VK, Chen YR. Orthognathic surgery in craniomaxillofacial fibrous dysplasia. J Craniofac Surg 1999;10:155–9.

41. Derham C, Bucur S, Russell J, et al. Frontal sinus mucocele in association with fibrous dysplasia: review and report of two cases. Childs Nerv Syst 2011;27:327–31.

42. MacNally SP, Ashida R, Williams TJ, et al. A case of acute compressive optic neuropathy secondary to aneurysmal bone cyst formation in fibrous dysplasia. Br J Neurosurg 2010;24:705–7.

43. Ruggieri P, Sim FH, Bond JR, et al. Malignancies in fibrous dysplasia. Cancer 1994;73:1411–24.

44. Kim YH, Song JJ, Choi HG, et al. Role of surgical management in temporal bone fibrous dysplasia. Acta Otolaryngol 2009;129:1374–9.

45. Bajwa MS, Ethunandan M, Flood TR. Oral rehabilitation with endosseous implants in a patient with fibrous dysplasia (McCune-Albright syndrome): a case report. J Oral Maxillofac Surg 2008;66:2605–8.

46. Frodel JL, Funk G, Boyle J, et al. Management of aggressive midface and orbital fibrous dysplasia. Arch Facial Plast Surg 2000;2:187–95.

47. Choi JW, Lee SW, Koh KS. Correction of proptosis and zygomaxillary asymmetry using orbital wall decompression and zygoma reduction in craniofacial fibrous dysplasia. J Craniofac Surg 2009;20(2):326–30.

48. Gosain AK, Celik NK, Avdin MA. Fibrous dysplasia of the face: utility of three-dimensional modeling and ex situ malar recontouring. J Craniofac Surg 2004;15(6):909–15.

49. Akintoye SO, Chebli C, Booher S, et al. Characterization of gsp-mediated growth hormone excess in the context of McCune-Albright syndrome. J Clin Endocrinol Metab 2002;87:5104–12.

50. Hannon TS, Noonan K, Steinmetz R, et al. Is McCune-Albright syndrome overlooked in subjects with fibrous dysplasia of bone? J Pediatr 2003;142:532–8.

51. Collins MT. Spectrum and natural history of fibrous dysplasia of bone. J Bone Miner Res 2006;21(Suppl 2):P99–104.

52. Pletcher SD, Metson R. Endoscopic optic nerve decompression for nontraumatic optic neuropathy. Arch Otolaryngol Head Neck Surg 2007;133(8):780–3.

53. Simmen D, Jones N. Selected procedures. Orbital decompression. In: Simmen D, Jones N, editors. Manual of endoscopic sinus surgery and its extended uses. New York: George Thieme; 2005. p. 223–5, Chapter 14.

54. Amit M, Fliss DM, Gil Z. Fibrous dysplasia of the sphenoid and skull base. Otolaryngol Clin North Am 2011;44(4):891–902.

55. Tan YC, Yu CC, Chang CN, et al. Optic nerve compression in craniofacial fibrous dysplasia: the role and indications for decompression. Plast Reconstr Surg 2007;120:1957–62.

56. Whitt JC, Rokos JW, Dunlap CL, et al. Segmental odontomaxillary dysplasia: report of a series of 5 cases with long-term follow-up. Oral Surg Oral Med Oral Pathol Oral Radiol Endod 2011;112:e29–47.

57. Spini TH, Sargenti-Neto S, Cardoso SV, et al. Progressive dental development in regional odonto-dysplasia. Oral Surg Oral Med Oral Pathol Oral Radiol Endod 2007;104:e40–5.

58. Sarode SC, Sarode GS, Waknis P, et al. Juvenile psammomatoid ossifying fibroma: a review. Oral Oncol 2011;47:1110–6.

59. Heggie AA, Shand JM, Aldred MJ, et al. Juvenile mandibular chronic osteomyelitis: a distinct clinical entity. Int J Oral Maxillofac Surg 2003;32:459–68.

60. Kadom N, Egloff A, Obeid G, et al. Juvenile mandibular chronic osteomyelitis: multimodality imaging findings. Oral Surg Oral Med Oral Pathol Oral Radiol Endod 2011;111:e38–43.

61. Hata T, Irei I, Tanaka K, et al. Macrognathia secondary to dialysis-related renal osteodystrophy treated successfully by parathyroidectomy. Int J Oral Maxillofac Surg 2006;35:378–82.

Vascular Anomalies in Children

Shelly Abramowicz, DMD, MPH[a,b,*],
Bonnie L. Padwa, DMD, MD[a,b]

KEYWORDS

- Vascular anomaly • Hemangioma • Lymphatic malformation • Capillary malformation
- Vascular malformation

KEY POINTS

- Most vascular anomalies are diagnosed by history and physical examination.
- Treatment of patients with vascular anomalies has been hampered by confusing and incorrect terminology. Correct diagnosis (tumor or malformation) is critical to caring for these patients because it dictates medical and/or surgical management.
- Patients with vascular anomalies are best treated by a multidisciplinary team made up of several surgical, radiologic, and medical specialists.
- Hemangioma is a benign vascular tumor; a vascular malformation is composed of abnormally formed lymphatics and/or blood vessels.

INTRODUCTION

Treating patients who have vascular anomalies has been hampered by confusing and incorrect terminology. In 1982, Mulliken and Glowacki[1] proposed a biologic classification system based on endothelial cell kinetics and clinical behavior. They described 2 types of vascular anomalies: hemangiomas and vascular malformations. In 1996, the International Society for the Study of Vascular Anomalies adopted an expanded classification system and categorized vascular anomalies into tumors and malformations.[2] More than 90% of vascular anomalies can be diagnosed based on history and physical examination.[3] Ultrasound (US), magnetic resonance imaging (MRI), and computed tomography (CT) can be used to confirm the clinical diagnosis, and to document the extent and flow characteristics.

Hemangioma is a benign vascular tumor; approximately one-third are present at birth and two-thirds appear after birth. The defining feature is rapid growth in infancy. In contrast, a vascular malformation occurs as the result of abnormal embryonic development. Vascular malformations are present at birth and expand commensurately with growth of the child. Vascular malformations are categorized as slow-flow (capillary malformations [CM], lymphatic malformation [LM], and venous malformation [VM]) and fast-flow lesions (arterial malformations and arteriovenous malformations [AVMs]). Histologically, hemangiomas show endothelial hyperplasia and glucose transporter-1 protein (GLUT1) immunopositivity, whereas vascular malformations have slow endothelial turnover and are GLUT1 negative.[4] Hemangiomas rarely cause skeletal hypertrophy or deformation of adjacent bone, whereas slow-flow vascular malformations can cause bony deformation, and fast-flow lesions typically cause osteolysis.[5]

HEMANGIOMAS

The infantile hemangioma (IH) is a common tumor of infancy occurring in 4% to 10% of white

Disclosures: The authors have nothing to disclose.
[a] Department of Oral and Maxillofacial Surgery, Harvard School of Dental Medicine, Boston, MA, USA;
[b] Department of Plastic and Oral Surgery, Children's Hospital Boston, 300 Longwood Avenue, Boston, MA 02115, USA
* Corresponding author. Department of Plastic and Oral Surgery, Children's Hospital Boston, 300 Longwood Avenue, Boston, MA 02115.
E-mail address: shelly.abramowicz@childrens.harvard.edu

Oral Maxillofacial Surg Clin N Am 24 (2012) 443–455
doi:10.1016/j.coms.2012.05.001
1042-3699/12/$ – see front matter © 2012 Elsevier Inc. All rights reserved.

newborns.[6] However, the incidence is 23% in premature infants weighing less than 1200 g.[7] The tumor occurs more commonly in girls, with a gender ratio of 2.4:1. Approximately 60% of IHs occur in the head and neck region,[3] and 20% of infants with IH have multiple lesions that can occur in the liver, brain, and/or gastrointestinal tract.[6]

IHs have a life cycle consisting of 3 phases that can be distinguished clinically, microscopically, and immunohistochemically.[8] Most IHs are not present at birth but appear during the first 2 weeks of life, although 30% to 50% of IHs are seen at birth as a telangiectatic stain or ecchymotic area.[9] The IH grows during the first 6 to 9 months (proliferating phase) (**Fig. 1**). After 12 months of age, the tumor begins to shrink and flatten and the color fades (involution phase). By age 5 years, complete resolution occurs in more than 50% of children, with continued improvement until age 10 to 12 years (involuted phase). However, nearly one-half of children have a residual abnormality, including redundant atrophic skin, yellow discoloration, residual fibrofatty tissue, and/or telangiectasia (**Fig. 2**).[10]

IHs can occur in association with other anomalies to make up an association that consists of plaquelike IH in a segmental or trigeminal dermatomal distribution of the face with at least 1 of the following anomalies: posterior fossa brain malformation, hemangioma, arterial cerebrovascular anomalies, coarctation of the aorta and cardiac defects, eye/endocrine abnormalities (PHACE).[11] Because 8% of children with PHACE have a stroke in infancy and 42% have a structural brain anomaly, patients with PHACE should have a brain MRI.[12] PHACE association affects approximately 2% of patients with IH.

There are rare vascular tumors that occur fully grown at birth and do not exhibit the expected postnatal course and life cycle of IH. The congenital hemangioma (CH) consists of 2 subtypes: rapidly involuting congenital hemangioma (RICH) and the noninvoluting congenital hemangioma (NICH). RICH commonly occurs on the trunk and extremities but also in the head and neck and liver. They are raised, with a characteristic red-vilaceous color, central telangiectasias, superficial ulceration, and a peripheral pale halo. RICH involutes rapidly during the first few weeks or months of life.[13–15] NICH are typically well circumscribed, slightly raised, averaging 5 to 6 cm in diameter. They are light gray in color with prominent coarse telangiectasias, warmth on palpation, and a predisposition for the mandibular border.[15]

Management

Most IHs are small, localized, and do not involve aesthetically or functionally important areas. These IHs can be managed by observation and waiting for involution.[9] Infants should be followed on a monthly basis during the proliferative phase and yearly during the involuting stage. Spontaneous ulceration can occur in 20% of cutaneous hemangiomas, possibly causing infection or local tissue destruction.[16] Therapy is indicated for hemangiomas that cause destruction, distortion, or obstruction (eg, subglottic narrowing, blockage of visual axis). Intralesional corticosteroid injection (triamcinolone 3 mg/kg) has antiangiogenic properties that accelerate involution[17]; it stabilizes the growth of the lesion in at least 95% of patients, and 75% of tumors decrease in size.[18] Thus, it is best for a small, well-localized IH that is less than 2 cm in diameter.[19] The corticosteroid lasts 4 to 6 weeks and therefore multiple injections during the proliferative phase may be necessary.[9] Daily oral prednisolone is recommended for an IH that is large, rapidly growing, and causing distortion of facial features, ulceration, and/or impinging on anatomic structures. When the tumor is no longer proliferating, the dose can be decreased slowly to prevent rebound tumor growth and adrenal crisis.

Propranolol has also been successfully used in some centers to treat IHs. Oral or intravenous administration of 2 mg/kg per day in divided doses reduced the volume, color, and elevation of IHs.[20,21] Thorough pretreatment evaluation, inpatient monitoring of vital signs and blood glucose levels at initiation of therapy, and frequent reassessments are necessary since propranolol can cause bradycardia, hypotension, and hypoglycemia,[22,23] although cardiovascular side effects have been infrequent and minor.[20,24]

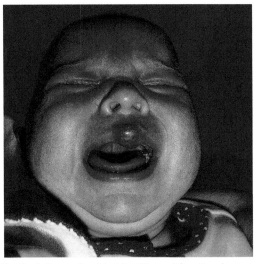

Fig. 1. A 3-month-old girl with proliferating hemangioma of upper lip.

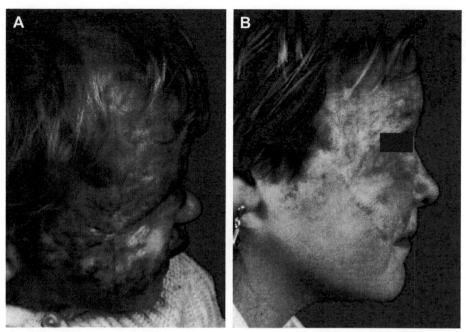

Fig. 2. (*A*) Involuting IH at age 3 years. (*B*) Age 9 years with involuted and regressed IH with residual discolored and scarred tissues.

Side effects seem to be primarily minor gastrointestinal disturbances and are easily managed. Although promising, propranolol's efficacy and safety compared with corticosteroids in this patient population is still unknown. **Fig. 3** shows management of an enlarging and bleeding IH that did not respond to steroid injections. Propranolol administration was initiated when the lesion continued to enlarge and, after 2 weeks, shows some shrinkage. Next-line therapy (vincristine, interferon-α) is indicated if the patient fails to respond to first-line agents and/or there are contraindications to prolonged systemic use of corticosteroids.[25,26]

Resection is a consideration at any time during the hemangioma life cycle. If there is obstruction of a vital structure, recurrent bleeding, and/or ulceration, excision can take place early during the proliferative

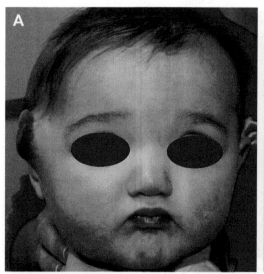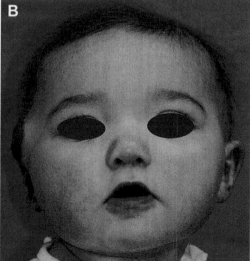

Fig. 3. (*A*) Large, progressive IH lesion measured 7 cm by 6 cm before propranolol administration. (*B*) Two weeks after initiation of propranolol the IH is blanched, softer, and measures 4 cm by 3 cm.

or involuting stage (**Fig. 4**). After involution, there may be residual fibrofatty tissue, redundant or damaged skin that can be removed.[27] Although waiting until the hemangioma has involuted ensures that the least amount of tissue is resected, leaving the smallest possible scar, this must be weighed against the psychosocial morbidity of having a deformity until late childhood. The conventional method of excision is in a lenticular format with linear closure in the axis of the relaxed cutaneous tension lines, either as a single or a staged procedure. However, a circular excision and purse-string closure converts a circular lesion into a small circular or ellipsoid scar. A second excision results in the smallest possible scar with minimal distortion of surrounding structures (**Fig. 5**).[28]

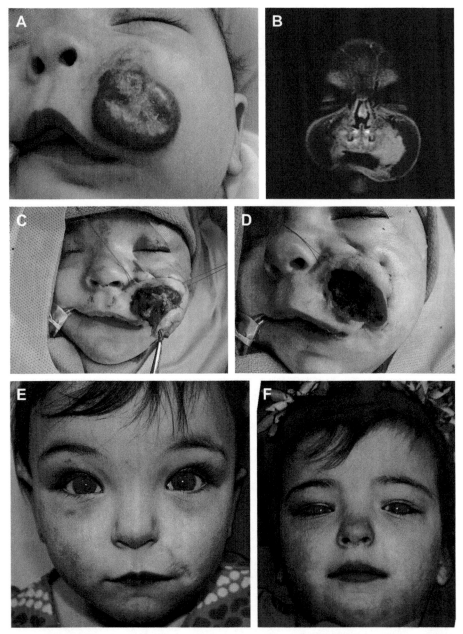

Fig. 4. (*A*) One-year-old girl with IH affecting nasal patency and chewing. (*B*) MRI coronal image showing hemangioma of right lip and cheek. (*C*) Excision of lesion through nasolabial approach. Note the circumferential purse-string suture. (*D*) Defect after excision. (*E*) One year after excision of IH. (*F*) Age 5 years (four years post excision).

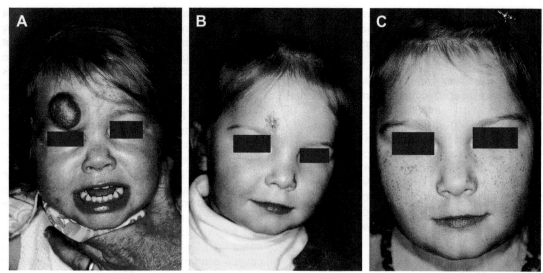

Fig. 5. (*A*) Two-year-old girl with hemangioma of right forehead. (*B*) Age 8 years, after involution of hemangioma with evidence of residual tissue before excision. (*C*) Patient at age 12 years, with minimal scarring after excision. (*Courtesy of* Dr John B. Mulliken, Boston, MA.)

VASCULAR MALFORMATIONS

Vascular malformations are abnormally formed lymphatics or blood vessels. They are characterized by the affected vasculature (capillaries, arteries, veins, and/or lymphatics), flow characteristics (slow or fast), and number of involved vessels (single or multiple). US helps to distinguish arterial malformations, VMs, and LMs.[29] MRI is the gold standard to determine the type and extent of the lesion. Vascular malformations can cause disfigurement and local complications (ie, destruction of anatomic structures, infection, obstruction, pain, thrombosis, ulceration). They can also lead to, disseminated intravascular coagulation, pulmonary embolism, and thrombocytopenia, and congestive heart failure.

Slow-Flow Vascular Malformations

Capillary Malformation

CMs, also known as port-wine stains, are present at birth and persist throughout life (**Fig. 6**). They are found in approximately 0.3% of newborns, with an equal sex distribution.[30] They appear as macular pink stains that blanch with pressure and they can occur anywhere on the body.[31] Facial CMs often occur in a dermatomal distribution: 45% are restricted to 1 of the 3 trigeminal dermatomes, whereas 55% overlap sensory dermatomes, cross the midline, or occur bilaterally.[32] Facial CMs tend to gradually darken to an intense red hue during young adulthood and to a deep purple during middle age. The skin thickens and becomes raised

with multiple nodular fibrovascular lesions. There can be associated overgrowth of soft tissue, gingiva, and skeleton in the area of the stain. Gingival overgrowth and intraoral pyogenic granulomas are common; prevention includes good oral hygiene and regular dental cleanings. Procedures in the oral cavity (eg, gingivectomy, extractions, osteotomies) can be done without concern for excessive bleeding.[33]

Sturge-Weber syndrome is defined as a CM in the ophthalmic and/or maxillary (trigeminal) distributions associated with leptomeningeal capillary and venous anomalies and vascular lesions of the ocular choroid. The leptomeningeal vascular lesions can cause refractory seizures, hemiplegia, and variable delayed motor and cognitive development. Anomalous choroidal vascularity can result in

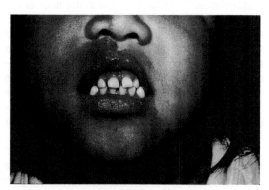

Fig. 6. Port-wine stain (CM) involving the right maxillary and mandibular dermatome distributions.

retinal detachment, glaucoma, and blindness.[34] Some patients exhibit major maxillary and/or mandibular overgrowth with evidence of vascular changes in bone.[35]

Management Management of CM consists of pulsed dye laser and multiple treatments are often needed in yearly intervals,[36,37] with 50% of patients achieving approximately 70% improvement.[38] Other laser modalities such as long pulsed laser and photodynamic therapy, are being studied.[31] Labial hypertrophy, a common problem in patients with facial CM, can be managed by contour resection. Orthognathic correction may be safely performed for occlusal canting caused by asymmetrical maxillary overgrowth or mandibular prognathism.[33]

Lymphatic Malformation

LMs result from an error in the embryonic development of the lymphatic system. Sprouting lymphatics may become separated from the primitive lymph sacs or main lymphatic channels,[39] or lymphatic tissue can form in an abnormal location.[40] LM is characterized by the size of the malformed channels: microcystic, macrocystic, or combined.[1] Isolated tiny mucosal or cutaneous blebs that are not radiographically detectable are microcystic LMs; large channel blebs that cannot be manually compressed are macrocystic LMs.[33] LMs can occur anywhere in the body; those in the head and neck region occur in the neck, cheek, and the cervicofacial region (incorrectly termed cystic hygroma) with extension into the mediastinum or orbit (**Fig. 7**).[41]

Prenatal US in the second trimester can detect large lesions.[42] Most LMs are noted at birth or within the first year of life. LMs enlarge commensurate with the child's growth, but can suddenly expand as a result of cellulitis secondary to an upper respiratory tract infection or intralesional hemorrhage from injury to small vessels within the malformation.[33,43] If there is LM in the floor of the mouth and tongue, the inflamed tissue can lead to macroglossia with dark-stained vesicles that tend to bleed.[33,42] This has the potential to cause airway obstruction. Cervicofacial LMs are associated with overgrowth of the mandible and can result in a severe malocclusion and open bite (**Fig. 8**).[41,42] Two-thirds of patients with cervicofacial LM require tracheostomy to maintain their airways.[44]

Management Small or asymptomatic lesions are observed. Intralesional bleeding is treated with pain medication, rest, and/or antibiotics. Because LMs are at risk for infection, good oral hygiene should be maintained.[33,39] Patients with more than 3 infections in 1 year are typically given daily prophylactic antibiotics. Symptomatic lesions that cause pain, significant deformity, or encroach on vital structures require treatment.[41] Vesicles of the mucous membranes and dorsal tongue can be treated by laser or radiofrequency ablation.[38] Persistent or larger LMs of the dorsal tongue may have to be treated surgically. Most patients require a combination of interventions to adequately treat LM of the lingual base and floor of mouth.[32,41] Local trauma and/or infection can cause vesicular bleeding that can be controlled by embolization.[42] Sclerotherapy is useful for large or problematic macrocystic/combined LM. Aspiration followed by an injection of an inflammatory agent (eg, ethanol, bleomycin, doxycycline) causes scarring of the cyst walls and the lesion shrinks.[45–48] More than 90% of macrocystic LMs that are treated with sclerotherapy do not regrow.[46]

Resection is indicated if sclerotherapy is no longer possible because all the macrocysts have been treated or if it will be curative because the lesion is small and well localized. Intraoral resection of the floor of mouth and tongue base should be avoided because of the high likelihood of postoperative functional problems. Aggressive debulking of an enlarged and protruding tongue can negatively affect speech and feeding secondary to insufficient functional lingual mass; however, to provide for optimal speech development, some surgical reduction or control of LMs may have to be undertaken. Many children have speech problems related to not only tongue bulk and reduced lingual mobility but also early tooth loss, palatal immobility, and poor oral competence.[41,42] Cervicofacial LMs can be disfiguring because of tissue hypertrophy, bony enlargement, and malocclusion. Patients develop progressive mandibular overgrowth and prognathism, causing a class III malocclusion, steep mandibular plane angle, and anterior open bite (**Fig. 8**). Orthognathic surgery can take place once the tongue size and position are acceptable; postoperative antibiotics (2–3 weeks) are warranted. Preoperative antibiotics are not typically necessary for extractions or resection but the airway must be appropriately managed.

Facial LMs that are amenable to resection, either because of their size or location (nonairway or nonorbital), or have been reduced and/or scarred by sclerotherapy, may be excised. As in hemangiomas, access incisions are placed in an anatomic margin or relaxed tension line. The parents should be informed that LMs are difficult to eradicate and that regrowth is possible. Also,

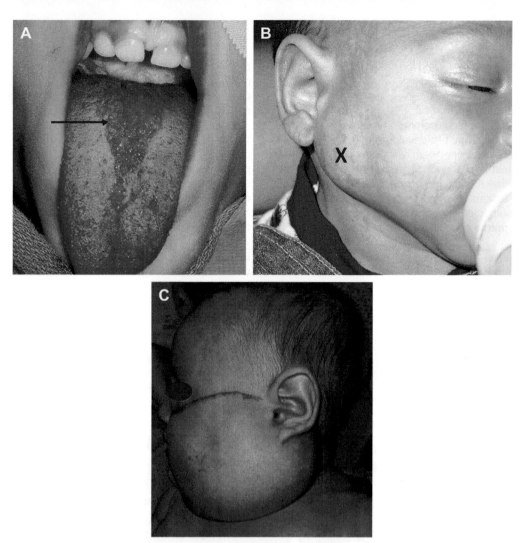

Fig. 7. (*A*) Mucosal blebs and microcystic LM of tongue. (*B*) Combined microcystic-macrocystic LM of right parotid and cheek. The lesion expands during feeding. (*C*) Cervicofacial LM of the neck and upper mediastinum.

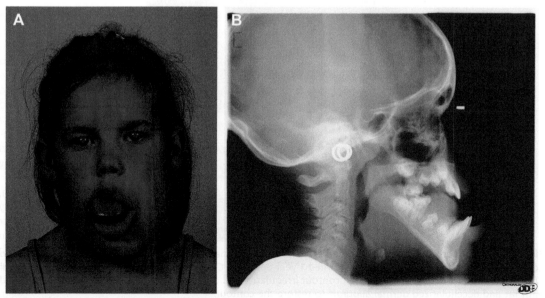

Fig. 8. (*A*) Frontal view of 10-year-old girl with obvious open bite and protruding tongue. (*B*) Lateral cephalograph shows mandibular prognathism with steep angle and open bite deformity.

postoperative scarring may alter the overlying soft tissue contour (**Fig. 9**).

Venous Malformation

VMs are the most common type of vascular malformation. They are developmental abnormalities of veins composed of thin-walled, dilated channels of variable size and mural thickness with normal endothelial lining and deficient smooth muscle.[6,40] The lesions expand, flow stagnates, and, as a result, clotting can occur. These lesions are blue-purple in color, soft, compressible, and nonpulsatile (**Fig. 10**). A phlebolith is occasionally palpable and may cause pain, distention, and tenderness.[49] In 90% of patients, VMs are solitary[50]; multifocal forms should raise the suspicion

that there is a hereditary basis (eg, glomuvenous malformation,[51] cutaneomucosal VM,[50] cerebral cavernous malformation,[52] blue rubber bleb nevus syndrome[53]).

Although VMs usually grow in proportion with the child, enlargement can occur with trauma, puberty, and/or pregnancy.[54] VMs can cause progressive distortion of facial features by causing skeletal alteration and hypertrophy without intraosseous involvement.[5] Oral VMs can cause malocclusion as a result of the mass effect on the dentoalveolus. They rarely interfere with speech and feeding.[49] Spontaneous and significant bleeding or life-threatening thrombosis is uncommon, although reports of life-threatening hemorrhage have occurred.[52,54] Patients are

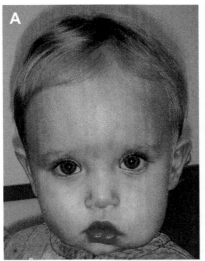
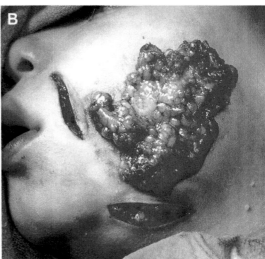
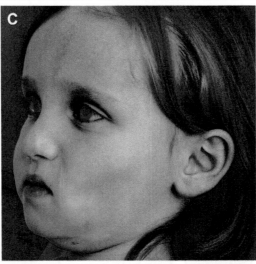

Fig. 9. (A) Before surgery and before administration of intralesional (saline) sclerosant to LM of left cheek. Two courses of intralesional therapy were performed 1 year apart. (B, C) Two years after excision through nasolabial and submental approaches. Note the skin contour irregularity and dimpling after healing. This was later grafted with fat and decellularized dermal allograft to restore the contour.

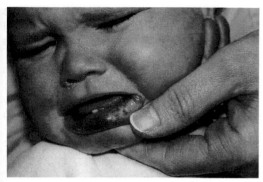

Fig. 10. An 8-month-old girl with VM of left lower lip and buccal mucosa. (*Courtesy of* Dr John B. Mulliken, Boston, MA.)

usually not at risk for thromboemboli because the deep venous system is rarely affected. However, stasis in large or extensive venous anomalies is frequently associated with localized or generalized intravascular coagulopathy,[55] which must be corrected before any surgical intervention.

Management The first-line treatment of problematic VMs is sclerotherapy. The injected sclerosing agent causes cellular destruction, thrombosis, and intense inflammation. Scarring shrinks the lesion in 75% to 90% of patients and it often alleviates symptoms.[55–58] However, VMs usually reexpand via recanalization[59] and thus may require multiple treatments. Resection is indicated to reduce bulk and to improve contour and function. Resection without preoperative sclerotherapy is indicated for small, solitary VMs in anatomic sites that are dangerous to sclerose because of immediate proximity to vital structures like the eye or major nerves.[33] Resection should usually take place following completion of sclerotherapy. Although complete excision of the VM is the therapeutic goal, this is often not possible because of the extent of the lesion and proximity to vital anatomic structures. In this case, only subtotal resection or contour resection is possible. Jaw surgery can be undertaken following preoperative treatment of localized coagulopathy, protection of the airway with tracheostomy, and the use of preoperative sclerotherapy.[33]

Fast-Flow Vascular Malformations

Arteriovenous Malformation

AVMs of the head and neck are less common than slow-flow anomalies. They result from an error in vascular development during embryogenesis.[60] An AVM is composed of abnormal communications between arteries and veins without the normal intervening capillary bed.[33] AVMs enlarge because of increased blood flow, collateralization, and recruitment (ie, dilatation of vessels and thickening of adjacent arteries and veins secondary to increased pressure).[61,62] AVMs are present at birth, but rarely expand in infancy or early childhood. They usually grow proportionately, starting in late childhood (**Fig. 11**). AVMs in the maxilla and mandible constitute 4% to 5% of all craniofacial AVMs.[62] AVMs in the jaws may be asymptomatic or present as a pulsatile swelling, with localized throbbing pain, toothache or earache, or unexpected hemorrhage following tooth exfoliation or extraction.[33]

The Schobinger clinical staging system for AVMs is used for documenting presentation and evolution of AVMs (**Table 1**).[63] AVMs can remain stable for years (stage I). The onset of pain, pruritus, or enlargement indicates progression. Rapid expansion can occur following local trauma, attempted excision or ligation, or hormonal changes associated with puberty or pregnancy.[62] Ninety percent of AVMs are diagnosed by history and physical examination.[1] Doppler examination or US show fast flow. MRI with contrast enhancement shows dilated feeding arteries, draining veins, and flow voids.[64] Angiography shows

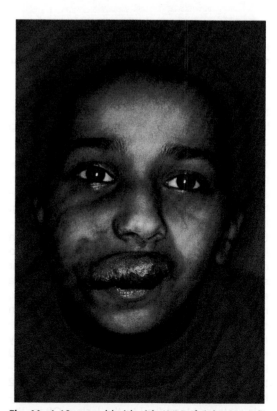

Fig. 11. A 10-year-old girl with AVM of right upper lip and maxilla. (*Courtesy of* Dr John B. Mulliken, Boston, MA.)

Table 1
Schobinger clinical staging system for AVM

Stage		Description
I	Quiescence	Pink-bluish stain, warmth, arteriovascular shunting by Doppler
II	Expansion	Same as stage I Plus enlargement, pulsations, thrill, bruit, and tortuous, tense veins
III	Destruction	Same as stage II Plus either dystrophic skin changes, ulceration, bleeding, persistent pain, or tissue necrosis
IV	Decompensation	Same as stage III Plus cardiac failure

From Mulliken JB, Fishman SJ, Burrows PE. Vascular anomalies. Curr Probl Surg 2000;37(8):566; with permission.

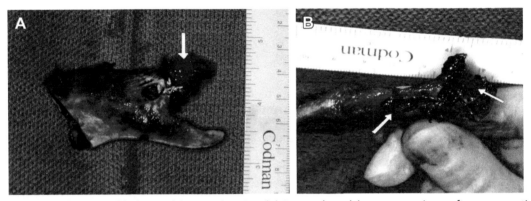

Fig. 12. AVM of the mandibular condylar-ramal region. (*A*) Resected condyle-ramus specimen after preoperative embolization; note the thrombosis in the venous sinusoid (*arrow*). (*B*) Intrabony evidence of osseous destruction and clot (*arrows*).

tortuous, dilated arteries with arteriovenous shunting and enlarged draining veins, often surrounding a nidus.[60]

Management The mainstays of AVM management are selective embolization, sclerotherapy, surgical resection, and reconstruction.[65] Intervention is necessary for treatment of pain, bleeding, ischemic ulceration, or cardiac failure. Embolization or direct transosseous puncture delivers an inert substance (onyx, ethanol, coil, or glue) to occlude the blood flow and/or fill the vascular space.[66] Embolization is almost never curative and only allows temporary control. Eventually, recanalization and reexpansion occur.[67] When excision or dental extraction is planned, preoperative embolization facilitates the procedure by reducing the size of the AVM, minimizing blood loss, and creating scar tissue to aid the dissection.[60] Surgical resection should occur 48 to 72 hours later, before recanalization and angiogenesis restores blood flow to the lesion. Often, the postembolization image indicates lesion inflow abruption with stagnation and the possibility of

resection with possible immediate reconstruction can take place. Complete resection is often not feasible (**Fig. 12**) because of the extent of the lesion, persistent inflow, venous runoff, difficulty controlling blood loss, and absence of tissue planes. Furthermore, the need to preserve blood supply to neighboring structures makes complete resection challenging.[33] As a result, most recurrences occur within the first year after intervention, and more than 86% reexpand within 5 years following resection.[62]

SUMMARY

The process of understanding and treating children with vascular anomalies has been hampered by confusing and occasionally incorrect terminology. The most important step when evaluating a maxillofacial vascular anomaly is to determine whether it is a tumor or a malformation. In most cases, this diagnosis can be made by history and physical examination. Selective radiographic imaging is helpful in differentiating vascular malformations or the extent of bony involvement and/or destruction. Children with vascular anomalies should be managed by an interdisciplinary team of trained providers who are committed to following, treating, and studying patients with these complex problems.

ACKNOWLEDGMENTS

This work was supported in part by a Faculty Educator Development Award sponsored by the Oral and Maxillofacial Surgery Foundation and the American Association of Oral and Maxillofacial Surgeons (S.A.).

REFERENCES

1. Mulliken JB, Glowacki J. Hemangiomas and vascular malformations in infants and children: a classification based on endothelial characteristics. Plast Reconstr Surg 1982;69:412–22.

2. Enjolras O, Mulliken JB. Vascular tumors and vascular malformations (new issues). Adv Dermatol 1997;13:375–423.

3. Finn MC, Glowacki J, Mulliken JB. Congenital vascular lesions: clinical application of a new classification. J Pediatr Surg 1983;18:894–900.

4. North PE, Waner M, Mizeracki A, et al. GLUT1: a newly discovered immunohistochemical marker for juvenile hemangiomas. Hum Pathol 2000;31(1): 11–22.

5. Boyd JB, Mulliken JB, Kaban LB, et al. Skeletal changes associated with vascular malformations. Plast Reconstr Surg 1984;74:789–97.

6. Marler JJ, Mulliken JB. Current management of hemangiomas and vascular malformations. Clin Plast Surg 2005;32:99–116.

7. Amir J, Metzker A, Krikler R, et al. Strawberry hemangioma in preterm infants. Pediatr Dermatol 1986;3:331–2.

8. Takahasi K, Mulliken JB, Kozakewich HP, et al. Cellular markers that distinguish the phases of hemangioma during infancy and childhood. J Clin Invest 1994;93:2357–64.

9. Greene AG. Management of hemangiomas and other vascular tumors. Clin Plast Surg 2011; 38:45–63.

10. Mulliken JB, Enjolras O. Congenital hemangiomas and infantile hemangiomas: missing links. J Am Acad Dermatol 2004;50:875–82.

11. Freiden IJ, Reese V, Cohen D. PHACE syndrome. The association of posterior fossa brain malformations, hemangiomas, arterial anomalies, coarctation of the aorta and cardiac defects, and eye abnormalities. Arch Dermatol 1996;132:307–11.

12. Metry DW, Dowd CF, Barkovich AJ, et al. The many faces of PHACE syndrome. J Pediatr 2001;139: 117–23.

13. Boon LM, Enjolras C, Mulliken JB. Congenital hemangioma evidence of accelerated involution. J Pediatr 1996;128:329–33.

14. Berenguer B, Mulliken JB, Enjolras O, et al. Rapidly involuting congenital hemangioma clinical and histopathologic features. Pediatr Dev Pathol 2003;6: 495–510.

15. Enjolras O, Mulliken JB, Boon LM, et al. Non-involuting hemangioma: a rare cutaneous vascular anomaly. Plast Reconstr Surg 2001;107:1647–54.

16. Achauer BM, Chang CJ, Vander Kam VM. Management of hemangioma of infancy: review of 245 patients. Plast Reconstr Surg 1997;99:1301–8.

17. Crum R, Szabo S, Folkman J. A new class of steroids inhibits angiogenesis in the presence of heparin or a heparin fragment. Science 1985;230:1375–8.

18. Sloan GM, Renisch JF, Nichter LS, et al. Intralesional corticosteroid therapy for infantile hemangiomas. Plast Reconstr Surg 1989;83:459–67.

19. Chen MT, Yeong EK, Horng SY. Intralesional corticosteroid therapy in proliferating head and neck hemangiomas: a review of 155 cases. J Pediatr Surg 2000;35:420–3.

20. Hogeling M, Adams S, Wargon O. A randomized controlled trial of propranolol for infantile hemangiomas. Pediatrics 2011;128:e259–66.

21. Holmes WJ, Mishra A, Gorst C, et al. Propranolol as first-line treatment for rapidly proliferating infantile haemangiomas. J Plast Reconstr Aesthet Surg 2011;64:445–51.

22. Lawley LP, Siegfried E, Todd JL. Propranolol treatment for hemangioma of infancy: risks and recommendations. Pediatr Dermatol 2009;26:610–4.

23. Frieden IL, Drolet BA. Propranolol for infantile hemangiomas: promise, peril, pathogenesis. Pediatr Dermatol 2009;26:642–4.

24. Buckmiller LM, Munson PD, Dyamenahalli U, et al. Propranolol for infantile hemangiomas: early experience at a tertiary vascular anomalies center. Laryngoscope 2010;120:676–81.

25. Perez J, Pardo J, Gomez C. Vincristine – an effective treatment of corticoid-resistant life-threatening infantile hemangioma. Acta Oncol 2002;41:197–9.

26. Ezekowitz RA, Mulliken JB, Folkman J. Interferon alpha-2a therapy for life-threatening hemangiomas of infancy. N Engl J Med 1992;326:1456–63.

27. Mulliken JB, Fishman SJ, Burrows PE. Vascular anomalies. Curr Probl Surg 2000;37:517–84.

28. Mulliken JB, Rogers GF, Marler JJ. Circular excision of hemangioma and purse string closure: the smallest possible scar. Plast Reconstr Surg 2002;109: 1544–54.

29. Paltiel HJ, Burrows PE, Kozakewich HP, et al. Soft-tissue vascular anomalies: utility of US for diagnosis. Radiology 2000;214:747–54.

30. Jacobs AH, Walton RG. The incidence of birthmarks in the neonate. Pediatrics 1976;58:218–22.

31. Maguiness SM, Liang MG. Management of capillary malformations. Clin Plast Surg 2011;38:66–73.

32. Enjolras O, Riché MC, Merland JJ. Facial port-wine stains and Sturge-Weber syndrome. Pediatrics 1985;76:48–51.

33. Padwa BL, Mulliken JB. Vascular anomalies of the oral and maxillofacial region. In: Fonseca RJ, Marciani RD, Turvey T, editors. Oral and maxillofacial surgery, vol. 2. St Louis (MO): Saunders; 2008. p. 577–91.

34. Thomas-Sohl KA, Vaslow DF, Maria BL. Sturge-Weber syndrome: a review. Pediatr Neurol 2004; 30:303–10.

35. Greene AK, Taber SF, Ball KL, et al. Sturge-Weber syndrome: soft-tissue and skeletal overgrowth. J Craniofac Surg 2009;20(Suppl):617–21.

36. Pence B, Aubey B, Ergenekon G. Outcomes of 532nm frequency-doubled Nd:YAG laser use in the treatment of port-wine stains. Dermatol Surg 2005; 31:509–17.

37. Lanigan SW, Taibjee SM. Recent advances in laser treatment of port-wine stains. Br J Dermatol 2004; 151:527–33.

38. Jasim ZF, Handley JM. Treatment of pulsed dye laser-resistant port-wine stain birthmarks. J Am Acad Dermatol 2007;57:677–82.

39. Greene AK, Perlyn CA, Alomari AI. Management of lymphatic malformations. Clin Plast Surg 2001;38: 75–82.

40. Young AE. Pathogenesis of vascular malformations. In: Mulliken JB, Young AE, editors. Vascular birthmarks: hemangiomas and malformations. Philadelphia: Saunders; 1988. p. 107–13.

41. Padwa BL, Hayward PG, Ferraro NF, et al. Cervicofacial lymphatic malformation: clinical course, surgical intervention, and pathogenesis of skeletal hypertrophy. Plast Reconstr Surg 1995;95:951–60.

42. Edwards PD, Rahbar R, Ferraro NF, et al. Lymphatic malformation of the lingual base and oral floor. Plast Reconstr Surg 2005;115:1906–15.

43. Ninh T, Ninh T. Cystic hygroma in children: report of 126 cases. J Pediatr Surg 1974;9:191–5.

44. Greinwald J Jr, Cohen AP, Hemanackah S, et al. Massive lymphatic malformations of the head, neck, chest. J Otolaryngol Head Neck Surg 2008; 37:169–73.

45. Alomari AI, Karian VE, Lord DJ, et al. Percutaneous sclerotherapy for lymphatic malformations: a retrospective analysis of patient-evaluated improvement. J Vasc Interv Radiol 2006;17:1639–48.

46. Smith ML, Zimmerman B, Burke DK, et al. Efficacy and safety of OK-432 immunotherapy of lymphatic malformations. Laryngoscope 2009; 119:107–15.

47. Kim KH, Sung MW, Roh JL, et al. Sclerotherapy for congenital lesions in the head and neck. Otolaryngol Head Neck Surg 2004;131:307–16.

48. Greene AK, Alomari AI. Management of venous malformations. Clin Plast Surg 2001;38:83–93.

49. Marler JJ, Fishman SJ, Upton J, et al. Prenatal diagnosis of vascular anomalies. J Pediatr Surg 2002;37: 318–26.

50. Vikkula M, Boon LM, Carraway KL 3rd, et al. Vascular dysmorphogenesis caused by an activating mutation in the receptor tyrosine kinase TIE2. Cell 1996;87:1181–90.

51. Brouillard P, Ghassibe M, Penington A, et al. Four common glomulin mutations cause two thirds of glomuvenous malformations ("familial glomangiomas"): evidence for a founder effect. J Med Genet 2005;42:e13.

52. Gunel M, Awad IA, Finberg K, et al. A founder mutation as a cause of cerebral cavernous malformation in Hispanic Americans. N Engl J Med 1996; 334:946–51.

53. Oranje AP. Blue rubber bleb nevus syndrome. Pediatr Dermatol 1986;3:304–10.

54. Kaban LB, Mulliken JB. Vascular anomalies of the maxillofacial region. J Oral Maxillofac Surg 1986; 44:203–13.

55. Dompmartin A, Acher A, Thibon P, et al. Association of localized intravascular coagulopathy with venous malformations. Arch Dermatol 2008;144:873–7.

56. Choi DJ, Alomari AI, Chaudry G, et al. Neurointerventional management of low-flow vascular malformations of the head and neck. Neuroimaging Clin North Am 2009;19:199–218.

57. Berenguer B, Burrows PE, Zurakowski D, et al. Sclerotherapy of craniofacial venous malformations: complications and results. Plast Reconstr Surg 1999;104:1–11.

58. Burrows PE, Mason KP. Percutaneous treatment of low flow vascular malformations. J Vasc Interv Radiol 2004;15:431–45.

59. Yomaki T, Nozki M, Sakurai H, et al. Prospective randomized efficacy of ultrasound-guided foam sclerotherapy compared with ultrasound-guided liquid sclerotherapy in the treatment of symptomatic cavernous malformations. J Vasc Surg 2008;47: 578–84.

60. Green AK, Orbach DB. Management of arteriovenous malformations. Clin Plast Surg 2011;38:96–106.

61. Young AE, Mulliken JB. Arteriovenous malformations. In: Mulliken JB, Young AE, editors. Vascular birthmarks: hemangiomas and malformations. Philadelphia: Saunders; 1988. p. 228–45.

62. Kohout MP, Hansen M, Pribaz JJ, et al. Arteriovenous malformations of the head and neck: natural history and management. Plast Reconstr Surg 1998;102:643–54.

63. Mulliken JB. Vascular anomalies. In: Aston JJ, Beasley RW, Thorne CHM, editors. Grabb and Smith's plastic surgery. Philadelphia: Lippincott-Raven; 1977.

64. Wu IC, Orbach DB. Neurointerventional management of high-flow vascular malformations of the head and neck. Neuroimaging Clin North Am 2009;19:219–40.

65. Shapiro NL, Shapiro NL, Cunningham MJ, et al. Osseous craniofacial arteriovenous malformations in the pediatric population. Arch Otolaryngol Head Neck Surg 1997;123:101–5.

66. Kademani D, Costello BJ, Ditty D, et al. An alternative approach to maxillofacial arteriovenous malformations with transosseous direct puncture embolization. Oral Surg Oral Med Oral Pathol Oral Radiol Endod 2004;97:701–6.

67. Persky MS, Yoo HG, Bernstein A. Management of vascular malformations of the mandible and maxilla. Laryngoscope 2003;113:1885–92.

Pediatric Neck Masses

Michael R. Goins, MD[a],*, Michael S. Beasley, MD[b]

KEYWORDS

- Pediatric • Neck masses • Cervical adenitis • Neoplasms

KEY POINTS

- Children with neck masses require a thorough clinical examination and follow-up to determine the biological nature and course of the abnormality. Malignancy must always be considered, as it occurs in 11% to 15% of all pediatric cervical masses.
- Inflammatory disease represents the most common cause of neck masses or lumps in children, with cervical adenitis being the most common entity of the inflammatory processes.
- The second branchial arch represents about 90% of all branchial cleft/arch-related cysts and sinuses.
- Cysts of the thyroglossal sinus tract should be preoperatively studied for remnant thyroid tissue along its track of descent from the base of tongue. All thyroglossal sinus tract excisions should include the mid portion of the hyoid using the Sistrunk technique to ensure eradication.

INTRODUCTION

Primary care physicians often see a child with a neck mass or an enlarging mass of several weeks' duration. The possible entities are many; however, it is important to be able to make an early distinction based on history and presentation and to subsequently make an appropriate referral to a pediatric specialist. Depending on the suspected lesion, imaging modalities are obtained to better define the nature and extent of the mass before definitive diagnosis and treatment.

Most neck masses are congenital or inflammatory in origin, although 5% of all pediatric neoplasms occur in the head and neck.[1] The initial investigation must include a very precise history as to time of appearance, duration and changes of the mass, prior occurrence or multiple lesions, associated pain or dysphagia, leakage of fluid from the mass, associated injury, illness or systemic condition, and exposure to animals and travel. A careful examination of the head and neck will help to further narrow the possible etiology. These aspects of the workup and diagnosis of the cervical mass in children are presented in this article, with proper surgical management outlined for each category of lesion.

The differential diagnosis of pediatric neck masses is broad. Although the majority are benign, approximately 1 in 10 of biopsied masses were malignant in a review from the Children's Hospital of Pennsylvania. In this review, Torsiglieri and colleagues[1] examined 445 pediatric neck masses and classified them into congenital, inflammatory, noninflammatory benign lesions, benign neoplasms, and malignant neoplasms.

Not surprisingly, congenital lesions were the most common mass based on Torsiglieri's review, with inflammatory lesions the second most common. However, many inflammatory lesions resolve with conservative therapy and are never removed or biopsied, and are likely the most common pediatric neck mass seen in clinical practice. This review[1] also likely overestimates the frequency of malignant masses, as the Children's Hospital of Pennsylvania is a tertiary care facility

[a] Ear, Nose and Throat Associates of Charleston, 500 Donnally Street, Suite 200, Charleston, WV 25301, USA;
[b] Private Practice of Otolaryngology, Eye and Ear Clinic Physicians, 1306 Kanawha Boulevard East, Charleston, WV 25301, USA
* Corresponding author.
E-mail address: mgoins8@yahoo.com

Oral Maxillofacial Surg Clin N Am 24 (2012) 457–468
doi:10.1016/j.coms.2012.05.006
1042-3699/12/$ – see front matter © 2012 Published by Elsevier Inc.

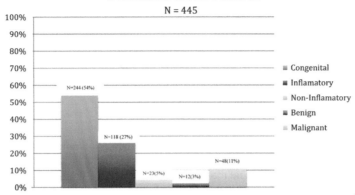

Fig. 1. Categories of neck masses presenting in children. (*Data from* Torsiglieri AJ Jr, Tom LW, Ross AJ 3rd, et al. Pediatric neck masses: guidelines for evaluation. Int J Pediatr Otorhinolaryngol 1988;16(3):199–210.)

for referred complex pediatric patients. However, Torsiglieri's survey provides the most comprehensive review of pediatric neck masses.

EMBRYOLOGY AND ANATOMY

A review of fetal development of the cervical region helps in understanding the nature and pathogenesis of some cervical masses.[2–4] During the latter part of the third week of craniocervical development, the buccopharyngeal membrane begins to break down into 6 paired pharyngeal arches. The fifth arch is small and disappears in the fourth week. The external surfaces are covered by ectoderm and internally by pharyngeal derived endoderm. Each pharyngeal (branchial) arch contains musculoskeletal, vascular, and neural elements, which contribute to future corresponding entities.

The first arch contains 2 cartilaginous structures: a maxillary process and a mandibular projection known as Meckel cartilage. Lateral ossification around Meckel cartilage forms the mandible, sphenomandibular, and anterior mallear ligaments. The nerve component is the trigeminal (fifth cranial nerve), and the arterial elements give rise to some portions of the internal maxillary artery. The muscles of mastication, tensor palatini and tensor tympani, anterior digastric and mylohyoid musculature, are all derived from the first arch.

The second branchial arch, also called Reichert cartilage, primarily forms musculoskeletal elements: muscles of facial expression, posterior digastric, stylohyoid, stapedius, and platysma muscles, and portions of the hyoid and the styloid process. The facial (seventh cranial nerve) nerve is derived from the second arch. Very little remains of the arterial component except for the stapedial artery.

The third arch gives rise to the remainder of the hyoid, the stylopharyngeus, upper constrictors,

and portions of the carotid vasculature. It also forms the inferior parathyroids, thymic duct, and thymus. The cranial nerve is the glossopharyngeal (ninth).

The fourth arch forms the inferior constrictor and cricothyroid muscles. Its nerve is the superior laryngeal, and vascular elements contribute to the right subclavian and on the left, the aortic arch. The superior parathyroids form from the fourth arch.

The remaining sixth arch gives rise to most of the laryngeal intrinsic musculature supplied by the recurrent laryngeal nerve. The arterial portion forms the ductus arteriosus and parts of the pulmonary artery. The fourth and sixth arches fuse to form the laryngeal cartilages.

The thyroid gland forms from descending endoderm at the tuberculum impar at the end of the third week. It travels to and around the developing hyoid bone to take up position in the lower anterior neck.

BACKGROUND

History and physical examination are paramount in the evaluation of the pediatric neck mass. The history and physical examination produce the differential diagnosis of the mass and often allow the differentiation of lesions into congenital, inflammatory, benign, or malignant, if a definite diagnosis cannot be made.

Certain caveats of the history and physical examination are crucially important. Location helps to narrow down the differential diagnosis. A midline neck mass may represent a thyroglossal duct cyst, dermoid and epidermoid cysts, cervical clefts, or teratomas.[3,4] Lateral neck masses are more likely to be branchial cleft anomalies, lymphatic or vascular malformations, and thyroid nodules. Congenital anomalies are more likely to present early, whereas malignancies are more frequently encountered in older children.[5]

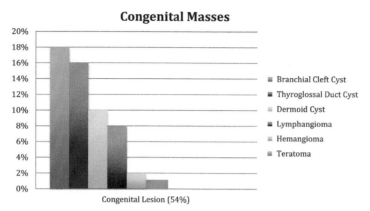

Fig. 2. Categories of congenital neck masses in children. (*Data from* Torsiglieri AJ Jr, Tom LW, Ross AJ 3rd, et al. Pediatric neck masses: guidelines for evaluation. Int J Pediatr Otorhinolaryngol 1988;16(3):199–210.)

Neck masses in children can be generally categorized by their location in the cervical anatomy.[6]

Anterior Triangle

Lymphadenopathy
> Infectious/Inflammatory: lymphadenitis, mycobacterial
> Neoplastic: lymphoma, secondary spread

Thyroglossal duct cysts
Branchial cleft cysts
Dermoids and lipomas
Thyroid masses (adolescent females), goiter.

Posterior Triangle

Lymphadenopathy
Vascular malformations (lymphatic)
Fibromatosis colli (pseudotumor of infancy)
Glandular (parotid).

Once the likely cause is determined by history and physical examination, further testing can be used to confirm the clinical suspicion. Laboratory testing, fine-needle aspiration (FNA) biopsy, and imaging of pediatric neck masses are often carried out to further classify the lesion.

CONGENITAL LESIONS

Congenital masses are the most common noninflammatory neck mass in children. Each type has a typical location and presentation in the neck. Children with congenital malformation of the neck require comprehensive pediatric evaluation to ensure it is not a manifestation of a systemic syndrome, which could modify the treatment plan.

Branchial Cleft Anomalies

During embryologic development, the tissues of the neck are derived from branchial arches that are separated externally by grooves and internally by pharyngeal pouches. Incomplete or aberrant fusion of 2 adjacent arches can result in the formation of branchial cleft anomalies that include cysts, internal sinuses, external sinuses, and fistulas.[2–4] Anomalies can arise from each embryologic groove and have characteristic locations and anatomic boundaries based on the structures derived from the adjacent embryologic arches.

Cysts arising from the first branchial arch comprise about 8% of cervical sinus tracts and

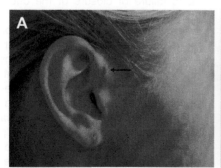
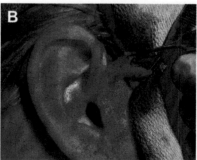

Fig. 3. A type I first branchial arch sinus and cyst presenting in the preauricular region. (*A*) Type I fistula (*arrow*) and cystic swelling preoperatively. (*B*) Sinus tract and cyst being delivered from its attachment to the external auditory canal cartilage.

cysts.[6] These cysts often present with recurrent swelling and drainage with secondary infection. Type I first-arch cysts typically open in the preauricular or postauricular region (**Figs. 1–3**). The sinus tract usually courses parallel to the external auditory canal to the middle ear or deep portion of the cartilaginous canal (**Fig. 4**).[7] Surgical excision is undertaken when no infection is present.

Type II cysts of the first arch are classically located in the anterior neck, superior to the hyoid. Sinuses course anteriorly to the hyoid, often through and around the parotid and facial nerve, respectively (**Fig. 5**).[4–7] Great care must be exercised in the surgical exposure of the area through superficial parotidectomy to avoid damage to the facial nerve.

Cysts of the second branchial arch are the most common branchial entity, accounting for about 90% of the cervical cysts.[3,4,6] If a skin opening is present, it is found along the anterior border of the sternocleidomastoid muscle (**Fig. 6**). As the cyst passes into the deep neck, it travels deep and posterior to the submandibular gland and between the internal and external carotid arteries to terminate in the tonsillar fossa (**Fig. 7**).[7] Imaging to delineate its course and endoscopy to visualize the pharynx for sinus openings are requisites before surgery (**Fig. 8**).

Cysts of the third and fourth branchial arches are uncommon (<2%) and represent sinus tracts, which course deep into the anterior cervical

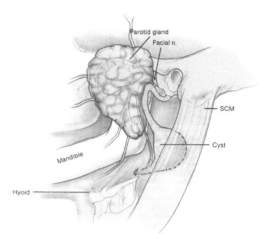

Fig. 5. Pathway of type II first branchial cleft anomalies. (*From* Drake A, Hulka G. Congenital neck masses. In: Shockley W, Pillsbury H, editors. Neck: diagnosis and surgery: Mosby; 2004. p. 98; with permission.)

structures and thyroid gland (**Fig. 9**). Imaging is important, as is endoscopic examination of the pyriform fossa, to identify the internal sinus opening. The unusual presentation of suppurative thyroiditis in children may be due to secondarily infected third- or fourth-arch sinuses.

Thyroglossal Duct Cyst

Thyroglossal duct cysts are the second most common congenital pediatric neck mass and form as a result of the thyroid's embryologic "journey" to the anterior neck.[7,8] The thyroid gland begins to develop in the third week in utero at the foramen cecum and then descends into the anterior neck to overlie the larynx. Occasionally, a remnant of embryologic ductal tissue persists following this process and can later develop into an epithelial lined tract (**Fig. 10**). In fact, the presence of the pyramidal lobe of the thyroid represents failure of closure of the duct at its most inferior location.[8]

Thyroglossal duct cysts primarily present in the midline, and can occur anywhere between the base of the tongue and the thyroid gland (**Fig. 11**). The cysts may lie dormant in a similar fashion to branchial cleft anomalies until they become swollen and painful, which can occur after an upper respiratory infection. Clinical diagnosis, based on a thorough history and physical examination, is usually accurate. Thyroglossal duct cysts are most easily seen with the neck in an extended position, and they will elevate with swallowing and tongue protrusion because of their fixation to the hyoid bone.

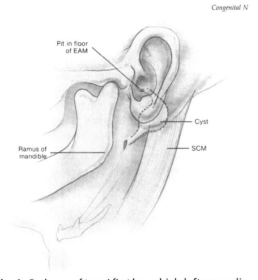

Fig. 4. Pathway of type I first branchial cleft anomalies. EAM, external auditory meatus; SCM, sternocleidomastoid muscle. (*From* Drake A, Hulka G. Congenital neck masses. In: Shockley WW, Pillsbury HC, editors. Neck: diagnosis and surgery: Mosby; 2004. p. 97; with permission.)

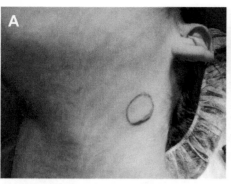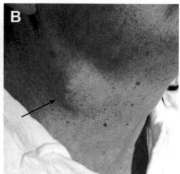

Fig. 6. (*A, B*) Second branchial arch cysts in 2 patients, both presenting anterior to the sternocleidomastoid muscle (*arrow*).

During the preoperative evaluation, additional imaging and thyroid uptake studies may be indicated. The best modality of imaging in children is ultrasonography, which can adequately document the presence and configuration of the thyroid gland or any derivatives in the descent route. It is important to confirm the presence of normal thyroid tissue outside of the thyroglossal duct cyst before excision, as well as identification and distinction from lingual thyroid tissue.

Complete excision of a thyroglossal duct cyst is performed by the Sistrunk procedure, first described in 1920.[9] This procedure requires removal of the cyst and any associated tract as well as the middle portion of the hyoid bone. Failure to remove the middle portion of the hyoid bone will often lead to recurrence and infection. Patients at greater risk of recurrence are those with infected, draining sinuses. Excision of sinus, anterior hyoid,

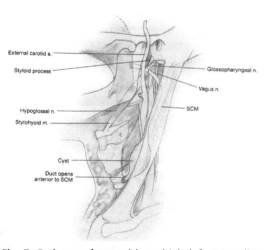

Fig. 7. Pathway of second branchial cleft anomalies. (*From* Drake A, Hulka G. Congenital neck masses. In: Shockley W, Pillsbury H, editors. Neck: diagnosis and surgery: Mosby; 2004; with permission.)

and investing scarred infrahyoid musculature may be necessary to achieve eradication.

Dermoid Cysts and Teratomas

The term dermoid cyst is often used in a generic sense to describe 3 separate entities that include epidermoid cysts, true dermoid cysts, and teratomas.[10] These pathologic entities are distinguished by their derivation. Epidermoid cysts arise from ectodermal tissue alone and are normally found superficially in the subcutaneous tissues. Histologically they have a squamous epithelial lining and often contain keratinaceous debris (**Fig. 12**). True dermoid cysts are composed of both ectodermal and mesodermal components including hair follicles, sebaceous glands, and/or sweat glands.

Both epidermoid and dermoid cysts may be congenital or acquired. Congenital lesions are thought to arise from the sequestration of ectoderm or endoderm within the deeper tissues along embryologic "folds."[11] In this respect they are similar to branchial cleft cysts, although they typically do not have sinus tracts nor do they arise from deep structures in the neck. Acquired cysts are commonly termed inclusion cysts because they are believed to result from traumatic implantation of a portion of the skin into the underlying layers,[10,11] which can result in the ectopic formation of a dermal cyst lined with squamous epithelium in any associated location. Depending on the size and depth of these lesions, preoperative imaging with ultrasonography, computed tomography (CT) or magnetic resonance imaging (MRI) may be indicated for diagnosis and surgical planning (**Fig. 13**).[12] The majority are amenable to direct surgical excision, and every effort should be made to remove the cysts without rupture of the cyst and spillage of contents. Epidermoid excision should include the overlying skin, whereas

A   **B**

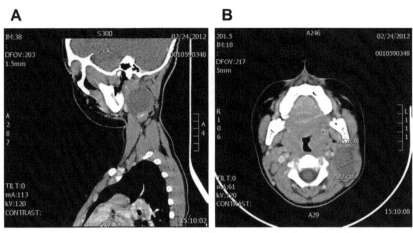

Fig. 8. Sagittal (*A*) and axial (*B*) computed tomography (CT) images of a branchial cleft cyst of the left neck.

dermoids are often attached to the underlying periosteum and require removal of the involved segment of periosteal attachment.[10]

Teratomas of the head and neck are rare tumors that are composed of all 3 embryologic layers: ectoderm, mesoderm, and endoderm.[13] These tumors may include any type or combination of tissues normally found within the human body. Although they are benign, they tend to grow more rapidly than other dermoid cysts.[13,14] In addition, their location is less predictable, and proximity to vital structures can make surgical excision difficult. Preoperative imaging with CT or MRI is normally indicated for diagnosis and surgical planning. Teratomas can present as an epignathus that may impinge on the airway. In the developed world, these are normally diagnosed prenatally with ultrasonography. If peripartum respiratory compromise is feared, the obstetric plan should include options for airway control including intubation or tracheotomy. An Ex Utero Intrapartum Therapy (EXIT) procedure may be indicated depending on the size and location of the mass, and should be considered and coordinated in advance of delivery.[15]

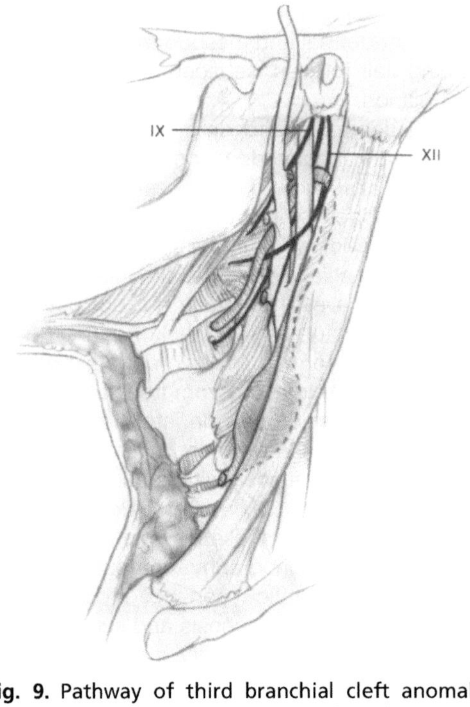

Lymphatic Malformations

Lymphatic malformations, previously termed lymphangiomas or cystic hygromas, are presently classified as vascular malformations, and occur in 1 out of every 2000 to 4000 births.[16] These malformations are more commonly found as isolated lymphatic lesions that tend to be of low flow in character, but can be seen in combination with arterial or venous vasculature as mixed lymphovascular lesions.[17] Lymphatic malformations are thought to arise as a benign growth of the lymphatic system; however, they can have significant local impact because of their growth potential and infiltrative nature.

Embryologically the lymphatic system develops from vascular endothelial cells.[18] The system is composed of thin-walled channels with limited basement membrane structure, allowing for increased permeability. The lymphatic system acts to drain extravascular fluid, direct antigens to regional lymph nodes, and absorb ingested fat.

Fig. 9. Pathway of third branchial cleft anomalies. (*From* Drake A, Hulka G. Congenital neck masses. In: Shockley W, Pillsbury H, editors. Neck: diagnosis and surgery: Mosby; 2004; with permission.)

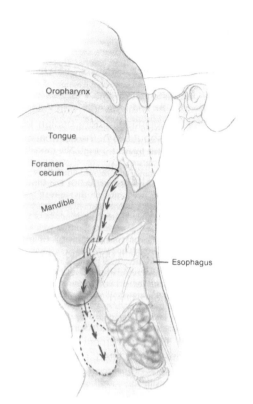

Fig. 10. Pathway of the thyroglossal duct with depiction of the typical cyst anterior to the hyoid. (*From* Drake A, Hulka G. Congenital neck masses. In: Shockley W, Pillsbury H, editors. Neck: diagnosis and surgery: Mosby; 2004; with permission.)

Lymphatic malformations are most commonly seen in the neck, but can be found anywhere in the soft tissues of the face and oral cavity; they are classically noted as a soft and compressible cystic mass that can be transilluminated. Lymphatic malformations can range in size and severity from small isolated lesions to extensive cervicofacial lesions (**Fig. 14**). The malformations may cause both cosmetic and functional

disturbances, including airway compromise and long-term distortion of facial growth. Although smaller lesions have been reported to regress without intervention, all of such lesions have the potential for rapid expansion secondary to hemorrhage, trauma, or infection.

Clinical diagnosis is confirmed with CT and/or MRI for complete characterization (**Fig. 15**). This imaging includes identification of microcystic and macrocystic components as well as delineation of anatomic location and extent of disease in relation to the surrounding vital structures.[19] The mainstay of treatment is surgical resection or debulking. Timing is debatable, and depends on the extent and impact of the lesion. Complete excision may be difficult without sacrifice of vital structures, and often multiple debulking procedures are performed. Multiple protocols regarding timing of surgical intervention and potential reconstruction are reported in the literature. Nevertheless, patients must be monitored for recurrence and long-term growth disturbances.

Sclerotherapy has been increasingly studied and used as a viable option to surgical resection, particularly in macrocystic lesions. Multiple protocols and sclerosant agents are currently being evaluated, including OK-432 (Picinabil), bleomycin, alcohol, and hypertonic saline.[20] Consideration must be given to the technique and control of infiltration as well as potential postoperative edema and pain.

For more in-depth discussion of lymphatic malformations, the reader is referred to the article on vascular malformations by Abramowicz and Padwa elsewhere in this issue.

INFLAMMATORY LESIONS

Inflammation and enlargement of the cervical lymph nodes represent the most common cause of neck masses in children. The review by Torsiglieri and colleagues[1] demonstrated a high percentage

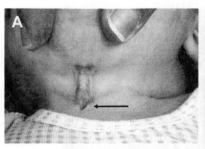
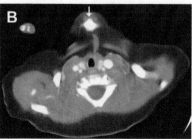
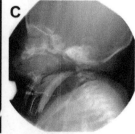

Fig. 11. Thyroglossal duct sinus and cyst. (*A*) Anterior neck of an infant with draining sinus tract (*arrow*). (*B*) Axial CT with contrast showing cystic cavity in fistula (*arrow*). (*C*) Fistulogram of thyroglossal sinus tract extending from tongue base to thyroid.

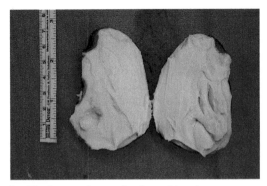

Fig. 12. Cut specimen of a dermoid cyst.

(27%) of neck masses as inflammatory in etiology (**Fig. 16**). Roughly half of all young children have palpable lymph nodes. The most common site for cervical adenitis is the submandibular and superior cervical nodes, although postauricular and occipital adenitis may result from chronic otitis and scalp infections (dermatitis, tinea, impetigo, and so forth). In general, a node larger than 2 cm^2 of longer than 2 months' duration should be sampled unless an infectious source can be documented. Vigilance through recall, examination, and systemic review is recommended.

History and physical examination are paramount in deciding whether to pursue further workup of a pediatric neck mass. One indication for FNA or open biopsy can be a mass that does not resolve after seemingly appropriate treatment. Others can be an enlarging mass, a suspicious clinical course, unusual imaging findings, or systemic symptoms. FNA can allow for Gram stain, culture, acid fast stain, immunocytochemistry, and cytogenetics. All FNAs have 2 inherent weaknesses: (1) the needle may miss the lesion of interest,

and (2) an FNA cannot appreciate histologic architecture.

NONINFLAMMATORY BENIGN LESIONS

The review by Torsiglieri and colleagues[1] grouped inclusion cysts, fibromatosis colli, and keloids into the category of noninflammatory benign lesions, which comprises about 5% of the cervical masses encountered in children. Inclusion cysts, which may develop from traumatically or iatrogenically induced means, and keloids are not be discussed here, as they make up only a very small component of the noninflammatory benign masses seen in children.

Fibromatosis colli, or pseudotumor of infancy, presents as torticollis with contracture of the sternocleidomastoid muscle (SCM).[21,22] The neck is flexed and foreshortened on the affected side with the child's head tilted ipsilaterally, with the chin deviated away. This firm mass typically follows a breech delivery with forceps, or a last trimester with little movement and the head engaged downward and tilted. Muscular damage to the SCM results in hematoma and fibrosis. Pseudotumor usually becomes evident soon after birth as the traumatized muscle is replaced with exuberant fibrosis tissue, which can be confirmed on ultrasonography (**Fig. 17**) or FNA or open biopsy.[21] On physical examination a firm, well-circumscribed, immobile soft-tissue mass may be felt in the belly of the sternomastoid muscle. Treatment of torticollis is primarily with aggressive physical therapy. In rare cases, the SCM may be surgically lengthened if torticollis persists beyond the first year of life. Physical therapy must resume immediately after the operation. Failure to treat can result in disfigurement of the craniofacial

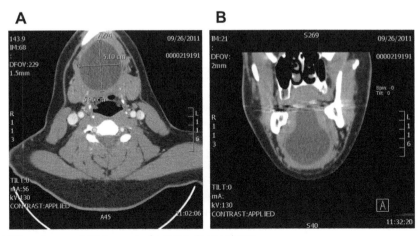

Fig. 13. Axial (*A*) and coronal (*B*) images of a large dermoid cyst.

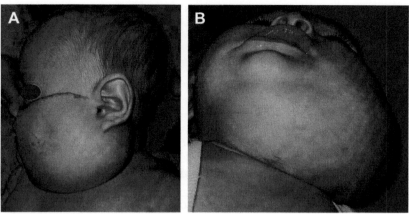

Fig. 14. An infant with a large cervical-facial lymphatic malformation of the left anterior neck. (*A*) Lateral view showing extent of lesion from a cephalad-caudal perspective. (*B*) Inferior view of large lymphatic malformation with mild external airway impingement.

skeleton through skewing of the cranial base, resulting in deformational plagiocephaly (**Fig. 18**).

BENIGN NEOPLASMS

Benign neoplasms are relatively uncommon pediatric neck lesions, accounting for only 3% of neck masses. Neurofibromas may present as either a solitary lesion or part of a generalized syndrome of neurofibromatosis (NFM). Neurofibromas, principally Schwann cells and melanocytes, are believed to arise from the neural crest.

Type I NFM or Recklinghausen disease is the most common form (90%) with an incidence of 1:4000 births.[23] It is an autosomal dominant disorder with variable expressivity. Type I NFM is diagnosed when any 2 of 9 inclusion criteria are met:

- Two or more neurofibromas or one plexiform (mass grouping) tumor
- Freckling of the groin or axilla
- Café-au-lait spots
- Skeletal deformity or scoliosis
- Lisch nodules (iritic hamartomas)
- Optic gliomas
- Macrocephaly ± hydrocephalus
- History of seizure
- Juvenile lenticular opacity.

When presumptive diagnosis of NFM is made, imaging (CT or MRI) may elucidate craniocervical involvement, particularly any tumor involvement of the airway (**Fig. 19**).[24] A central low T2 signal on MRI is a feature of NFM tumors.[25] Type II NFM is less common, and generally presents as a central nervous system disorder involving the

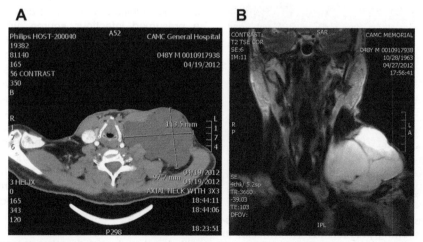

Fig. 15. (*A*) Axial CT image of a large lymphatic malformation. (*B*) Coronal magnetic resonance image of a large lymphatic malformation.

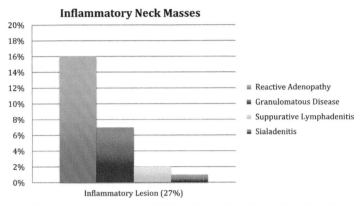

Fig. 16. Inflammatory neck masses of the neck in children. (*Data from* Torsiglieri AJ Jr, Tom LW, Ross AJ 3rd, et al. Pediatric neck masses: guidelines for evaluation. Int J Pediatr Otorhinolaryngol 1988;16(3):199–210.)

vestibular nerve (eighth cranial nerve) with subsequent hearing loss. Imbalance, headaches, facial palsies, and other craniospinal tumors accompany type II NFM.

Surveillance and selective tumor excision or debulking is the mainstay of management, as cure is not possible. A child with known NFM of the cervical region who begins to develop signs of airway obstruction (progressive snoring, stridor, and hoarseness) should undergo airway evaluation with endoscopy. Airway impingement from multiple or large tumors may necessitate prophylactic removal, if possible, with insurance of the airway

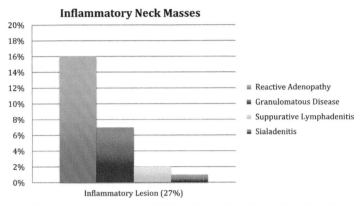

Fig. 17. Ultrasonogram of neck and sternocleidomastoid muscle showing pseudotumor (*arrowheads*) in the muscle belly. (*Courtesy of* http://pediatricimaging.wikispaces.com/; with permission.)

postoperatively, most likely with tracheostomy. Genetic counseling is encouraged.

Lipomas, though more common in the adult population, also occur in children. Lipomas are the most common benign mesenchymal tumors.[26,27] In children, lipomas typically arise before 8 years of age and have a rapid growth history. Lipomas are soft, compressible lesions, which may distort the neck and even compress the airway, although this is rare. Lipomas are one of the few lesions with anterior and posterior location in the neck, particularly with infiltrating masses. Multiple lipomas should alert the clinician to possible syndromic involvement with imaging, and FNA or open biopsy will confirm the diagnosis so that plans can be made for excision of the tumor.

MALIGNANT NEOPLASMS

In the child who first presents with a neck lump and who is sick, that is, febrile and lethargic, it is reasonable to initiate a course of antibiotics to treat a presumed infectious source, which is most common. However, if after 10 to 14 days of no improvement or worsening systemic signs and symptoms, a more serious condition should be entertained. Any child with a progressively enlarging neck mass and signs of systemic disease (fatigue, weight loss, fever/chills, night sweats, and so forth) should be highly suspect for malignancy.

Malignancy is a diagnosis that should be considered in the workup of all pediatric neck masses, as they represent 11% to 15% of all neck masses in children.[1,28,29] Lymphoma is the third most common pediatric cancer and is the most common malignancy presenting as a mass in the neck of a child.[29,30] In Torsiglieri's review,[1] 35% of patients with head and neck lymphoma presented with a supraclavicular mass. This finding confirms the

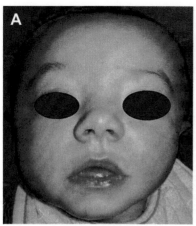
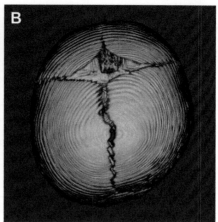

Fig. 18. Fibromatosis colli (pseudotumor) in an infant resulting in "twisted" face. (*A*) Infant with right facial fullness (and consequent flatness on the left side) and mandible deviated to the right, secondary to foreshortening of the sternocleidomastoid muscle. (*B*) Three-dimensional CT image demonstrating persistent deformational plagiocephaly caused by fibromatosis colli and torticollis.

need to have a high index of suspicion in the child who presents with a long-standing neck mass (>6 to 8 weeks) and has accompanying systemic signs of illness.

Because of accompanying involvement of the chest and abdomen, children may complain of shortness of breath, chest and abdominal discomfort, and gastrointestinal disorders. The workup consists of CT imaging, FNA or open biopsy for cellular type, blood panel, marrow biopsy, and surgical staging. Treatment is based on cellular type and corresponding clinical staging paradigms. Except for bony involvement and pathologic fracture or infection, surgical management does not play a role in the treatment of lymphoma in children.

SUMMARY

The differential diagnosis of the pediatric neck mass includes a wide array of congenital, inflammatory, benign, and malignant lesions in many locations of the neck. The initial history and physical examination is of utmost importance, and should be used to place the mass into one of these categories if a definitive diagnosis is not possible. The most common cervical masses are inflammatory in nature and represent a benign course, with little treatment other than watchful waiting. A mass that does not respond to seemingly appropriate treatment, and is accompanied by systemic symptoms or unusual imaging findings, should prompt the consideration of fine-needle aspiration and/or surgical biopsy.

Fig. 19. Coronal CT image of a neurofibroma in the left neck.

REFERENCES

1. Torsiglieri AJ Jr, Tom LW, Ross AJ 3rd, et al. Pediatric neck masses: guidelines for evaluation. Int J Pediatr Otorhinolaryngol 1988;16(3):199–210.
2. Carstens MH. Neural tube programming and craniofacial cleft formation. Eur J Paediatr Neurol 2004; 8(4):181–210.
3. Nicollas R, Guelfucci B, Roman S, et al. Congenital cysts and fistulas of the neck. Int J Pediatr Otorhinolaryngol 2000;55(2):117–24.
4. Schroeder JW Jr, Mohyuddin N, Maddalozzo J. Branchial anomalies in the pediatric population. Otolaryngol Head Neck Surg 2007;137(2):289–95.

5. Roh JL. Lymphomas of the head and neck in the pediatric population. Int J Pediatr Otorhinolaryngol 2007;71(9):1471–7.

6. Gross E, Sichel JY. Congenital neck lesions. Surg Clin North Am 2006;86(2):383–92.

7. Moir CR. Neck cysts, sinuses, thyroglossal duct cysts, and branchial cleft anomalies. Oper Tech Gen Surg 2004;6(4):281–95.

8. Rovet JF. Congenital hypothyroidism: an analysis of persisting deficits and associated factors. Child Neuropsychol 2002;8(3):150–62.

9. Sistrunk WE. The surgical treatment of cysts of the thyroglossal tract. Ann Surg 1920;71(2):121–2.

10. Pryor SG, Lewis JE, Weaver AL, et al. Pediatric dermoid cysts of the head and neck. Otolaryngol Head Neck Surg 2005;132(6):938–42.

11. Thomson HG. Common benign pediatric cutaneous tumors: timing and treatment. Clin Plast Surg 1990; 17(1):49–64.

12. Ahuja R, Azar NF. Orbital dermoids in children. Semin Ophthalmol 2006;21(3):207–11.

13. Wakhlu A, Wakhlu AK. Head and neck teratomas in children. Pediatr Surg Int 2000;16(5–6):333–7.

14. Bailey BJ. Congenital neck masses and cysts. In: Bailey BJ, Johnson JT, Newlands SD, editors. Head and neck surgery—otolaryngology. 3rd edition. Baltimore (MD): Lippincott Williams and Wilkins; 2001. p. 933–9.

15. Rahbar R, Vogel A, Myers LB, et al. Fetal surgery in otolaryngology. Arch Otolaryngol Head Neck Surg 2005;131:393–8.

16. Perkins JA, Manning SC, Tempero RM, et al. Lymphatic malformations: review of current treatment. Otolaryngol Head Neck Surg 2010;142(6):795–803.

17. Kennedy TL, Whitaker M, Pellitteri P, et al. Cystic hygroma/lymphangioma: a rational approach to management. Laryngoscope 2001;111:1929–37.

18. Perkins JA, Manning SC, Tempero RM, et al. Lymphatic malformations: current cellular and clinical investigations. Otolaryngol Head Neck Surg 2010;142(6):789–94.

19. MacArthur CJ. Head and neck hemangiomas of infancy. Curr Opin Otolaryngol Head Neck Surg 2006;14(6):397–405.

20. Smith ML, Zimmerman B, Burke DK, et al. Efficacy and safety of OK-432 immunotherapy of lymphatic malformations. Laryngoscope 2009;119: 107–15.

21. Lowry KC, Estroff JA, Rahbar R. The presentation and management of fibromatosis colli. Ear Nose Throat J 2010;89(9):E4–8.

22. Turkington JR, Paterson A, Sweeney LE, et al. Neck masses in children. Br J Radiol 2005;78:75–85.

23. Torpy JM, Burke AE, Glass RM. Neurofibromatosis Type I peripheral nerve tumors. JAMA 2008;300(3): 352–7.

24. Rahbar R, Litrovnik BG, Vargas SO, et al. The biology and management of laryngeal neurofibromas. Arch Otolaryngol Head Neck Surg 2004;130: 1400–6.

25. Steen RG, Taylor RS, Langston JW, et al. Prospective evaluation of the brain in asymptomatic children with NFM type I. Am J Neuroradiol 2001;22(5): 810–7.

26. de Jong AL, Park A, Taylor G, et al. Lipomas of the head and neck in children. Int J Ped Otolaryngol 1998;43(1):53–60.

27. Lerosey Y, Choussy O, Gruyer X, et al. Infiltrating lipoma of the head and neck. Int J Ped Otolaryngol 1999;47(1):91–5.

28. Neck masses. Publication of the American Academy of Otolaryngology—Head and Neck Surgery, Inc. One Prince Street. Alexandria (VA). 22314–23357. Available at: www.entnet.org/EducationAndResearch/Journal.cfm. Accessed April 27, 2012.

29. Smith MA, Seibel NL, Altekruse SF, et al. Outcomes for children and adolescents with cancer: challenges for the twenty-first century. J Clin Oncol 2010;28(15):2625–34.

30. Percy CL, Smith MA, Linet M, et al. Lymphomas and reticuloendothelial neoplasms. In: Ries LA, Smith MA, Gurney JG, editors. Cancer incidence and survival among children and adolescents: United States SEER program 1975-1995. Bethesda (MD): National Cancer Institute, SEER Program; 1999. p. 35–50. NIH Pub.No. 99-4649. Available at: http://seer.cancer.gov/publications/childhood/lymphomas.pdf. Accessed April 29, 2012.

Pediatric Infectious Disease
Unusual Head and Neck Infections

Kathryn S. Moffett, MD

KEYWORDS

• Pediatric • Sinusitis • Acute otitis media • Pharyngitis • Lymphadenitis

KEY POINTS

• Otoscopic findings are critical in making an accurate acute diagnosis of otitis media.
• In children, 80% to 90% of orbital or postseptal cellulitis is most commonly secondary to acute or chronic sinusitis.
• The syndrome of periodic fever, aphthous stomatitis, pharyngitis, and cervical adenitis is the most common periodic fever disease in children.
• Human papillomavirus is a causative agent of oropharyngeal cancer in 45% to 90% of cases.

Infections in children in the head and neck regions are common, leading to frequent use and overuse of antibiotics. Viral upper respiratory tract infection, pharyngitis, acute otitis media, and acute sinusitis comprise the majority of pediatric visits to primary care providers. This review includes common as well as diverse and unusual infectious diseases that occur in infants, children, and adolescents. In addition, the first available pediatric vaccines with the potential to prevent oropharyngeal cancers are reviewed.

SINUS/ORBIT/MIDDLE EAR INFECTIONS

In the United States, acute otitis media (AOM) is the most common condition for which antibiotics are prescribed for children. Clinical practice guidelines suggest observation without use of antibacterial agents in select children with uncomplicated AOM. The decision to observe or treat is based on a child's age, diagnostic certainty, and illness severity.[1] A recent systematic review on AOM diagnosis and treatment found that otoscopic findings are critical in making an accurate diagnosis of AOM. AOM microbiology has changed with use of pneumococcal conjugate vaccine—heptavalent (PCV7). The prevalence of Streptococcus pneumoniae as the cause of AOM has decreased from 48%

to 31% of isolates while that of Haemophilus influenzae has increased from 43% to 57% of isolates. Moraxella catarrhalis makes up 3% to 10% of isolates. Antibiotics are modestly more effective than no treatment, but cause adverse effects in 4% to 10% of children (rash and/or diarrhea). Most antibiotics have comparable clinical success, although data are absent regarding long-term effects on antimicrobial resistance.[2]

The treatment of AOM has become challenging with the emergence of pneumococcal resistance. Many penicillin-resistant strains of pneumococci have alterations in their penicillin-binding proteins that render them resistant to other β-lactam agents, such as ceftriaxone and cefotaxime. Nonsusceptible strains are further divided into intermediate and resistant isolates. This resistance can be overcome by using higher dosages of penicillin. Because antibiotic concentrations in nonmeningeal sites, such as the sinus and middle ear, are significantly greater than achievable concentrations in the meninges, definitions of susceptibility differ depending on whether the infection is in a meningeal or nonmeningeal site. For example, an isolate of S pneumoniae that has a minimal inhibitory concentration (MIC) of 2.0 μg/mL isolated from the middle ear is considered intermediately resistant to ceftriaxone. The same isolate

Pediatric Infectious Diseases, West Virginia University, HSC-9214, Morgantown, WV 26506-9214, USA
E-mail address: kmoffett@hsc.wvu.edu

Oral Maxillofacial Surg Clin N Am 24 (2012) 469–486
doi:10.1016/j.coms.2012.05.008
1042-3699/12/$ – see front matter © 2012 Elsevier Inc. All rights reserved.

found in the cerebrospinal fluid is considered resistant to ceftriaxone. These definitions take into account the antibiotic concentrations that can be achieved at different sites in order for the antimicrobial levels to be above the MIC for the treatment period. The use of high-dose oral amoxicillin (90 mg/kg/d) is commonly used as first-line therapy for treatment of AOM.[3,4]

Whereas *Mycoplasma pneumoniae* is a well-documented cause of atypical pneumonia as well as other respiratory syndromes such as bronchitis, bronchiolitis, pharyngitis, and croup,[5] it is an unlikely causative agent in bullous myringitis. A study of 49 middle-ear fluid samples from children with bullous and hemorrhagic myringitis were studied by polymerase chain reaction (PCR) for *M pneumoniae*; all samples were negative, suggesting that *M pneumoniae* is not an etiologic agent in acute bullous myringitis.[6]

Studies in children have shown that bullous myringitis accounts for less than 10% of AOM cases, and that the distribution of viral and bacterial pathogens in bullous myringitis is similar to that in AOM without bullous myringitis, except for a relative increase in the proportion of *S pneumoniae*.[5] In a study of 518 cases of AOM in children aged 6 months to 12 years, 41 cases (7.9%) were complicated by bullous myringitis. Children with bullous myringitis had more severe symptoms at the time of diagnosis and were more likely to have bulging of the tympanic membrane in the quadrants that were not obscured by the bulla. These children also required more aggressive pain management. Although parents and clinicians may agree that a watchful-waiting approach is appropriate for older children with mild AOM and may be acceptable, children experiencing painful AOM with bullous myringitis may not be successful candidates for a watchful-waiting approach.[7]

Treating a child with a draining ear is a common occurrence, and a multitude of factors must be considered in arriving at a diagnosis, including a history of the frequency, duration, and characteristics of the drainage. Cleansing of the external auditory canal is vital before the tympanic membrane can be accurately visualized for accurate diagnosis and treatment. The differential diagnoses of a draining ear include acute suppurative otitis media, otitis externa, granuloma, bullous myringitis, and a retained foreign body; most patients will respond well to a regimen of aural hygiene and topical therapy. Young children and those with a chronically draining ear may require more aggressive therapy, with systemic antimicrobials and culture; examination under anesthesia may be necessary to properly debride and visualize the canal. Children with tympanostomy tubes are especially at high risk for suppurative complications, and may require removal of the tube if drainage persists.[8]

Like AOM, *S pneumoniae*, *H influenzae*, and *M catarrhalis* are the most common bacterial pathogens causing uncomplicated acute sinusitis. Complications from sinusitis include preseptal or periorbital cellulitis, orbital cellulitis, epidural abscess, and venous sinus thrombosis. Intracranial complications of sinusitis such as epidural or subdural empyema are most commonly caused by microaerophilic or anaerobic streptococci, and such infections are often polymicrobial. Streptococci recovered on culture are commonly from the *Streptococcus anginosus* group (also known as *milleri* streptococci). *S aureus* can cause subdural or epidural empyema, but is more commonly isolated in combination with other pathogens such as streptococci.

Swelling of or around the eye may be due to infectious and noninfectious causes. Noninfectious causes of eye swelling include: (1) blunt trauma for which the history provides the key to the diagnosis—in these cases, bruising and eyelid swelling increase over 48 hours and then resolve over a several-day period; (2) allergic inflammation, which includes contact hypersensitivity or angioneurotic edema; (3) local edema whereby there is bilateral, boggy, nontender, nondiscolored soft-tissue swelling that may be caused by hypoproteinemia or congestive heart failure; and (4) tumors of the eye such as hemangiomas of the lid, ocular tumors (retinoblastoma, choroidal melanoma), and orbital neoplasms (neuroblastoma, rhabdomyosarcoma). These conditions usually cause a gradual onset of proptosis in the absence of inflammation.

Infectious causes of eye swelling may be periorbital or orbital. Cellulitis is defined as an infection that is either anterior to the orbital septum (preseptal or periorbital), or as an infection that is posterior to the orbital septum (orbital or postseptal). The orbital septum is a thin connective tissue extension of the orbital periosteum that is reflected into the upper and lower tarsal plates of the eyelids. It serves as a barrier between the superficial lids and the orbit.[9,10]

The eye and the paranasal sinuses are closely contiguous structures that share common elements. The venous system that drains the orbit, the ethmoid and maxillary sinuses, and the skin of the eye and periorbital tissue provide opportunities for spread of infection from one anatomic site to another and predisposes to involvement of the cavernous sinus. These veins represent an anastomosing and valveless network. The orbit is surrounded by the frontal sinus (roof of the orbit) and the maxillary sinus (the floor of the orbit). The medial wall of the orbit is formed by the frontal maxillary process, the lacrimal bone, the lamina papyracea of the ethmoid bone, and a small part of the sphenoid bone (**Fig. 1**). Therefore, an infection of the mucosa of the paranasal sinuses can spread to involve the bone and the intraorbital contents. Involvement of the intraorbital contents occurs through bony dehiscence in the lamina papyracea of the ethmoid or frontal bones or via foramina through which the ethmoid arteries pass.

Periorbital (Preseptal) Cellulitis

Periorbital or preseptal cellulitis (**Fig. 2**) may occur secondarily to a localized infection or inflammation of the conjunctiva, eyelids, or adjacent structures (conjunctivitis, hordeolum, acute chalazion, dacryocystitis, dacroadenitis, or impetigo, **Fig. 3**). It also may result from traumatic bacterial cellulitis at the site of local skin trauma (including insect bites), or spread of infection from a focus of impetigo. The overlying skin can be intensely erythematous and swollen. Most patients are afebrile; rarely is bacteremia present. The most common causative organisms are S aureus, group A β-hemolytic streptococci (GABHS), nontypeable H influenzae, and S pneumoniae.

Periorbital cellulitis may occur secondarily to hematogenous dissemination of nasopharyngeal pathogens to the periorbital tissue; however, in the era of universal H influenzae type b and pneumococcal vaccination, this is rare. Bacteremic periorbital cellulitis is most often seen in infants younger than 18 months who have had a preceding

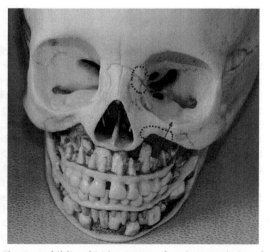

Fig. 1. A child's orbital anatomy, showing proximity of ethmoid air cells and maxillary dentition with regard to ascending infections into the orbit through the lamina papyracea (*cross*).

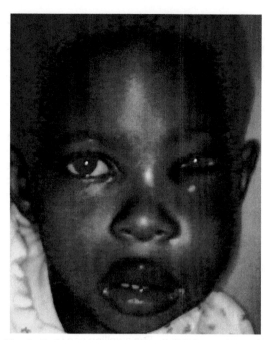

Fig. 2. Periorbital (preseptal) cellulitis in a 4-year-old child.

viral upper respiratory tract infection (URI). Patients develop a sudden increase in fever, accompanied by the acute and rapid progression of eyelid swelling. Swelling usually begins in the inner canthus of the upper and lower eyelid, and can obscure the eyeball within 12 hours. Periorbital tissues are usually erythematous; however, if the swelling has been rapidly progressive, the tissues may have a violaceous discoloration. Tenderness is usually mild, the globe is normal, and extraocular eye movements are intact. The pathogenesis of these infections is hematogenous dissemination from a portal of entry in the nasopharynx. Before universal immunization against H influenzae type b, this organism caused 80% of

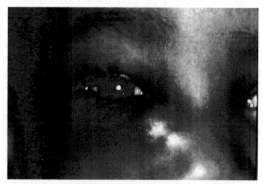

Fig. 3. Dacryocystitis in a 5-year-old child with spread to the preseptal tissues.

cases of bacteremic periorbital cellulitis, with *S pneumoniae* accounting for the remaining 20%. With the use of universal vaccination for *H influenzae* type b and *S pneumoniae*, there has been a substantial decline in the number of cases of bacteremic periorbital cellulitis. Less common pathogens include nontypeable *H influenzae* and GABHS.[11]

Most commonly periorbital cellulitis occurs as a manifestation of inflammatory edema or a sympathetic effusion in patients with acute sinusitis. The venous drainage of the upper and lower eyelid and surrounding structures include the inferior and superior ophthalmic veins, which pass through or next to the ethmoid sinus. If the sinuses are completely congested, venous drainage is physically impeded, resulting in soft-tissue swelling of the eyelids; this is usually most prominent at the medial aspect of the lids. Often, there may be intermittent periorbital swelling (early-morning or after awakening from a nap) that resolves after a few hours. Often however, the swelling can be persistent and progressive. Eye swelling can have significant degrees of erythema; tenderness is variable. Periorbital cellulitis has no displacement of the globe (proptosis) or impairment of extraocular eye movements. The peripheral white blood cell count is usually normal and blood culture results are negative, and sinus radiographic studies show ipsilateral ethmoiditis or pansinusitis. The infecting organisms are the same as those that cause uncomplicated acute sinusitis, namely *S pneumoniae*, nontypeable *H influenzae*, and *M catarrhalis*.[12]

Orbital (Postseptal) Cellulitis

In children, 80% to 90% of orbital or postseptal cellulitis is most commonly secondary to acute or chronic sinusitis.[12,13] The infection may result in the development of a subperiosteal abscess, orbital abscess and cellulitis, or cavernous sinus thrombosis. Patients with orbital disease caused by sinusitis usually develop the sudden onset of erythema and swelling of the eye after several days of a viral URI, although eye pain can precede the swelling and is often significant. Infection of the orbit is suggested by the presence of proptosis with the globe displaced anteriorly and downward, impairment of and pain with extraocular eye movements, usually upward or lateral gaze, loss of visual acuity, and chemosis (edema of the bulbar conjunctiva0 (**Fig. 4**). Fever and other systemic signs are variable.

Among young children, the subperiosteal abscess results from ethmoiditis and ethmoid osteitis, whereas in adolescents the subperiosteal abscess may be a complication of frontal sinusitis and osteitis

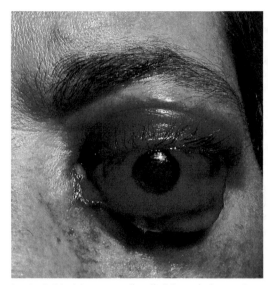

Fig. 4. Orbital (postseptal) cellulitis and abscess in an 18-year-old male patient. Note proptosis, conjunctival injection, chemosis, and dilated pupil.

(Pott puffy tumor). Most commonly in all ages, an abscess is located along the medial wall of the orbit. The most common organisms causing infection include *S pneumoniae*, nontypeable *H influenzae*, *M catarrhalis*, GABHS, *S aureus*, and anaerobic bacteria of the upper respiratory tract (anaerobic cocci, group C *Streptococcus*, *Bacteroides*, *Eikenella*, *Prevotella*, *Fusobacterium*, or *Veillonella* spp). Polymicrobial infection with a mixture of aerobic and anaerobic organisms is common. In patients with diabetic ketoacidosis, severe dehydration, and metabolic acidosis, and those with immunosuppression, *Aspergillus fumigatus*, *Aspergillus flavus*, *Mucor*, and other endemic fungi may rarely be the cause of disease (**Fig. 5**).[13]

Less commonly, orbital cellulitis may occur secondarily to hematogenous dissemination and the development of endophthalmitis, or may occur through traumatic inoculation of the orbit, penetrating trauma, open periorbital fracture, or orbital surgery. The most common organisms causing infection are those found on the skin, the sinuses, and the lacrimal mucosa, and include the same bacterial pathogens as occur in sinus-related orbital cellulitis. In cases of penetrating trauma where there is concern for a soil-contaminated foreign body, gas-forming anaerobic bacteria such as *Clostridium* species and aerobic, gram-positive *Bacillus cereus* may cause infection.[14]

LYMPHADENITIS AND LYMPHADENOPATHY

Lymphadenopathy, most commonly a reactive process, frequently occurs in the regional area of

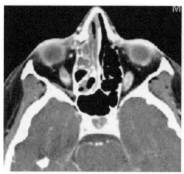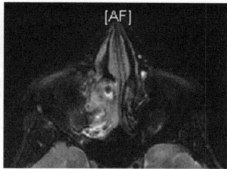

Fig. 5. Axial magnetic resonance imaging of *Mucor* infection of the right orbit and ethmoid sinus: flair images (*left*) and fast spin-echo (FSE) T2-weighted images (*right*). A 12-year-old girl receiving azathioprine and corticosteroid treatment for autoimmune hepatitis presented with rapidly progressive right facial numbness, right ear pain, and deviation of the tongue to the right with otalgia. Ophthalmology findings included a right VI nerve palsy; right cranial nerves V1, V2, V3 palsy; and anisocoria. She required urgent debridement of the sinus and orbit, along with antifungal treatment, and a reduction in the immunosuppression.

the neck, as a result of GABHS pharyngitis, viral URI, or a cutaneous inoculation leading to skin or soft-tissue infection. In most instances, bilateral cervical adenopathy is part of a localized response to acute pharyngitis. Viral cervical adenitis (**Fig. 6**) may be part of either a local response to viruses from the oropharynx or respiratory tract (adenovirus, coxsackievirus) or a more generalized reticuloendothelial response to systemic viral-associated infection (cytomegalovirus, human immunodeficiency virus [HIV], human herpes virus 6, or Epstein-Barr virus), toxoplasmosis and, less commonly in children, histoplasmosis and sporotrichosis. A lymph node biopsy may need to be performed to exclude lymphoma, especially in those patients who have an atypical presentation or who have delayed resolution of systemic symptoms. Other noninfectious causes include congenital and acquired cysts, Kawasaki disease, PFAPA (Periodic Fever, Aphthous stomatitis, Pharyngitis, cervical Adenitis) syndrome, Kikuchi disease, and sarcoidosis.

The differential diagnosis of lymphadenitis in children primarily includes infectious and malignant causes of lymphadenopathy. The presence of tender lymph nodes suggests an infectious cause. The most common bacterial cause of cervical adenitis is *S aureus* or GABHS (**Table 1**). The other 2 common causes of adenitis in infants and children are cat-scratch disease (CSD) and nontuberculous mycobacterium (NTM) infection. Medical management of bacterial adenitis with oral or intravenous antimicrobial management is often sufficient, along with pain management. In a child with a rapidly enlarging lymphadenitis, radiographic imaging with ultrasonography or computed tomography (CT) may be helpful in determining whether there is an abscess requiring surgical management (**Fig. 7**).

Less common bacteria causing bacterial lymphadenitis include anaerobic bacilli, *Haemophilus parainfluenzae*, *Haemophilus aphrophilus*, *Streptococcus anginosus*, and *Streptococcus agalactiae* (in a neonate). Rare causes include *Actinomyces israelii*, *Nocardia* species, *Francisella tularensis*, *Erysipelothrix rhusiopathiae*, *Bacillus anthracis*, *Yersinia pestis*, or *Borrelia burgdorferi*. *Streptococcus agalactiae* (group B *Streptococcus*)

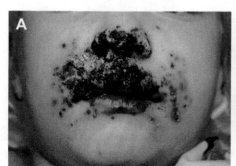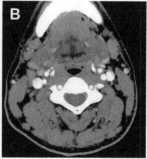

Fig. 6. A young child with viral aphthae (*A*) and associated lymphadenitis on computed tomography (CT) (*B*).

Table 1
Clinical presentation of bacterial lymphadenitis

Etiology, 53%–89% of bacterial isolates	*Staphylococcus aureus*; GABHS Acute onset most common *S aureus* has longer duration of symptoms before diagnosis
Pathophysiology	Entry to Cervical Lymphatics Oropharynx (GABHS) Anterior nares (*S aureus*)
Age	1–4 y
Sex	Male = female
Primary site	Submandibular (50%–60%); upper cervical (25%–30%); submental (5%–8%); occipital (3%–5%); lower cervical (2%–5%)
Size	2.0–6.0 cm
Fluctuant	25%–30%
Time to suppuration	86% Within 2 wk of Onset *S aureus* more likely to have suppuration
Unilateral	Common Concomitant lymphadenopathy at another site: 33%
History of:	Upper respiratory tract infection, including pharyngitis (40%) Earache or coryza (16%) Impetigo (32%)
Fever	Minimal or Absent Young infants more likely to have fever Fever accompanied by cellulitis, metastatic focus of infection, bacteremia
Tenderness	Common

Abbreviation: GABHS, Group A β-hemolytic streptococci.

is a cause of unilateral cervical adenitis and sepsis in neonates and young infants. *Staphylococcus mucilaginosus* is an opportunistic organism that rarely causes serious disease in otherwise normal patients. However, it may complicate head and neck surgery or cause sepsis in patients with underlying immune dysfunction or malignancy.

CSD is a common cause of lymphadenitis in children (**Table 2**). The lymph node affected depends on the site of skin inoculation. *Bartonella henselae* is the etiologic agent in most cases of CSD. Cats serve as the natural reservoir for *B henselae*; CSD occurs following the scratch or bite from a cat, especially from a young cat/kitten or a cat with

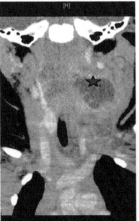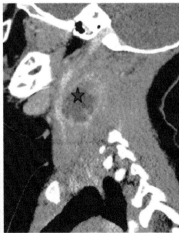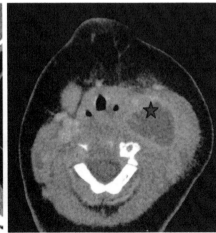

Fig. 7. (*Left to right*) Coronal, sagittal, and axial CT images of left neck lymphadenitis (*star*) complicated by a 35 × 35 × 24-mm lymph nodal abscess in previously healthy 10-month-old infant. Culture from the incision and drainage of the abscess grew methicillin-resistant *Staphylococcus aureus*.

Table 2
Summary of clinical and diagnostic features of cat-scratch disease

Etiology	*Bartonella henselae*
Transmission	Scratch, bite, or lick from kitten or cat, less commonly dog
Vector	Cat flea, *Ctenocephalides felis*
Pathophysiology	Inoculation of Organism in Skin/Mucous Membrane Causes a localized cutaneous skin lesion Lymph node enlargement near the site of organism inoculation
Location of adenitis	43% (Neck), 37% (Axilla), 20% (Groin) 37% of cases reported having multiple lymphadenopathy sites
Ocular involvement	Parinaud Oculoglandular Syndrome Granulomatous nonsuppurative conjunctivitis Ipsilateral preauricular lymphadenopathy Follows direct inoculation of the bacteria into the eye
Other manifestations	Systemic, blood-borne disseminated infection, infecting the liver, spleen, eye, or central nervous system (aseptic meningitis); prolonged fever; neuroretinitis; facial nerve palsy; encephalitis; mastoiditis; endocarditis; pneumonia; osteomyelitis; peliosis hepatis; bacillary angiomatosis
Initial finding	Granulomatous, nontender skin papule at site of inoculation
Duration skin papule	1–3 wk (range several d to mo)
Onset of lymphadenopathy	Regional Lymphadenopathy Proximal to the inoculation site 2 wk (range, 7–60 d) after the organism is inoculated into the skin
Lack of history of preceding skin papule	10%–15%
Clinical features	Lymph nodes are often tender, with erythema of the overlying skin; only 10%–15% of infected lymph nodes suppurate
Geographic distribution	Broad Worldwide Seasonal distribution in North America, and peak in fall and early winter
Diagnosis	Suspected from the Typical Clinical Findings, Confirmation From: Positive serologic test (positive *B henselae* antibody titer) Tissue biopsy of skin inoculum site or lymph node reveals a noncaseating granuloma with chronic inflammatory changes Polymerase chain reaction of the tissue *B henselae* cannot be cultured from tissue specimens Warthin-Starry stain is strongly suggestive of CSD; CSD skin test is no longer used
Treatment	Azithromycin Shown to decrease the size of lymphadenopathy if administered within the first 30 d of illness
Prevention	Hand washing after close contact with animals and control of vector (flea) infestation

Abbreviation: CSD, cat-scratch disease.
Data from Refs.[15–21]

fleas, and less commonly from a dog. The cat flea, *Ctenocephalides felis*, plays a critical role in as a vector in transmission.[15] Following inoculation of *B henselae* into humans, the organism typically causes a localized cutaneous skin lesion and lymph node enlargement near the site of organism inoculation (**Figs. 8** and **9**). Parinaud oculoglandular syndrome follows direct inoculation of the bacteria into the eye, resulting in a granulomatous nonsuppurative conjunctivitis and ipsilateral preauricular lymphadenopathy (**Fig. 10**).

When there is no reported history of animal contact or if the primary papule infection site has healed, diagnosis of this infection is challenging. Papules and pustules along cat scratches can easily be overlooked, especially when the enlarging lymph nodes appear 3 to 4 weeks after the primary infection. Of proven cases of CSD, 10% to 15% have no history of a preceding skin papule. The diagnosis of CSD may be suspected from the typical clinical findings, and laboratory evaluation can confirm the diagnosis based on a positive serologic test. Most cases of CSD are self-limited and require no surgical intervention. It is estimated that the annual incidence of CSD is 3.7 per 100,000 persons; however, the highest age-specific attack rate of 9.3 per 100,000 per year is seen in children younger than 10 years.[15] In a study of primary head and neck masses, CSD was identified in 13%. Other diagnoses included primary lymphadenopathy caused by other infectious agents in 11.9%, lymphadenopathy that occurred in association with primary infections of other organs in 9.0%, malignant neoplasm in 11.5%, benign neoplasm in 3.2%, and autoimmune disease in 3.3%. No cause of the cervical lymph node enlargement could be found in 37.7%.[17]

Pediatric NTM lymphadenitis is a common infection in healthy young children (toddlers and preschoolers) in the United States and worldwide. Surgical excision has been recommended as the treatment of choice for this condition. The incidence of NTM lymphadenitis infection is poorly understood, particularly in regions where *Mycobacterium tuberculosis* (TB) is endemic.[22] A Texas study conducted over 5 years found 34 children with mycobacterial lymphadenopathy disease: 30 children with NTM infection and 4 with infection from tuberculosis.[23] Cervical lymph nodes (84%) were most frequently involved (**Fig. 11**), and patients with NTM infection had a median age of 3.0 years. *Mycobacterium avium* complex is usually the most common organism isolated, by tissue culture or PCR, in children with NTM lymphadenitis. Often an etiologic organism is not identified. A recent survey of pediatric infectious disease specialists and otolaryngologists reported that surgical excision followed by adjunctive antibiotic therapy was favored in the majority (59%) of cases where a treatment method was reported. The use of surgical excision alone or antibiotic therapy alone was reported respectively in 24% and 17% of cases. Antibiotics were prescribed without diagnostic confirmation of infectious organisms in 28% of cases.[23] Several observational studies of NTM lymphadenitis in healthy children whose parents opted for conservative treatment showed total resolution within 6 to 12 months without surgical or antimicrobial intervention.[23,24] Fine-needle aspiration biopsy or incision and drainage of the involved lymph nodes, without complete surgical excision of the involved node, may be followed by formation of fistulas with chronic drainage, and should be avoided.[25]

Tuberculous lymphadenitis accounts for approximately 10% of TB cases in the United States. The epidemiologic characteristics include a 1.4:1 female-to-male ratio, a peak age range of 30 to 40 years, and dominant foreign birth, especially East Asian.[26] A child with cervical lymphadenitis and abnormal findings on a chest radiograph, especially born in a TB-endemic region, is more likely to have TB lymphadenitis than non-TB lymphadenitis. Surgical excision with culture confirmation deserves consideration for both optimal diagnosis and management when the diagnosis is not clear.[27–29] **Table 3** is a comparison of the clinical and diagnostic features of TB and NTM lymphadenitis.

PHARYNGITIS

GABHS pharyngitis is a common diagnosis. Up to 20% of school-aged children can be colonized with GABHS during the winter and spring in temperate climates, which may make it difficult to determine whether a child is experiencing a true streptococcal infection. The first step in

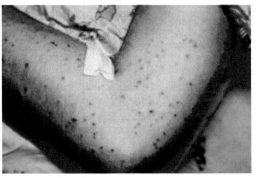

Fig. 8. Numerous scratches on the left arm of a child with cat-scratch disease.

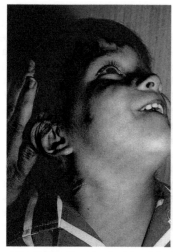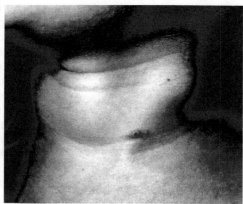

Fig. 9. Cat-scratch disease lymphadenitis with visible skin papules. (*Left*) papule on the face and right cervical lymphadenitis. (*Right*) Posterior cervical lymphadenitis with papule on the left neck.

management is to carefully review the individual episodes to ascertain whether the patient has actually had recurrent streptococcal pharyngitis. Moreover, the isolation of GABHS on throat culture, during asymptomatic intervals (and when symptoms of cough, coryza, and/or sneezing are present) suggests pharyngeal carriage and not infection.

The most frequent reason for recurrent GABHS pharyngitis is the acquisition of new strains from family or school contacts. There is a limited role for testing family members for streptococcal colonization, but this approach can be considered if recurrent episodes are occurring in multiple family members. There is no evidence that pets are a reservoir for streptococcal colonization. True relapse of GABHS pharyngitis after antibiotic treatment (bacteriologic failure) occurs rarely and can be due to poor compliance, or to macrolide (erythromycin or clarithromycin) or azalide (azithromycin) resistance. Macrolide or azalide resistance is found in approximately 5% of GABHS isolates in the United States, and penicillin resistance has never been documented. Therefore, a recurrence can be treated with the same β-lactam agent that was used previously. Intramuscular penicillin G benzathine is an alternative if noncompliance is suspected. Cocolonization by commensal flora has been proposed as a reason for true bacteriologic failures. The argument is that β-lactamase–producing organisms that reside in the tonsils (such as nontypeable *H influenzae* or *M catarrhalis*) prevent penicillin or amoxicillin from eradicating GABHS. However, evidence is lacking to justify the use of these broad-spectrum agents, such as a second (cefuroxime) or third (cefixime or cefdinir) cephalosporin, to treat recurrent GABHS pharyngitis, and is not recommended.

An attempt to eradicate carriage is usually not recommended, unless there is a family or personal history of acute rheumatic fever or, as a last resort, if tonsillectomy is being considered as a modality for preventing recurrences. Tonsillectomy may decrease the number of recurrent episodes in the

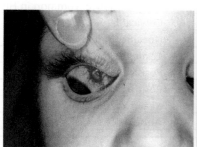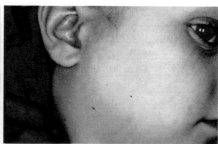

Fig. 10. A child with Parinaud oculoglandular syndrome. A papule is noted on the superior medial aspect of the right eye with ipsilateral preauricular lymphadenopathy.

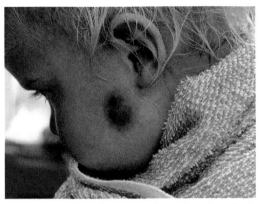

Fig. 11. Nontuberculous *Mycobacterium* lymphadenitis of the left face in a young child. Note the reddish-blue/violet discoloration. Fine-needle aspiration and incision should be avoided because fistula formation is common. Surgical excision is the recommended treatment of choice.

short term, but recurrences will inevitably happen because of reacquisition of strains. The efficacy of daily prophylactic oral penicillin V in prevention of recurrences of GABHS pharyngitis is unproven and is not recommended except to prevent relapses of rheumatic fever. An end-of-treatment throat culture is not recommended if the child is asymptomatic, unless he or she has a history of rheumatic fever.

The occurrence of a case of GABHS infection in a school or child care attendee is not an indication for laboratory screening of other students, staff, or attendees, unless they are symptomatic, because the prevalence of GABHS pharyngeal carriage in healthy children can be as high as 20%. Chemoprophylaxis of contacts in these settings is also not recommended. The index case should be excluded from school or child care until at least 24 hours of appropriate antibiotic therapy has been completed. Similarly, although there is a higher rate of transmission (upto 50%) to immediate family contacts than to other contacts, routine screening or chemoprophylaxis is not indicated, with a few exceptions. If the index case has acute rheumatic fever or acute glomerulonephritis, all household contacts should be screened, because they have potentially been exposed to a rheumatogenic or nephritogenic strain. In both situations they should be treated prophylactically if they are positive. Very rarely, if a cluster of cases is deemed to be an outbreak by health authorities, screening of all asymptomatic household contacts may be considered. Severe invasive GABHS disease or streptococcal toxic shock syndrome in the index case is associated with a slightly elevated risk of invasive GABHS disease in household contacts. Such patients need only be monitored for signs of illness, but chemoprophylaxis should be considered for selected high-risk persons: those

Table 3
Comparison of features of lymphadenitis caused by nontuberculous mycobacterium (NTM) infection and *Mycobacterium tuberculosis* (TB)

	NTM	TB
Age range (y)	1–6	20–40
Sex	Female = male	Female > male
Birth country	Non–TB-endemic	TB-endemic
HIV infection status	Rare	Common in HIV-endemic countries, rare in developed countries
Clinical features	Indolent, painless swelling Uncommon systemic symptoms	Indolent, painless swelling Uncommon systemic symptoms in HIV-negative; common in HIV-positive
Location	Cervicofacial	Cervical
Bilateral involvement	Uncommon	Not uncommon
Pulmonary disease	Absent	Common
Tuberculin skin test	Occasionally positive	Positive
IGRA	Negative	Positive
Histology	Caseating granuloma	Reactive adenitis
Treatment	Excision ± antibiotics	Antibiotics ± excision

Abbreviations: HIV, human immunodeficiency virus; IGRA, interferon-γ release assay.
Data from Fontanilla JM, Barnes A, von Reyn CF. Current diagnosis and management of peripheral tuberculous lymphadenitis. Clin Infect Dis 2011;53(6):555–62.

who are elderly or immunocompromised, and those with active varicella.[30]

Untreated GABHS pharyngitis can lead to local suppurative complications, lymphadenitis in the cervical lymph nodes, and infection of the tonsillar and parapharyngeal tissue space. Lymphadenitis is unilateral, markedly tender to palpation, and characterized by necrosis that can be identified on imaging. This condition is clinically distinct from the bilateral reactive lymphadenopathy that accompanies pharyngitis. For prevention of rheumatic fever, erythromycin is no longer recommended, nor are sulfonamides and trimethoprim, tetracyclines, or quinolones; once-daily amoxicillin or twice-daily penicillin are the preferred treatment options, and intramuscular benzathine penicillin is a third choice.[31]

Tonsillectomy is one of the most common surgical procedures in the United States, with more than 530,000 procedures performed annually in children younger than 15 years. Recent guidelines provide evidence-based recommendations on the preoperative, intraoperative, and postoperative care and management of children 1 to 18 years old under consideration for tonsillectomy, which include a strong recommendation for watchful waiting for recurrent throat infection if there have been fewer than 7 episodes in the past year or fewer than 5 episodes per year in the past 2 years; assessing the child with recurrent throat infection for modifying factors that may nonetheless favor tonsillectomy, which may include but are not limited to multiple antibiotic allergy/intolerance, periodic fever, aphthous stomatitis, pharyngitis and adenitis, or history of peritonsillar abscess; and asking caregivers of children with sleep-disordered breathing and tonsil hypertrophy about comorbid conditions that might improve after tonsillectomy, including growth retardation, poor school performance, enuresis, and behavioral problems.[32]

The syndrome of periodic fever, PFAPA, first described in 1987, is the most common periodic-fever disease in children.[33] PFAPA syndrome is sporadic, and appears to be a disorder of innate immunity and Th1 activation responsive to interleukin-1 blockade.[34] Attacks typically begin in a preschool-aged child and are characterized by abrupt onset of fever, malaise, chills, aphthous stomatitis, pharyngitis, headache, and tender cervical adenopathy, which occur at 3- to 6-week intervals over periods of years. These episodes of illness resolve spontaneously in 4 to 5 days. Affected children grow normally, usually are not susceptible to infection, and exhibit no long-term sequelae. Attacks may be aborted by short courses of prednisone but do not respond to nonsteroidal anti-inflammatory agents. Tonsillectomy or adenotonsillectomy in the management of affected children with PFAPA should be reserved for the child who has failed corticosteroid management. The precise role of surgery remains to be clarified.[32,35]

Arcanobacterium haemolyticum is a gram-positive bacillus that commonly causes pharyngitis, tonsillitis, and anterior cervical adenitis; 40% to 70% of cases are accompanied by an exanthematous rash. The peak age for developing pharyngitis is during the second decade of life. Tonsils may demonstrate exudate in 50% to 70% of patients, and nearly half of patients have a fever and cough that is nonproductive. In both normal and immune-compromised hosts, *A haemolyticum* can cause cutaneous abscesses and wound infections and, rarely, invasive disease such as sepsis, endocarditis, and meningitis. Infection is transmitted from human to human. Horse or sheep agar, generally used to isolate GABHS, is not satisfactory for the growth and identification of this organism; culture of *A haemolyticum* requires rabbit or human agar. Therefore, unless this organism is specifically requested from the microbiology laboratory, it is rarely isolated. No specific treatment studies have been performed, although consensus for treatment is the use of a macrolide (erythromycin, clarithromycin) or azilide (azithromycin) antibiotic. Although *A haemolyticum* is sensitive to penicillin, treatment failures have occurred. This organism is resistant to trimethoprim-sulfamethoxazole.[36]

Corynebacterium diphtheriae primarily causes respiratory infections, and is historically the most important member of the genus known as diphtheroids. Respiratory diphtheria is manifested by membranous nasopharyngitis or obstructive laryngotracheitis caused by infection with toxigenic strains. Sore throat is universal in tonsillar or pharyngeal diphtheria. Dysphagia, hoarseness, and headache occur in fewer than 50% of cases. The characteristic dense, necrotic, and adherent pseudomembrane, which consists of sloughed epithelial cells, microbes, fibrin, leukocytes, and erythrocytes, can extend from the soft palate to the glottic areas (**Fig. 12**). Associated soft-tissue edema and regional cervical adenopathy can become severe, resulting in the bull-neck appearance (**Fig. 13**). Airway obstruction also can occur and can mimic croup, epiglottis, or bacterial tracheitis. Humans are the only reservoir of *C diphtheriae*.

Carriage remains endemic in eastern Eurasian territories of the former Soviet Union, Africa, Latin America, the Middle East, and other parts of Asia. There has been no locally acquired respiratory

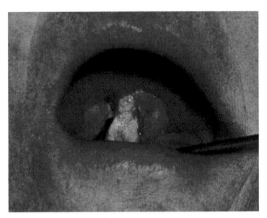

Fig. 12. Pseudomembrane in a patient with respiratory diphtheria. (*Courtesy of* Dr Peter Strebel, Centers for Disease Control and Prevention, Atlanta, GA.)

diphtheria in the United States since 2003. Fully immunized persons may have mild sore throat or be asymptomatic carriers. Respiratory diphtheria is most common in autumn and winter months. Summer outbreaks can occur in warm climates. When diphtheria infection of any site is suspected, the clinical laboratory should be notified because special culture medium is required; all isolates of *C diphtheriae* should be tested for toxin production by a laboratory determined by state or local public health authorities. All isolates also should be sent to state health departments and forwarded to the Centers for Disease Control and Prevention.

A prolonged febrile episode in an ill adolescent may be due to Lemierre syndrome or Lemierre disease, caused by the anaerobe *Fusobacterium necrophorum*, and was originally described in the literature by Lemierre in 1936 as "postanginal septicemia." Lemierre syndrome may occur at any age, but is seen most commonly in adolescents and young adults and has been reported to

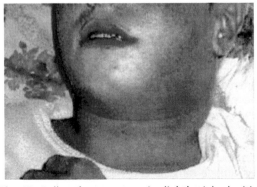

Fig. 13. Bull-neck appearance in diphtherial adenitis. (*Courtesy of* the Centers for Disease Control and Prevention/Barbara Rice.)

complicate odontogenic infections, mastoiditis, and otitis media, leading to a necrotizing pharyngotonsillitis, peritonsillar abscess, parapharyngeal, or posterior pharyngeal space infection. Local septic thrombophlebitis of the jugular vein results in sepsis and metastatic spread of abscesses throughout the body, most commonly in the lungs and large joints. In addition to *F necrophorum*, Lemierre syndrome has been caused by *Streptococcus pyogenes*, *A haemolyticum*, *S aureus*, including methicillin-resistant *S aureus*, and oral gram-positive anaerobic bacteria. Frequently seen in the preantibiotic era, incidence of Lemierre syndrome diminished with the use of penicillin for the treatment of pharyngitis. As antibiotic treatment patterns of nonspecific pharyngitis have changed in the recent decades to more use of cephalosporin and macrolide antibiotics, an increase in the incidence of Lemierre syndrome has been noted.[37]

The diagnosis often is overlooked, and must be considered in an ill patient with severe pharyngitis or tonsillitis. The patient's age, antecedent progressively worsening sore throat, unilateral tonsillar abscess, and negative Rapid Strep Test result all provide clues to the diagnosis.[38] CT scan or magnetic resonance imaging (MRI) of the head, neck, and chest should be performed in patients with suspected Lemierre syndrome to delineate the extent of the thrombosis and extension to deep neck structures and mediastinum. Comprehensive testing for thrombophilia should also be performed. Management includes antibiotics directed against the most likely organisms and drainage of abscesses. Some experts suggest anticoagulation.[37]

Invasive bacterial infections of the deep neck structures are not uncommon complications in children and adolescents, and result from direct invasion of bacteria from the tonsils and nasopharynx. The anatomy of the deep neck spaces is vital for understanding how these infections can spread.

Tonsillar and peritonsillar abscess (also known as quinsy) can occur at any age but is seen most often in preadolescents, adolescents, and young adults, especially those who have a history of recurrent tonsillitis. It presents as severe odynophagia with difficulty swallowing solids and liquids and in advanced disease the patient will drool and be unable to swallow saliva. Patients may speak with a muffled voice and trismus (the inability to open the mouth widely) may occur Deviation of the uvula will be apparent. Peritonsillar abscess is almost always unilateral, and the ipsilateral cervical nodes are usually also enlarged and tender. The abscess is most often in the superior aspect of the tonsil.

Complications of untreated peritonsillar abscess include dehydration, sepsis, spontaneous rupture with aspiration of abscess contents, aspiration pneumonia, and Lemierre syndrome with metastatic abscesses. The bacterial organisms most often associated with peritonsillar abscess include GABHS, S aureus, Fusobacterium species, Peptostreptococcus species, Bacteroides species, Prevotella species, A haemolyticum, and H influenzae. Management includes antibiotics with activity against gram-positive organisms and oral anaerobes, administered intravenously or orally. In some patients, local aspiration of the abscess or surgical drainage is indicated. Tonsillectomy may be performed at presentation to drain the abscess or after the acute episode resolves to prevent recurrences.

Retropharyngeal abscess may occur at any age but is more common in infancy and early childhood. It occurs less commonly than a peritonsillar abscess. Retropharyngeal abscess may begin as a cellulitis or phlegmon that complicates pharyngitis, pharyngeal trauma or puncture wounds, dental infection, or procedures involving the cervical vertebrae. A retropharyngeal abscess is located between the posterior pharynx and the prevertebral fascia. On presentation, the patient may appear to have a stiff neck or torticollis, and will be ill-appearing and febrile; an infant may have stridor and be unable to swallow food, liquids, or saliva. On examination, there may be anterior bulging of the posterior pharyngeal wall. Complications include rupture of the abscess contents with aspiration, as well as contiguous spread to the posterior mediastinum, carotid sheath, or lateral pharyngeal space.

Plain lateral radiograph of the neck may show a retropharyngeal space mass, and CT will differentiate retropharyngeal cellulitis from a mature abscess cavity (**Fig. 14**) and determine whether septic thrombophlebitis or extension into the mediastinum has occurred. The organisms most often associated with retropharyngeal abscess include S aureus, GABHS, F necrophorum, Eikenella corrodens, Bacteroides species, Peptostreptococcus, and other gram-positive oral anaerobes. Rarely, gram-negative enteric organisms, such as Escherichia coli and Klebsiella pneumoniae, have been isolated from children with retropharyngeal abscesses. In immune-compromised hosts, unusual organisms and fungi may be isolated. Management includes monitoring of the patient's airway, and if airway compromise is imminent, intubation and surgical drainage of the abscess should be performed. Prompt initiation of intravenous antibiotic therapy against the likely organisms is vital; surgical drainage is indicated if an organized abscess cavity develops.[39]

A parapharyngeal abscess is the least common of the deep neck abscesses, but potentially the most serious and life threatening. It results from extension of a peritonsillar or retropharyngeal abscess, parotitis, mastoiditis, or dental abscess. Oral trauma from blunt object or puncture may precipitate a parapharyngeal space infection. Most patients will appear febrile and toxic, and will have severe neck pain and pain with swallowing, as well as cervical lymphadenitis and torticollis. Patients may also have decreased gag reflex and ipsilateral paralysis of vocal cords.

The complications of parapharyngeal space infection often involve the structures contained within this space, which may involve the carotid artery. Erosion into the carotid sheath may produce fatal hemorrhage, and thrombosis may produce stroke with hemiplegia. Extension of the infection may cause suppurative intracranial complications, such as cavernous or lateral sinus thrombosis and brain abscess. Dissemination of the infection may result in sepsis and septic pulmonary emboli. CT scan or MRI of the head, neck, and chest are indicated to delineate the involvement of vital structures and to assess for complications. The microbiology of parapharyngeal abscesses is less well described than that of peritonsillar and retropharyngeal abscesses, but because the infection extends from the oral cavity, the microbiology is likely to be similar. Management includes intravenous antibiotics, surgical incision if abscess is present, and airway monitoring.

Ludwig angina is a rapidly progressive "brawny" cellulitis of the floor of the mouth, tongue, and submandibular, sublingual, and submental spaces of the oral cavity (**Fig. 15**). It has been reported in young children to occur in approximately 15% of all cases.[40] Ludwig angina most often develops after trauma to the mouth, infection of the lower molar teeth, or procedures such as frenuloplasty and tongue piercing. It also may develop in complicated herpetic gingivostomatitis in toddlers or in children predisposed to infections, for example, sickle cell disease or a compromised immune system. Complications associated with Ludwig angina are mostly related to airway obstruction, which is of great concern in young children from an airway management perspective. The infection also may extend to the neck and mediastinum or may produce septic thrombophlebitis with sepsis. Patients with Ludwig angina will present with drooling and forward posture with the mouth held open. Children often are unable to eat, drink, swallow, or talk. Decreased oral intake with dehydration, high fever, and airway compromise necessitates hospitalization and medical and surgical management. Ludwig angina may be the presenting illness for

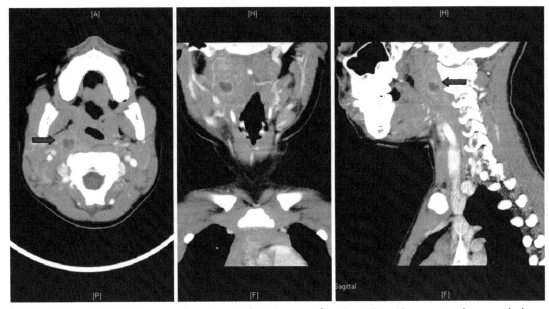

Fig. 14. (*Left to right*) Axial, coronal, and sagittal CT images of a 10 × 10 × 10-mm retropharyngeal abscess (*arrows*) in a 7-year-old child. The abscess has resulted in some airway narrowing. Culture from the abscess grew Group A β-hemolytic streptococci.

disorders associated with immune dysfunction, such as primary immune deficiency, diabetes mellitus, or malignancy, which should trigger investigations accordingly. The organisms associated with Ludwig angina include *Streptococcus* species, *S aureus*, *Peptostreptococcus* species, *Bacteroides* species, *Prevotella* species, *Fusobacterium* species, and *Actinomyces* species. Management of Ludwig angina includes intravenous antibiotics directed against gram-positive and

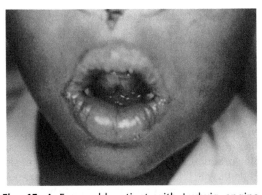

Fig. 15. A 5-year-old patient with Ludwig angina. Note floor-of-mouth induration causing elevation of the tongue. (*From* Britt JC, Josephson GD, Gross CW. Ludwig's angina in the pediatric population: report of a case and review of the literature. Int J Pediatr Otorhinolaryngol 2000;52(1):79–87; with permission.)

anaerobic bacteria, surgical drainage or dental extraction if an abscess develops, and airway monitoring to prevent obstructive asphyxiation.[41] Intravenous dexamethasone is helpful in reducing the cellulitic component of the infection and relieving airway obstruction.

Deep-space and parapharyngeal infections in children require prompt investigations through imaging, cultures and laboratory tests, and quick management. Children are more susceptible to airway compromise, tire more easily under metabolic demand and stress in advanced infections or sepsis, and have limited reserve. Children who do not favorably respond to initial management with rehydration, antibiotics, and surgical drainage should be investigated for underlying immunodeficiency, new-onset diabetes, and malignancy.

OTHER INFECTIOUS DISEASES
Lyme Disease

Lyme disease in children is manifested by clinical infection in 3 stages: early localized, early disseminated, and late disease. The distinctive rash erythema migrans (**Fig. 16**), accompanies the early localized stage, usually also with fever, malaise, headache, myalgia, mild neck stiffness, and arthralgia. Early disseminated disease manifests the same systemic symptoms as occur in early localized disease, with multiple erythema migrans lesions in approximately 15% of patients. In

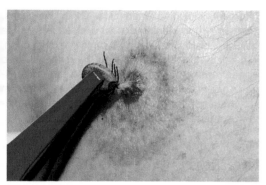

Fig. 16. Erythema migrans of back of the leg at the area of a tick bite. This manifestation closely followed high fever, generalized arthralgia, and headache.

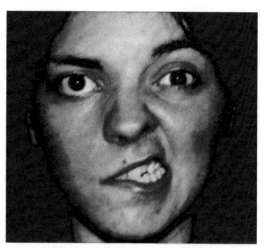

Fig. 17. Unilateral right facial palsy (neuroborreliosis) after a tick bite, indicating early disseminated disease.

addition, palsies of cranial nerves (especially cranial nerve VII), lymphocytic meningitis, conjunctivitis, and carditis (characterized by heart block) may occur. Among children who do not receive appropriate antimicrobial therapy approximately 50% develop arthritis, 10% develop central nervous system disease, and fewer than 5% develop cardiac involvement. Late disease is characterized by recurrent arthritis that is usually pauciarticular and affects large joints.

Lyme disease occurs in mainly 3 geographic regions of the United States: southern New England and the mid-Atlantic states, the Midwest, especially Wisconsin, and less commonly, Northern California. A clinical diagnosis is best made by recognizing the characteristic rash. Antibody diagnosis is recommended using a 2-step approach for serologic diagnosis of B burgdorferi. Patients with early localized disease may not have detectable antibodies against B burgdorferi initially; however, most patients with early disseminated disease and virtually all patients with late disease have antibodies against B burgdorferi.

The neurologic feature of Lyme disease in children manifests most commonly as peripheral facial palsy (**Fig. 17**), found in 55% of all cases of neuroborreliosis.[42] Bilateral facial nerve palsy is nearly pathognomonic for neuroborreliosis in children in epidemic areas. B burgdorferi infection in children is rarely complicated by the neuralgic radicular pain seen in adults. Children also are less likely to have clinical signs of meningeal irritation, despite cerebrospinal fluid pleocytosis.[42] The location of tick bites in children with Lyme disease are located more commonly in the head and neck region (49%), compared with only 2% for adults.[43] Treatment consists of oral amoxicillin or doxycycline for 14 to 28 days; parenteral treatment with ceftriaxone or penicillin is recommended for treatment of carditis, meningitis, or recurrent arthritis.

Human Papillomavirus

In developing countries, human papillomavirus (HPV) is a causative agent of oropharyngeal cancer in 45% to 90% of cases. Case-control studies show that patients with oropharyngeal cancer have a higher average number of lifetime sexual partners, which is a surrogate marker for oral HPV exposure, and are more likely than controls to have oral HPV infection.

The epidemiology of head and neck squamous cell carcinoma has decreased in the last 2 decades in the United States, which is thought to be related to the concurrent decrease in tobacco use. However, the incidence of HPV-associated oropharyngeal cancer is increasing, despite the decrease in tobacco use. In Sweden, only 23% of oropharyngeal cancers in the 1970s were associated with HPV. That number has steadily increased over the decades: 28% in the 1980s, 57% in the 1990s, and most recently 93% in 2007.[44] Similarly a 4-fold increase in HPV-related oropharyngeal cancers has been observed in the United States: 16% in the 1980s to 73% in 2000-2004.[45] This increase does not seem to be related to the integrity of the tumor samples, but instead reflects an actual change in the etiology of the disease.

The increasing incidence of HPV-associated oropharyngeal cancers is likely related to the changes in sexual behavior observed over the past decades in Europe and the United States: younger age at sexual debut and an increase in lifetime sexual partners. Because HPV infection usually must be present 10 years or longer for infection to progress to malignancy, the temporal change in sexual behavior could explain the observed increase in these cancers one to more decades later.

HPV DNA can be detected in exfoliated oral cells from an oral rinse or swab. Oral HPV infection is uncommon in children (<1%),[46] and seems to increase around the sexual debut, with oral HPV detected in 1.2% of 12- to 15-year-olds and 3.3% of 16- to 20-year-olds.[46,47] The highest detection is among healthy adults, at 4.5%.[48] Higher oropharyngeal prevalence is found in persons with HIV infection and women with cervical infection. The clinical usefulness of testing a patient for oral HPV is unknown, not readily clinically available, and not recommended at present.

Infection with HPV types 6 and 11 within the larynx or vocal cords can lead to recurrent respiratory papillomatosis (RRP). Characterized by multiple benign growths or papillomas in the middle and lower respiratory tract, RRP causes significant morbidity, requiring multiple surgeries and mortality if respiratory obstruction occurs. RRP has an incidence of 0.5 to 4 per 100,000[49] and has a bimodal age distribution: juvenile onset (<5 years, due to vertical transmission from the mother to child) and adult onset (>12 years, usually in adults 20–40 years old). The risk of transmission of HPV to a child from a mother with genital condyloma is reported to be approximately 7 per 1000 vaginal births.[50]

At present there are 2 HPV vaccines available in the United States, both of which are licensed for the prevention of HPV infection.[51,52] The bivalent vaccine (HPV2 or Cervarix) provides protection against HPV types 16 and 18 and is licensed for the prevention of cervical cancer in girls and young women aged 9 to 26 years. The quadrivalent vaccine (HPV4 or Gardasil) protects against infection with HPV types 6, 11, 16, and 18, and is licensed for all aged 9 to 26 years: in females for the prevention of genital warts and cervical, vaginal, vulvar, and anal cancers, and in males for the prevention of anal cancer and genital warts. Clinical trials have demonstrated high efficacy for the prevention of HPV in vaccine-type-naïve individuals. Although the HPV vaccines are not licensed for the prevention of oral pharyngeal infection or cancer, the potential for benefit in the coming decades is immense.[53]

SUMMARY

Infections in children must be quickly diagnosed and managed to avoid complications of dehydration, airway compromise, progression of disease, and sepsis. Although most pediatric maxillofacial infections will respond favorably to removal of the infected tooth, ear and sinus disease, tonsillitis, and so forth, some of these processes become chronic in nature, requiring vigilance and long-term treatment, including antibiotics. Other infections, such as lymphadenitis or Lyme disease, require thorough history taking and clinical examination, with selected testing to confirm the diagnosis and proper treatment. As in many disease states in children, prevention and education are important in early treatment and successful long-term management of many head and neck infections.

REFERENCES

1. American Academy of Pediatrics and American Academy of Family Physicians. Diagnosis and management of acute otitis media. Pediatrics 2004;13:1451–65.
2. Coker TR, Chan LS, Newberry SJ, et al. Diagnosis, microbial epidemiology, and antibiotic treatment of acute otitis media in children: a systematic review. JAMA 2010;304(19):2161–9.
3. American Academy of Pediatrics. Pneumococcal infections. In: Pickerington LK, Baker CJ, Kimberlin DW, et al, editors. Red book: 2009 report of the Committee on Infectious Diseases. 28th edition. Elk Grove Village (IL): American Academy of Pediatrics; 2009. p. 524–35.
4. Weinstein MP, Klugman KP, Jones RN. Rationale for revised penicillin susceptibility breakpoints versus Streptococcus pneumoniae: coping with antimicrobial susceptibility in an era of resistance. Clin Infect Dis 2009;48:1596–600.
5. Cherry JD, Welliver RC. Mycoplasma pneumoniae infections of adults and children. West J Med 1976;125(1):47–55.
6. Kotikoski MJ, Kleemola M, Palmu AA. No evidence of Mycoplasma pneumoniae in acute myringitis. Pediatr Infect Dis 2004;23(5):465–6.
7. McCormick DP, Saeed KA, Pittman C, et al. Bullous myringitis: a case-control study. Pediatrics 2003; 112(4):982–6.
8. Ramsey AM. Diagnosis and treatment of the child with a draining ear. J Pediatr Health Care 2002; 16(4):161–9.
9. Givner LB. Periorbital versus orbital cellulitis. Pediatr Infect Dis J 2002;21(12):1157–8.
10. Wald ER. Periorbital and orbital infections. Pediatr Rev 2004;25(9):312–20.
11. Ambati BK, Ambati J, Azar N, et al. Periorbital and orbital cellulitis before and after the advent of Haemophilus influenzae type B vaccination. Ophthalmology 2000;107:1450–3.
12. Hauser A, Fogarasi S. Periorbital and orbital cellulitis. Pediatr Rev 2010;31(6):242–9.
13. Jain A, Rubin PA. Orbital cellulitis in children. In Ophthalmol Clin 2001;41:71–86.
14. Rumelt S, Rubin PA. Potential sources for orbital cellulitis. Int Ophthalmol Clin 1996;36:207–21.

15. Hamilton DH, Zangwill KM, Hadler HL, et al. Cat-scratch disease—Connecticut, 1992-1993. J Infect Dis 1995;172:570–3.

16. Gerd J, Ridder GH, Boedeker CC, et al. Role of cat-scratch disease in lymphadenopathy in the head and neck. Clin Infect Dis 2002;35:643–9.

17. Ridder GH, Boedeker CC, Technau-Ihling K, et al. Cat-scratch disease: otolaryngologic manifestations and management. Otolaryngol Head Neck Surg 2005;132:353–8.

18. Munson PD, Boyce TG, Salomao DR, et al. Cat-scratch disease of the head and neck in a pediatric population: surgical indications and outcomes. Otolaryngol Head Neck Surg 2008;39:358–63.

19. Chui AG, Hecht DA, Prendiville SA, et al. Atypical presentations of cat scratch disease in the head and neck. Otolaryngol Head Neck Surg 2001;125: 414–6.

20. Cheung VW, Moxham JP. Cat scratch disease presenting as acute mastoiditis. Laryngoscope 2010; 120(Suppl 4):S222.

21. Bass JW, Freitas BC, Freitas AD, et al. Prospective randomized double blind placebo controlled evaluation of azithromycin for treatment of cat-scratch disease. Pediatr Infect Dis J 1996;17:447–52.

22. Tremblay V, Ayad T, Lapointe A, et al. Nontuberculous mycobacterial cervicofacial adenitis in children: epidemiologic study. J Otolaryngol Head Neck Surg 2008;37(5):616–22.

23. Cruz AT, Ong LT, Starke JR. Mycobacterial infections in Texas children: a 5-year case series. Pediatr Infect Dis J 2010;29(8):772–4.

24. Pilkington EF, MacArthur CJ, Beekmann SE, et al. Treatment patterns of pediatric nontuberculous mycobacterial (NTM) cervical lymphadenitis as reported by nationwide surveys of pediatric otolaryngology and infectious disease societies. Int J Pediatr Otorhinolaryngol 2010;74(4):343–6.

25. Zeharia A, Eidlitz-Markus T, Haimi-Cohen Y, et al. Management of nontuberculous mycobacteria-induced cervical lymphadenitis with observation alone. Pediatr Infect Dis J 2008;27(10):920–2.

26. Lindeboom JA. Conservative wait-and-see therapy versus antibiotic treatment for nontuberculous mycobacterial cervicofacial lymphadenitis in children. Clin Infect Dis 2011;52(2):180–4.

27. Fontanilla JM, Barnes A, von Reyn CF. Current diagnosis and management of peripheral tuberculous lymphadenitis. Clin Infect Dis 2011;53(6):555–62.

28. Carvalho AC, Codecasa L, Pinsi G, et al. Differential diagnosis of cervical mycobacterial lymphadenitis in children. Pediatr Infect Dis J 2010;29(7):629–33.

29. Griffith DE, Aksamit T, Brown-Elliott BA, et al, ATS Mycobacterial Diseases Subcommittee; American Thoracic Society; Infectious Disease Society of America. An official ATS/IDSA statement: diagnosis, treatment, and prevention of nontuberculous mycobacterial diseases. Am J Respir Crit Care Med 2007;175(4):367–416 Review.

30. Gerber MA. Pharyngitis. In: Long S, Pickering LK, Prober CG, editors. Principles and practice of pediatric infectious diseases. 3rd edition. Philadelphia: Churchill Livingstone Elsevier; 2008.

31. Gerber MA, Baltimore RS, Eaton CB, et al. Prevention of rheumatic fever and diagnosis and treatment of acute streptococcal pharyngitis: a scientific statement from the American Heart Association Rheumatic Fever, Endocarditis, and Kawasaki Disease Committee of the Council on Cardiovascular Disease in the Young, the Interdisciplinary Council on Functional Genomics and Translational Biology, and the Interdisciplinary Council on Quality of Care and Outcomes Research: endorsed by the American Academy of Pediatrics. Circulation 2009;119: 1541–51.

32. Baugh RF, Archer SM, Mitchell RB, et al. American Academy of Otolaryngology-Head and Neck Surgery Foundation. Clinical practice guideline: tonsillectomy in children. Otolaryngol Head Neck Surg 2011;144(Suppl 1):S1–30.

33. Marshall GS, Edwards KM, Butler J, et al. Syndrome of periodic fever, pharyngitis, and aphthous stomatitis. J Pediatr 1987;110(1):43–6.

34. Stojanov S, Lapidus S, Chitkara P, et al. Periodic fever, aphthous stomatitis, pharyngitis, and adenitis (PFAPA) is a disorder of innate immunity and Th1 activation responsive to IL-1 blockade. Proc Natl Acad Sci U S A 2011;108(17):7148–53.

35. Garavello W, Pignataro L, Gaini L, et al. Tonsillectomy in children with periodic fever with aphthous stomatitis, pharyngitis, and adenitis syndrome. J Pediatr 2011;159(1):138–42.

36. Karpathios T, Drakonaki S, Zervoudaki A, et al. *Arcanobacterium haemolyticum* in children with presumed streptococcal pharyngitis or scarlet fever. J Pediatr 1992;121:735–7.

37. Goldenberg NA, Knapp-Clevenger R, Hays T, et al. Lemierre's and Lemierre's-like syndromes in children: survival and thromboembolic outcomes. Pediatrics 2005;116(4):e543–8.

38. Ridgway JM, Parikh DA, Wright R, et al. Lemierre syndrome: a pediatric case series and review of the literature. Am J Otolaryngol 2010;31(1):38–45.

39. Goldstein N, Hammerschlag M. Peritonsillar, retropharyngeal and parapharyngeal abscesses. In: Feigin RD, Cherry JD, Demmler-Harrison GJ, et al, editors. Textbook of pediatric infectious diseases. 6th edition. Philadelphia: Saunders; 2009. p. 177–85.

40. Kurien M, Mathew J, Job A, et al. Ludwig's angina. Clin Otolaryngol 1997;22(3):263–5.

41. Britt J, Josephson G, Gross C. Ludwig's angina in the pediatric population: report of a case and review of the literature. Int J Pediatr Otorhinolaryngol 2000; 52(1):79–87.

42. Christen HJ. Bacterial meningitis and Lyme neuro-borreliosis in childhood. Curr Opin Neurol Neurosurg 1993;6:403–9.

43. Berglund J, Eitrem R, Ornstein K, et al. An epidemiologic study of Lyme disease in southern Sweden. N Engl J Med 1995;333:1319–24.

44. Nasman A, Attner P, Hammarstedt L, et al. Incidence of human papillomavirus (HPV) positive tonsillar carcinoma in Stockholm, Sweden: an epidemic of viral-induced carcinoma? Int J Cancer 2009;125:362–6.

45. Chaturvedi A, Engels E, Pfeiffer R, et al. Human papilloma virus (HPV) and rising oropharyngeal cancer incidence and survival in the United States. J Clin Oncol 2011;29(32):4294–301.

46. Smith EM, Swarnavel S, Ritchie JM, et al. Prevalence of human papilloma virus in the oral cavity/oropharynx in a large population of children and adolescents. Pediatr Infect Dis J 2007;26:836–40.

47. D'Souza G, Agrawl Y, Halpern J, et al. Oral sexual behaviors associated with prevalent oral human papillomavirus (HPV) infection. J Infect Dis 2009;199:1–7.

48. Kreimer AR, Alberg AJ, Daniel R, et al. Oral human papillomavirus infection in adults is associated with sexual behavior and HIV serostatus. J Infect Dis 2004;189:686–98.

49. Larson DA, Derkey CS. Epidemiology of recurrent respiratory papillomatosis. APMIS 2010;118:450–4.

50. Silverberg MJ, Thorsen P, Lindeberg H, et al. Condyloma in pregnancy is strongly predictive of juvenile-onset recurrent respiratory papillomatosis. Obstet Gynecol 2003;101:645–52.

51. Centers for Disease Control and Prevention (CDC). FDA licensure of quadrivalent human papillomavirus vaccine (HPV4, Gardasil) for use in males and guidance from the Advisory Committee on Immunization Practices (ACIP). MMWR Morb Mortal Wkly Rep 2010;59(20):630–2.

52. Markowitz LE, Dunne EF, Saraiya M, et al, Centers for Disease Control and Prevention (CDC); Advisory Committee on Immunization Practices (ACIP). Quadrivalent human papillomavirus vaccine: recommendations of the Advisory Committee on Immunization Practices (ACIP). MMWR Recomm Rep 2007;56(RR-2):1–24.

53. D'Souza G, Dempsey A. The role of HPV in head and neck cancer and review of the HPV vaccine. Prev Med 2011;53:S5–11.

Sinonasal Disease and Orbital Cellulitis in Children

Daniel J. Meara, MS, MD, DMD

KEYWORDS

- Sinonasal • Disease • Orbital • Cellulitis • Children

KEY POINTS

- Sinonasal disease is common in all age groups but is particularly common in children as a manifestation of many disease entities.
- As a result of the close anatomic proximity of the paranasal sinuses to the orbit and its contents, significant orbital disease can result from rhinosinusitis.
- Orbital cellulitis, if not treated promptly and aggressively, can result in vision loss, cavernous sinus thrombosis, and even intracranial abscess formation.
- History and physical examination, in conjunction with radiographic analysis, is critical to the diagnosis and institution of medical and/or surgical intervention.
- Prognosis is typically excellent as long as the diagnosis is accurate and treatment is initiated without delay.

Sinonasal disease is common in all age groups but is particularly common in children and can be a manifestation of many disease entities. However, the symptoms are often nonspecific and the differential diagnosis must initially include both infectious and noninfectious causes such as trauma, congenital defects, metabolic diseases, tumors, and immune-mediated processes such as Wegener granulomatosis and sarcoidosis.[1] Infectious causes such as rhinosinusitis are diagnosed when a child experiences symptoms of rhinorrhea, nasal congestion, postnasal drip, cough, headaches, and fever as a result of inflammation of the nose and paranasal sinuses.[2] As a result of the close anatomic proximity of the paranasal sinuses to the orbit and its contents, significant orbital disease can result from rhinosinusitis.[3] Orbital cellulitis can develop and, if not treated appropriately, vision loss, cavernous sinus thrombosis, and intracranial abscesses have been reported (Fig. 1).[4] Again, noninfectious causes of a red and swollen eye must be considered, such

as trauma, insect bites, and allergic reactions. Narrowing toward the correct diagnosis requires a detailed history in conjunction with a proper physical examination. Once an inflammatory cause is suggested, hordeolum, dacryocystitis, and conjunctivitis are typically less serious and are identified by their location and appearance. However, orbital cellulitis can be more difficult to diagnose but acute orbital inflammation is secondary to sinusitis in about 70% to 90% of cases.[5]

EPIDEMIOLOGY OF ORBITAL CELLULITIS

- No clear ethnicity differences[1]
- 2:1 prevalence in boys compared with girls[6]
- Suggestion of increased incidence in the late fall through the early spring months secondary to increased incidence of sinusitis[6]
- Greater incidence of acute sinusitis in younger children[7]

The author has nothing to disclose.
Oral and Maxillofacial Surgery Residency, Department of Oral and Maxillofacial Surgery, Christiana Care Health System, 501 West 14th Street, Suite 2W44, Wilmington, DE 19899, USA
E-mail address: dmeara@christianacare.org

Oral Maxillofacial Surg Clin N Am 24 (2012) 487–496
doi:10.1016/j.coms.2012.05.002

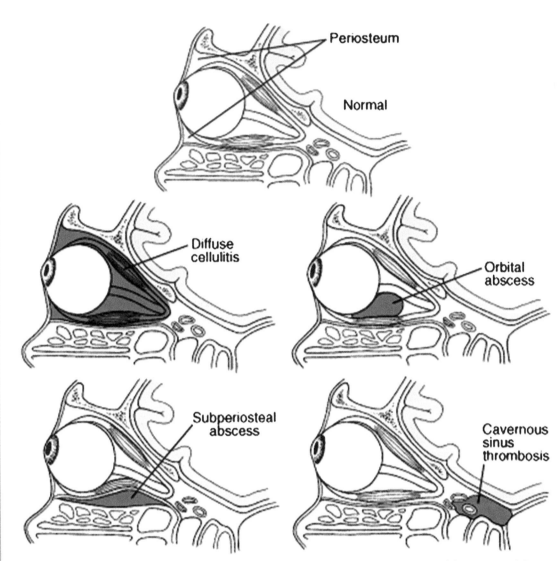

Fig. 1. Orbital cellulitis and its complications. (*From* Porter R, editor. The Merck manual of diagnosis and therapy Online Medical Library. Copyright 2004–2011 by Merck Sharp & Dohme Corp, a subsidiary of Merck & Co, Inc Whitehouse Station (NJ). Available at: http://www.merckmanuals.com. Accessed April 17, 2012; with permission.

- Rare presence of chronic sinusitis in patients younger than 16 years[7]
- Paranasal sinusitis frequency by site.[3]

Ethmoid>maxillary>frontal>sphenoid:

- Often patients have an infection in 2 or more sinuses, with the ethmoid-maxillary combination being the most common[3]
- Mean age at time of orbital cellulitis diagnosis is 7 years[6]
- Mean age at time of orbital cellulitis with subperiosteal abscess is 5.5 to 9 years[6]
- Preseptal cellulitis is more common than orbital cellulitis.[8]

ANATOMIC CONSIDERATIONS

Orbital cellulitis can occur as the result of exoge-nous causes such as penetrating trauma or via endogenous causes such as bacterial endocardi-tis, but the main source of disease in children is direct extension caused by the anatomic con-struction of the facial skeleton. The soft tissues of the orbit are distinct from the eyelids as a resul of the orbital septum. The orbital septum is ar extension of the orbital rim periosteum. The junc-tion of the periosteum with the septum is known as the arcus marginalis and the septal extension merges with the inferior aspect of the tarsal plate in the lower eyelid and the levator aponeurosis superior tarsal plate in the upper lid. The thinnest portion of the orbit is the medial orbital wall, also known as the lamina papyracea, which overlies the ethmoid sinus cavity. Further, the medial wall is often incomplete because defects, known as Zuckerkandl dehiscences, exist along with small neurovascular perforations. As a result of the basic anatomy at this site, the medial orbital wall is the most common location for acute sinusitis and is often associated with subperiosteal abscess formation in the orbit. This same anatomic design also can allow superior intracranial extension of bacteria. In addition, the paranasal sinuses drain primarily through the orbital venous channels that are without valves, allowing anterograde and retrograde infectious spread (**Fig. 2**).[9] In young children, the paranasal sinus ostia are wide relative to the sinus cavities requiring drainage and thus upper respiratory infections often involve the nose and sinuses as 1 collective structure, explaining the greater incidence of acute sinusitis in younger children. As growth occurs throughout childhood, the sinus ostia become narrower relative to the size of the increasing sinus cavities and nasal passageway. These changes promote chronic sinusitis, more complex infections, and slower resolution of disease.[3]

CLASSIFICATION SYSTEMS

Hubert[10] (NY State J Med 37:1559) was the first to categorize the orbital complications of acute sinusitis in 1937, and Chandler and colleagues[11] formalized the categories into a classification system in 1970 (**Table 1**). These historical classifications have been simplified by Jain and Rubin[9] into (1) preseptal cellulitis, (2) orbital cellulitis, and (3) orbital abscess (**Fig. 3**). The orbital abscess group is further divided into intraorbital abscess and subperiosteal abscess subgroups.

CLINICAL FINDINGS

Tables 2 and **3** present delineations of presentation, signs, and symptoms of preseptal and postseptal orbital cellulitis.

Preseptal cellulitis[12]:

- No eye pain
- No visual impairment
- Rarely fever
- No leukocytosis
- No radiographic evidence of sinusitis.

Postseptal cellulitis[12]:

- Positive for pain with eye movements
- Fever usually present
- Often irritability and toxic appearance
- Positive for erythema and induration of lids
- May develop limited extraocular movements, proptosis, decreased visual acuity, and papilledema
- Leukocytosis present
- Radiographic evidence of sinusitis noted.

MICROBIOLOGY

A systematic review by Nageswaran and colleagues[6] revealed the bacterial spectrum consistent with most cases of orbital cellulitis secondary to paranasal sinusitis. Most bacteria isolated were pathogens associated with acute sinusitis: *Streptococcus pneumoniae*, *Haemophilus influenzae*, *Moraxella catarrhalis*, *Streptococcus pyogenes*, *Staphylococcus aureus*, and anaerobes such as *Bacteroides*, *Peptostreptococcus*, *Prevotella*, and *Fusobacterium*. However, the incidence of *H influenzae*–related disease has diminished as a result of immunization, although untypeable *Haemophilus* may still cause disease. Polymicrobial infections are more often noted in children 9 years of age or older,[13] whereas the infections are typically caused by a single gram positive organism in younger children.[1]

Fungal

Mucormycosis, typically in the diabetic patient, and aspergillosis are the 2 main fungal or nonbacterial entities resulting in orbital infections. These 2 entities have distinguishing features and both are rare, with mucormycosis occurring mostly in the setting of underlying systemic disease, such as (1) diabetic ketoacidosis, (2) metabolic acidosis secondary to vomiting and dehydration, and

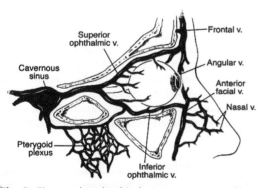

Fig. 2. Sinonasal and orbital venous anatomy. (*From* Steinkuller P, Jones D. Microbial preseptal and orbital cellulitis. In: Tasman W, Jaeger E, editors. Duane's ophthalmology (CD-ROM). Lippincott Williams & Wilkins; 2006; with permission.)

Table 1
Chandler classification of orbital extension of paranasal sinusitis

Chandler Class	Diagnosis	Clinical Signs
I	Inflammatory edema	Eyelid edema and erythema Normal extraocular movements Normal visual acuity
II	Orbital cellulitis	Diffuse edema of orbital contents No discrete abscess formation
III	Subperiosteal abscess	Collection of purulent exudate beneath periosteum of lamina papyracea Displacement of globe downward and lateral
IV	Orbital abscess	Purulent collection within orbit proper Proptosis, chemosis, and ophthalmoplegia Decreased visual acuity
V	Cavernous sinus thrombosis	Bilateral eye findings Prostration Meningismus

Modified from Sobol S, Marchand J, Tewfik T. Orbital complications of sinusitis in children. J Otolaryngol 2002;31:132; with permission.

(3) as a result of immune system modulation in the form of systemic steroid use or radiation therapy.[9] In addition, orbital aspergillosis can often be distinguished from mucormycosis and acute bacterial infections by its slowly progressive nature, with the disease propagation occurring over months to years.[14]

LABORATORY DATA IN ORBITAL CELLULITIS
Complete Blood Count

Increase can occur in both preseptal cellulitis and postseptal cellulitis but is most likely to be present in patients with postseptal (orbital) cellulitis.[15]

Blood Cultures

Bacteremia may be present in up to 33% of children less than the age of 4 years, although the yield for a positive culture is low.[14]

Sinus Cultures

Direct sinus aspiration provides the best culture medium, short of open surgery, for tailoring the antibiotic regimen and should be obtained in recurrent or recalcitrant sinusitis.[1]

Nasal Cultures

Nasal swab cultures may provide organism identification in the presence of purulent nasal discharge.[1] Preadmission or first-visit nasal swabs should be performed on all children to rule out methicillin-resistant *S aureus* carriers.

Conjunctival Cultures

Conjunctival swabs of the lacrimal puncta have limited diagnostic value because of low yield for specific organisms.[1] If associated dacryocystitis is highly suspected, then simultaneous lacrimal irrigation and culture may be both therapeutic and diagnostic.

Lumbar Puncture

Lumbar puncture for obtaining cerebrospinal fluid specimen is recommended only in the presence of meningeal signs or symptoms.[1]

IMAGING

Radiographic imaging for orbital infections is often a controversial topic in the work-up of a swollen eye. Ultrasonography, computed tomography (CT), and magnetic resonance imaging (MRI) may all be considered but the expected benefit must be clearly defined, to reduce patient angst, avoid unnecessary health care expenditures, and prevent unnecessary radiation exposure (CT).

Ultrasonography

Ultrasound may provide higher resolution for evaluation of soft tissue changes and the presence of a fluid collection but it is inadequate for imaging the bony anatomy, the paranasal sinuses, or the posterior one-third of the orbit.[9]

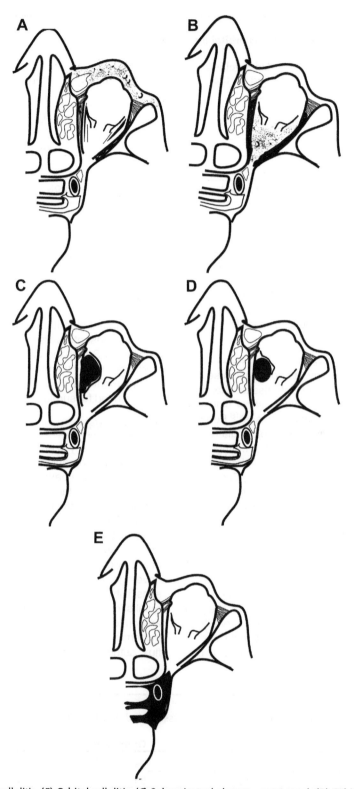

Fig. 3. (*A*) Preseptal cellulitis. (*B*) Orbital cellulitis. (*C*) Subperiosteal abscess – extraconal. (*D*) Orbital abscess – intraconal. (*E*) Cavernous sinus thrombosis. (*From* Dhariwal DK, Kittur MA, Farrier JN, et al. Post-traumatic orbital cellulitis. Br J Oral Maxillofacial Surg 2003;41:21–8; with permission.)

Table 2
Typical findings in periorbital versus orbital infections

Infection	Lid Swelling and Erythema	Ophthalmoplegia	Proptosis	Visual Acuity Changes
Periorbital cellulitis	Yes	No	No	No
Orbital cellulitis	Yes	Yes	Yes	Maybe
Subperiosteal abscess	Yes	Yes	Yes	Yes
Orbital abscess	Yes	Yes	Yes	Yes
Cavernous sinus thrombosis	Yes	Yes	Yes	Yes

Data from Teele D. Management of the child with a red, swollen eye. Pediatr Infect Dis J 1983;2:258–62.

MRI

MRI provides optimal evaluation of intracranial disease propagation such as cavernous sinus thrombosis. MRI is also effective for localization of fluid collections, especially on T2-weighted images, but provides limited bony detail.[3]

CT

CT is the imaging modality of choice because it is able to differentiate subtle soft tissue changes, localize abscess fluid collections, show sinusitis, and evaluate for intracranial processes.[16] Further, it shows the bony anatomy, particularly for obstructive sinusitis or destructive changes of the bony orbit. However, its use should be dictated by certain parameters, as suggested by Eustis and colleagues[16]: (1) visual acuity changes, (2) proptosis, (3) limitation of motility, (4) uncertainty of diagnosis, and (5) deterioration of overall condition despite treatment. Tole and colleagues[17] showed that up to 30% of patients with suspected preseptal cellulitis have evidence of orbital involvement on CT imaging, and Todman and colleagues[18] recently confirmed that the presence of large subperiosteal abscess formations are more likely to require and/or benefit from surgical intervention. Thus, CT imaging is often of great benefit even if the diagnosis is already known, because it can

guide treatment. However, in a growing child, there are concerns about cumulative radiation dosage.

MANAGEMENT

The treatment algorithm revolves around the decision of a preseptal versus postseptal infection, as detailed by Sobol and colleagues[19] (**Fig. 4**). Once orbital cellulitis is the prevailing diagnosis, medical management and adjunctive therapies commence and the need for surgical intervention is monitored.

Antimicrobials

Antibiotic therapy is empirically initiated based on the expected organisms present and taking into consideration the patient's age and comorbidities. Ampicillin-sulbactam is a reasonable starting choice in all patients because most organisms are odontogenic or sinus related.[20,21] Patients younger than 9 years may also be given ceftriaxone as a single agent and, in those patients 9 years of age or older, clindamycin may be added for dual coverage. Vancomycin is reserved for penicillin sensitivity.[9] Antibiotic therapy is tailored as culture results dictate. Recalcitrant sinusitis may signal anatomic (ostial) obstruction or nasal polyps, or systemic problems such as gastroesophageal reflux, asthma, and severe allergies.[21]

Table 3
Statistical analysis of clinical findings in sinusitis-associated postseptal infections

	Fever (%)	Ophthalmoplegia (%)	Proptosis (%)
Sensitivity	58	79	79
Specificity	40	99	99
Positive predictive value	27	97	97
Negative predictive value	72	93	93

Data from Sobol S, Marchand J, Tewfik T. Orbital complications of sinusitis in children. J Otolaryngol 2002;31:131–6.

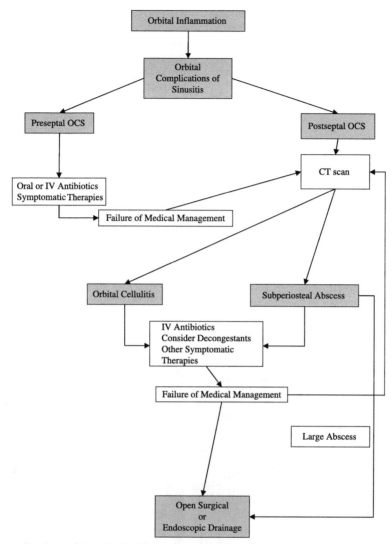

Fig. 4. Orbital complications of sinusitis (OCS) management algorithm. IV, intravenous. (*Modified from* Sobol S, Marchand J, Tewfik T. Orbital complications of sinusitis in children. J Otolaryngol 2002;31:135; with permission.)

Fungal-associated sinusitis that extends to the orbit is uncommon in children. Patients are often systemically ill and supportive treatments must be initiated, therefore pediatric infectious disease consultation is recommended. Antifungal therapy is initiated with intravenous amphotericin B. Orbital extension or erosive cases require surgical treatment, especially in the mucormycosis subset.[9] Overall prognosis in fungal-associated cases is poor, particularly in the immunocompromised patient.[22]

Adjunctive Therapy

Systemic or nasal-specific decongestants, warm compresses, and head-of-bed elevation along with generalized supportive care can be effective in improving patient comfort and facilitating recovery. Continuing with nasal hygiene management, like nasal saline lavage and immunotherapy, is important in speeding recovery and maintaining prophylaxis.

Surgery

Huang and colleagues[23] showed, in their 11-year study of sinus-related orbital infections, a nearly 6% surgical conversion rate. Indications for surgery exist in both absolute and relative categories:

Relative indications for surgery[7]

- No improvement or worsening is noted within 24 to 48 hours

- The patient is older than 9 years of age (more complex microbial forms of infection with increasing age)
- Immunocompromised patients
- Small subperiosteal abscess.

Surgery may then be warranted to enhance the therapy even if no significant abscess collection is delineated.

Absolute indications for surgery[7,18]

- Ophthalmoplegia
- Visual acuity loss
- Frontal sinusitis (Pott puffy tumor in frontal osteitis)
- Large subperiosteal abscess
- Frank orbital abscess
- Intracranial complications.

Such findings require immediate surgical intervention.

Long-standing sinusitis or previous penetrating trauma to the sinuses and orbit may initiate a chronic sinusitis condition that may later progress to acute infection with orbital perforation and abscess formation. **Fig. 5** shows a 16-year-old boy who had sustained penetrating trauma to the left maxillary sinus 2 years previously. Chronic sinusitis evolved to an acute condition with ultimate orbital cellulitis, orbital abscess, and ascending spread intracranially. Treatment consisted of multiple sinusotomies with sinus lavage, orbital drainage, and high-dose, broad-spectrum intravenous antibiotics. Long-term surveillance is necessary to ensure that sinus health and drainage are maintained.

CONTROVERSY

Controversy exists regarding the need for surgical treatment of subperiosteal abscess collections in patients with orbital cellulitis.[20,22] The orbital septum is thought to be a strong barrier to infectious spread and some have advocated intravenous antibiotics alone. However, a significant

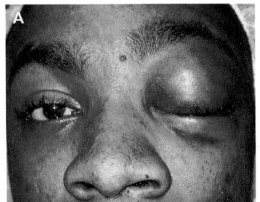
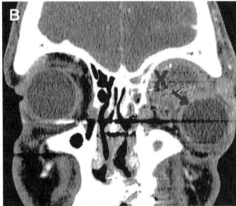
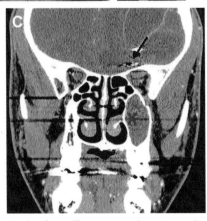

Fig. 5. A 16-year-old boy who had sustained maxillary trauma 2 years previously, now with evolving sinusitis and orbital and intracranial extension. (*A*) Left orbital cellulitis and abscess formation with proptosis. (*B*) Coronal CT with evidence of abscess and phlegmon formation (X) and globe displacement (*arrow*) inferiorly. (*C*) Coronal CT with evidence of sinusitis (X) and intracranial spread with gas formation (*arrow*).

complication rate of up to 20% was noted by Vairaktaris and colleagues,[20] and surgical principles support incision and drainage for definitive treatment in addition to systemic antibiotics. In addition, some think that the most important factor predicting the failure of antibiotic treatment is the presence of an abscess.[19,21,23] More specifically, Todman and colleagues,[18] in a 2011 investigation, suggested that the volume of a particular subperiosteal abscess is the most important criterion regarding the need for surgery. Volumes of less than 1.25 cm^3 did not require surgery, whereas those more than 1.25 cm^3 universally needed surgery and also were associated with more complications.

TECHNIQUE

Sinus surgery with traditional maxillofacial surgical or endoscopic (functional endoscopic sinus surgery [FESS]) approaches, can eradicate the abscess and improve sinus health and drainage patterns. Because most orbital abscesses initiate from the ethmoids, FESS procedures are generally performed to deroof and open infected air cells as well as to drain the abscess.[21] Concurrent sinus lavage during and after surgery may be required. Specific surgical technique is determined by the abscess site and the involved paranasal sinuses. Senior and colleagues[24] maintained that performing sinus surgery in children is safe, with minimal long-term impact on facial growth of the developing child. This view may further support or suggest a role for early surgical intervention in patients with orbital cellulitis as a result of sinonasal disease.

SUMMARY

Sinonasal disease is common in the pediatric population because of anatomic, environmental, and physiologic factors. Once paranasal sinusitis develops, orbital cellulitis is a concerning sequela that can result in loss of visual acuity and even intracranial disease. Thus, a clear history and physical examination in conjunction with radiographic studies are critical to a correct diagnosis and timely institution of treatment that may include hospitalization, serial ophthalmologic examinations, intravenous antibiotics, and surgery. The serious nature of orbital cellulitis in children cannot be overestimated but, if prompt and appropriate treatment is initiated, the prognosis is excellent and long-term sequelae should be limited.

REFERENCES

1. Hong E, Allen R. Orbital cellulitis in a child. Available at: http://www.EyeRounds.org/cases/103-Pediatric-Orbital-Celulitis.htm. 2010;1–8. Accessed January 12, 2010.

2. Rudnick E, Mitchell R. Long-term improvements in quality-of-life after surgical therapy for pediatric sinonasal disease. Otolaryngol Head Neck Surg 2007;137:873–7.

3. El-Sayed Y. Orbital involvement in sinonasal disease. Saudi J Ophthalmol 1995;9:29–37.

4. Teele D. Management of the child with a red, swollen eye. Pediatr Infect Dis J 1983;2:258–62.

5. Goodyear P, Firth A, Strachan D, et al. Periorbital swelling: the important distinction between allergy and infection. Emerg Med J 2004;21:240–2.

6. Nageswaran S, Woods C, Benjamin D, et al. Orbital cellulitis in children. Pediatr Infect Dis J 2006;25: 695–9.

7. Harris G. Subperiosteal abscess of the orbit: age as a factor in the bacteriology and response to treatment. Ophthalmology 1994;101:585–95.

8. Uzcategui N, Warman R, Smith A, et al. Clinical practice guidelines for the management of orbital cellulitis. J Pediatr Ophthalmol Strabismus 1998;35: 73–9.

9. Jain A, Rubin P. Orbital cellulitis in children. Int Ophthalmol Clin 2001;41:71–86.

10. Hubert L. Orbital infections due to nasal sinusitis. NY State J Med 1937;37:1559–64.

11. Chandler J, Langenbrunner D, Stevens E. The pathogenesis of orbital complications in acute sinusitis. Laryngoscope 1970;80:1414.

12. Clarke W. Periorbital and orbital cellulitis in children. Paediatr Child Health 2004;9:471–2.

13. Barone S, Aiuto L. Periorbital and orbital cellulitis in the *Haemophilus influenzae* vaccine era. J Pediatr Ophthalmol Strabismus 1997;34:293–6.

14. Steinkuller P, Jones D. Microbial preseptal and orbital cellulitis. In: Tasman W, editor. Foundations of clinical ophthalmology. Philadelphia (PA): Lippincott; 1999. p. 1–8, 17–29. Chapter 25.

15. Weiss A, Friendly D, Eglin K, et al. Bacterial periorbital and orbital cellulitis in childhood. Ophthalmology 1983;90:195.

16. Eustis H, Armstrong D, Buncic J, et al. Staging of orbital cellulitis in children: computerized tomography characteristics and treatment guidelines. J Pediatr Ophthalmol Strabismus 1986;23:246–51.

17. Tole DM, Anderton LC, Hayward JM. Orbital cellulitis demands early recognition, urgent admission and aggressive management. J Accid Emerg Med 1995;12:151–3.

18. Todman M, Enzer Y. Medical management versus surgical intervention of pediatric orbital cellulitis: the importance of subperiosteal abscess volume as a new criterion. Ophthal Plast Reconstr Surg 2011;27:255–9.

19. Sobol S, Marchand J, Tewfik T. Orbital complications of sinusitis in children. J Otolaryngol 2002;31:131–6.

20. Vairaktaris E, Moschos M, Vassiliou S, et al. Orbital cellulitis, orbital subperiosteal and intraorbital abscess. Report of three cases and review of the literature. J Craniomaxillofac Surg 2009;37:132–6.

21. Brook I. Acute and chronic bacterial sinusitis. Infect Dis Clin North Am 2007;21(2):427–48.

22. Georgakopoulos C, Eliopoulou M, Stasinos S, et al. Periorbital and orbital cellulitis: a 10-year review of hospitalized children. Eur J Ophthalmol 2010;6: 1066–72.

23. Huang S, Lee T, Lee Y, et al. Acute rhinosinusitis-related orbital infection in pediatric patients: a retrospective analysis. Ann Otol Rhinol Laryngol 2011;120:185–90.

24. Senior B, Wirtschafter A, Mai C, et al. Quantitative impact of pediatric sinus surgery on facial growth. Laryngoscope 2000;110:1866–70.

Facial Dermatologic Lesions in Children

Joli C. Chou, DMD, MD, FRCD(C)[a],*,
Bruce B. Horswell, MD, DDS, MS[b]

KEYWORDS

• Dermatologic • Pediatric • Facial

KEY POINTS

• Skin lesions of the face and neck are common in the pediatric population; however, most of these lesions are benign.
• Infectious and inflammatory lesions are the most common dermatologic conditions seen in children are primarily treated nonsurgically.
• Epidermal inclusion cyst, dermoid cyst, and pilomatricoma require surgical excision.
• Surgical excision of melanotic lesions may be required because of risk of dysplasia and the increasing rate of melanoma in children.

Skin lesions of the face and neck are common in the pediatric population. However, most of these lesions are benign. Recognition and identification of the more common skin lesions allows for timely treatment and detailed and thoughtful discussion of the necessary treatment with the child's parents. The cause, presentation, and treatment of the more common benign cutaneous lesions in the maxillofacial region in children are reviewed in this article.

INFECTIOUS LESIONS
Molluscum Contagiosum

Molluscum contagiosum is a viral infection of the skin caused by a human-specific poxvirus that induces epidermal cell proliferation. Infection is the result of contact with affected people and common in young children (ages 2–5) who bathe or swim together.[1] The infection is highly contagious and, as long as there are lesions, the virus can be spread. The incubation period ranges from 2 weeks to 6 months.[2] Children with atopic dermatitis or who are immune-compromised may have more severe presentations with associated dermatitis and masses of lesions (**Fig. 1**).[3]

The lesions are commonly found on the face, trunk or flexor surfaces and appear as dome-shaped, pearly or flesh-colored papules with central umbilication. The size of the lesions may vary from 1 mm to 1 cm. Lesions in the face are randomly distributed but are more commonly seen on eyelids and around the mouth.[4] Clusters of lesions that persist over years should alert the clinician to possible immune deficiency.

Molluscum contagiosum is a self-limiting infection and the lesions typically resolve spontaneously in 6 to 9 months but can persist up to 3 years.[2] Once diagnosis is confirmed with biopsy, watchful waiting may be an acceptable option. Skin hygiene, appropriate barrier use, and hand washing is important for children and families to

The authors have nothing to disclose.

[a] Department of Oral and Maxillofacial Surgery and Pharmacology, University of Pennsylvania School of Dental Medicine, Schattner Building, 240 South, 40th Street, Philadelphia, PA 19104, USA; [b] First Appalachian Craniofacial Deformity Specialists, Women and Children's Hospital, Charleston Area Medical Center, Suite 302, 830 Pennsylvania Avenue, Charleston, WV 25302, USA

* Corresponding author. 5 White, Department of Oral and Maxillofacial Surgery, Hospital of University of Pennsylvania, 3400 Spruce Street, Philadelphia, PA 19104.
E-mail address: jolichou@netscape.net

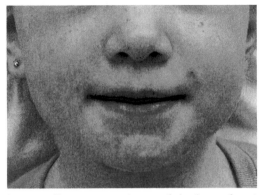

Fig. 1. Molluscum contagiosum of the lower face in a young girl.

implement. Treatments include curettage or cryotherapy but this may result in depressed scars. Topical treatment with 5% imiquimod, an immunomodulator, and cantharidin, a vesicant, have also been used but have not been thoroughly studied for use on the face.[5,6]

Warts

Warts are caused by the human papillomavirus (HPV), usually HPV 2 (a-e) 3a, 4, and 10a,b subtypes. HPV infects the stratified squamous epithelium which stimulates benign keratinocyte proliferation. Hence, warts can be found in any area of the body with stratified squamous epithelium. Although the prevalence of this lesion peaks in adolescence, it is not uncommon in childhood with 5% of children affected by age 10.[7] Warts are spread by direct or indirect contact and the incubation period varies from a few weeks to 2 years.[4]

Although there are several types of warts (common, plantar, mosaic, and planar or flat), the most prevalent in the head and neck area are the common and planar wart. On the face, warts are found most commonly on the cheek, nose, and lips.[4] Common warts (verruca vulgaris) present as smooth flesh-colored papules with a hyperkeratotic surface of grossly thickened keratin and often occur at sites with impairment of normal skin barrier function. Planar warts are flat-topped papules found generally on the face, arms, and legs. Warts can range from 1 mm to several millimeters in size, singly or in clusters.

In healthy children, most warts resolve within 2 to 4 years without treatment and two-thirds of lesions disappear earlier.[4,7] Multiple warty growths can be unsightly and more prone to irritation and discomfort; therefore, most children and parents seek treatment. Salicylic acid products available over the counter or higher-concentration formulations by prescription are the only treatment that has been proven to be effective. Although effective, caution must be taken when salicylic acid is used for the treatment of facial warts because of the risk of scarring. Cryotherapy has a proven track record in removing most common warts. Pulsed dye laser and photodynamic therapy with 5-aminolaevulinic acid seems to provide cosmetic results for facial lesions (**Fig. 2**).[8]

Tinea

Tinea is a fungal infection caused by dermatophytic fungi that invade the stratum corneum,

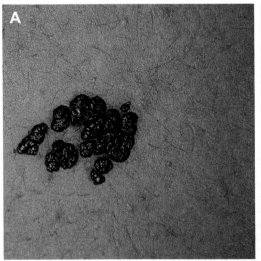
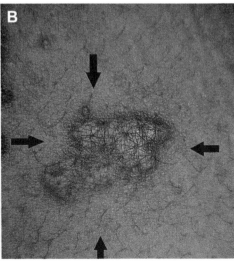

Fig. 2. (A) Common warts of the cheek. (B) Arrows point to the same area of involvement after pulsed dye laser treatment.

hair shaft, and nail beds. In the scalp, tinea capitis, the two most implicated fungal organisms are *Trichophyton tonsurans* (95% of tinea capitis) and *Microsporum canis*. Facial lesions, tinea corporis, are caused by a variety of fungal organisms and tinea faciei is most commonly caused by *M canis*.[9] Tinea is contracted from spores in soil, open lesions in other children, or from animals, typically pets or farm animals. Once inoculated, lesions generally develop within 1 to 3 weeks after contact with the spores or hyphae.[4]

Tinea capitis typically has a noninflammatory phase of 2 to 8 weeks followed by an inflammatory stage with itching, scaly erythematous lesions, and loss of hair. Infection from *T tonsurans* may be slightly delayed in onset and may mimic seborrheic dermatitis in pattern with some open lesions and pustular areas of alopecia.[9] Prolonged and untreated tinea capitis may lead to an intense inflammatory response with boggy, nodular, pustular lesions (kerion), scarring, and hair follicle necrosis.[9]

When found on the face, tinea lesions may present as single or multiple round scaly macules (**Figs. 3** and **4**). The lesions have a typical erythematous, raised border with central pallor or diminished pigmentation. Some children will manifest a butterfly-like pattern around the perinasal area, reminiscent of lupus. These lesions are variably pruritic and may be hypopigmented or hyperpigmented. Diagnosis is made by positive Wood lamp fluorescence of infected hair shafts, microscopic identification of hyphae and spores on hair shaft, or a scale sample taken from the edge of the lesion prepared with potassium hydroxide. Confirmation of the fungal organism is by culture that may take several weeks to manifest.

Topical 2% miconazole, 1% clotrimazole, imidazole, ciclopiroloxamine, or benzylamine are first-line treatments for tinea. Treatment takes up to 4 weeks and, in some forms, may take months to achieve eradication. Oral therapy with ketoconazole, itraconazole, terbinafine, or griseofulvin is reserved for widespread infection or tinea capitis or those resistant to topical treatment.[8] Widespread disease or persistence despite oral therapy should prompt the clinician to consider immunosuppression.

Impetigo

Impetigo is a superficial pyoderma caused by *Staphylococcus aureus* or *Streptococcus pyogenes*. It is the most common bacterial skin infection in children and the third most common skin disease in children with a peak incidence at 2 to 6 years of age.[10] Infections are the result of direct contact with lesions and are more common in children with atopic dermatitis, poor skin hygiene, and in cramped and humid living conditions.

Impetigo presents in two forms—bullous or nonbullous impetigo (contagiosum), which is the most common form of impetigo. Lesions initially present as vesicles or pustules then progress into gold-crusted plaques (**Fig. 5**). Impetigo is common in the face and extremities and heals without scarring. Bullous impetigo is caused by an epidermolytic toxin produced by *S aureus* and presents initially as flaccid blisters or vesicles often grouped in the oronasal area. Bullous impetigo is usually associated with fever and malaise. Culture of the exudate confirms the diagnosis.

In mild cases of impetigo, topical mupirocin ointment applied three times daily up to 10 days is usually effective. For systemic illness or in nonresponsive cases, antibiotics should be instituted once sensitivities have returned from the culture.[11] Excellent skin hygiene and strict hand washing protocols should be reviewed with the child and family during treatment to prevent self-inoculation or spread to family members. Generally, household members should be evaluated with nasal swabbing to rule out chronic carriers of *S aureus* (methicillin-resistant *S aureus* [MRSA] organisms).

ACNE VULGARIS

Acne vulgaris is most commonly seen in adolescence but it can also be found in neonates, infants, or young children.[12] Acne vulgaris is characterized by hyperkeratosis of the follicular epithelium with or without inflammation.[13] Several factors have been implicated: hyperkeratosis of the follicular epithelium, increased sebum production and excretion, and stimulation by androgens. In the neonate, maternal androgens are transferred via the placenta.[14] In addition, the neonatal adrenal gland consists of an enlarged zona reticularis, the

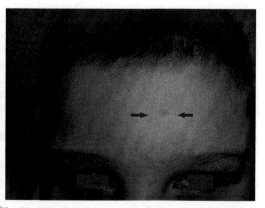

Fig. 3. Arrows point to tinea corporis in the forehead of a child.

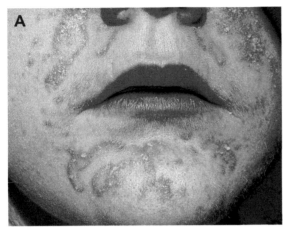
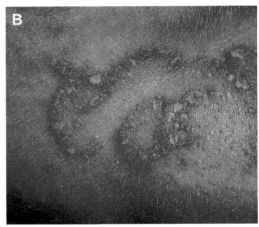

Fig. 4. (*A*) Tinea faciei in a fourteen year old girl. (*B*) Tinea faciei close-up.

androgen-producing zone, producing high levels of dehydroepiandrosterone (DHEA).[15] Neonatal acne may overlap with milia, a condition affecting the sebaceous glands as well. However, in acne the papules are red whereas milia is composed of small, white bumps (plugged glands) with little inflammatory component.[15,16] The differential diagnosis may include neonatal cephalic pustulosis, erythema toxicum neonatorum, transient neonatal pustular melanosis, milia, and miliaria.[15]

Increased levels of DHEA persist until around 1 year of age and may stimulate sebaceous glands. Also, during the first year of life, boys may have an early pubertal level of luteinizing hormone and testosterone that may stimulate the sebaceous glands, accounting for the higher incidence of neonatal acne in boys.[12] Infants and children up to the age of 7 are rarely affected by acne.[4] If severe acne persists despite treatment, then hyperandrogenism or oral-facial-digital syndrome, type I should be excluded.[15]

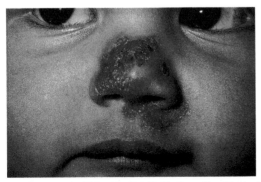

Fig. 5. Impetigo. (*From* Bacterial infections (pyodermas) and spirochetal infections of the skin. In: Weston WL, Lane AT, Morelli JG, editors. Textbook of pediatric dermatology. Philadelphia: Mosby, Elsevier; 2007.)

Similarly, in prepubertal children the increased level of DHEA during adrenarche may reactivate the sebaceous glands. In adolescence, genetics and *Propionibacterium acnes* are also implicated as key factors in the development of acne vulgaris. The predilection for follicular epidermal hyperproliferation in adolescence is inherited as an autosomal dominant pattern with variable penetrance.[13] *P acnes* is an anaerobe that will flourish deep in the sebaceous plug, resulting in an inflammatory response. Further propagation results in the more serious forms of acne in Grades III and IV (see later discussion). Aggravating factors that may augment acne formation include: cosmetic agents, steroids, lithium, some antiepileptics, congenital adrenal hyperplasia, polycystic ovary syndrome, and mechanical occlusion with headbands, shoulder pads, and constrictive clothing.[13] The differential diagnosis includes seborrheic dermatitis, keratosis pilaris, and rosacea. Up to 71% of premenarchal girls have been reported to be affected by acne. Most Americans are affected by acne at some time in their lives.[13]

Clinically, acne may present with closed comedones (whitehead) then progress to open comedones (blackheads), which may be precursors of papules and pustules (raised bumps with inflammation) (**Fig. 6**). Severity of the acne (Grades I–IV) depends on the ratio of comedones and inflammatory lesions present. The more papules and pustules present the more severe the acne and higher the grade (**Fig. 7**).[13] Grade IV or cystic acne (**Fig. 8**) is very difficult to manage and will result in scarring to some degree.

Neonatal acne may be treated with daily cleansing with a mild soap and water; it is usually mild and transient and resolves without scarring in 4 to 12 weeks.[15] Severe or persistent forms of infantile acne vulgaris is treated medically with

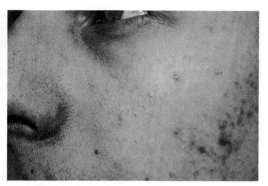

Fig. 6. Grade I to II acne with open and closed comedones.

topical or systemic agents after ruling out hyperandrogenesis.[16,17] Topical agents, including retinoids (adapalene, tazarotene, tretinoin), benzoyl peroxide, and topical antibiotics such as erythromycin or clindamycin, may adequately treat mild cases.[13,15]

Adolescent forms of acne vulgaris are treated according to the grade designation. Grades I and II are generally treated with over-the-counter products and benzoyl peroxide–containing agents with or without an antibiotic. It is better to use benzoyl peroxide and an antibiotic together (topical or oral) because this will kill all *P acne* and prevent

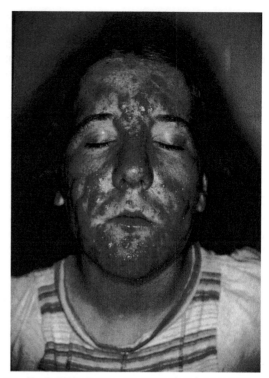

Fig. 8. Nodular cystic acne. (*From* Bacterial infections (pyodermas) and spirochetal infections of the skin. In: Weston WL, Lane AT, Morelli JG, editors. Textbook of pediatric dermatology. Philadelphia: Mosby, Elsevier; 2007.)

resistant forms.[18] Persistent infectious (pustules) lesions require systemic antibiotics for a longer period of time. Weaning onto a topical agent, such as clindamycin or erythromycin, will generally keep infection from recurring.[17,18]

For Grades II and III, a topical retinoid can be added to the regimen. Retinoids reduce the follicular hyperkeratinization, help to restore epithelial health and turnover, reduce the numbers of comedones, and are antiinflammatory.[15,17,19] The topical retinoids available for use are adapalene, tazarotene, and tretinoin. They are applied once daily to clean, dry skin. Generally it is better to begin at lower dosages until a response is obtained, which may take several weeks.[13,15] The patient should be informed of drying and irritation, which can be controlled with a water-based (noncomedogenic) moisturizer. Both benzoyl peroxide and topical antibiotics can be used in conjunction with a topical retinoid, but excessive drying may result and many teens will not wish to continue such a rigorous regimen.[15,18]

For severe pustular acne, systemic agents such as oral antibiotics (minocycline, doxycycline, sulfamethoxazole-trimethoprim), oral contraceptives, spironolactone, and isotretinoin may be used. If

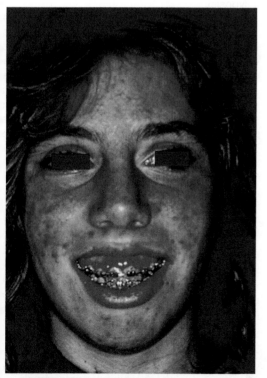

Fig. 7. Grade II to III with inflammatory acne with papulopustules.

pustular lesions persist despite first-line antibiotics with minocycline or doxycycline, the presence of resistant organisms like *S aureus* (MRSA) should be considered and the pustules cultured. Oral tetracyclines are not recommended in children younger than 8 years of age and should be cautiously prescribed to females of child-bearing age because of staining of the fetal dentition. Spironolactone reduces the androgen production by binding to androgen receptors; therefore, pregnancy must be avoided during its use owing to the risk of feminization of the male fetus.

Oral isotretinoin is a highly effective systemic retinoid that is reserved for severe, recalcitrant cases of pustular and cystic acne vulgaris.[17] Isotretinoin normalizes the epidermal differentiation, reduces sebum production, is antiinflammatory and may reduce bacterial colonization of plugged pores.[19,20] It is not recommended for children younger than 12 years of age and its use must be carefully weighed against the reported side effects of depression and potential hepatotoxicity.[15] Baseline laboratory data and suicide or depression screens should be obtained before beginning isotretinoin therapy and repeated periodically. Isotretinoin is a teratogen, so pregnancy must be avoided. Contraceptive counseling and two negative pregnancy test results are required by the US Food and Drug Administration for females of childbearing age before the initiation of oral isotretinoin

therapy. All individuals prescribing, dispensing, or taking isotretinoin are required to register with the US Food and Drug Administration. Finally, patients taking isotretinoin are at risk for abnormal cutaneous healing. Elective invasive procedures of the skin, such as dermabrasion or scar revision, should be deferred for at least 1 year after cessation of the drug.[13]

EPIDERMAL INCLUSION CYST

Epidermal inclusion cysts (formerly referred to as sebaceous cysts) are cysts of skin lined with keratinizing squamous epithelium and filled with keratin debris. These cysts form as a result of traumatic implantation of epithelium into the dermis, trauma or irritation of the pilosebaceous unit, or by embryonic inclusion.

Epidermal inclusion cysts more commonly present in adolescence and adults and less often in infants and children. It usually presents as an asymptomatic solitary mobile smooth intradermal swelling (**Fig. 9**).[21] Episodes of infection or inflammation can occur, often prompting medical attention. Differential diagnosis, depending on location, may include dermoid cyst, branchial cyst, lipoma, and nonspecific lymph node enlargement. Multiple cysts should prompt investigation to rule out Gardner syndrome (multiple cysts, osteomas, colonic polyposis).

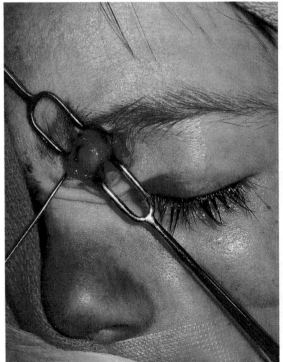
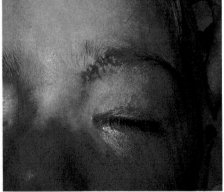
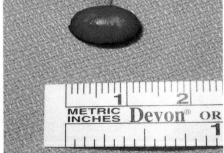

Fig. 9. Periorbital epidermoid cyst and surgical excision of cyst.

Treatment of epidermal inclusion cyst is surgical excision during a noninfected or noninflammatory stage. Inclusion of the overlying epidermis in the cystic specimen includes the offending pilosebaceous unit as well as provides for skin closure with a thicker and more easily approximated epidermis.[22] Should cystic contents spill into the wound, vigorous irrigation should follow to ensure removal of the keratinous material and attendant inflammatory response, which may compromise the cosmetic result.

DERMOID CYST

Dermoid cysts are benign neoplasms of ectodermal and mesodermal origin. In the head and neck area, dermoids form along the lines of embryologic fusion and contain both dermal and epidermal derivatives such as keratinizing squamous epithelium, hair follicles, smooth muscle, sweat and sebaceous glands, and fibroadipose tissue.[23]

Dermoid cysts are present at birth. They are slow growing but become evident in early childhood. Approximately 7% of all dermoid cysts are in the head and neck area.[23] The most common locations in the head and neck are periorbital and nasal (**Fig. 10**). In the nasal region, the cyst can present as a midline lesion, along the dorsum from the glabella to the tip, or at the columellar base. Intraorbital, intracranial, and intranasal dermoids may cause a mass effect with associated symptoms of pain, double vision, obstruction, and so forth if they are allowed to grow or become secondarily infected.[24] Clinically, the lesion may be mobile or fixed to the periosteum with associated scalloping of the underlying bone (**Fig. 11**).[22] It is important to obtain imaging studies such as CT scan or MRI to determine the full extent of the lesion. Neurosurgical consultation should be obtained when there is intracranial extension. Differential diagnosis of the lesion, depending on location, includes epidermal cyst, meningomyelocele, glioma, hemangioma, branchial cleft cyst, and benign lymphadenopathy.

Treatment of dermoids is complete surgical excision when the child is healthy. Attachment of the cyst wall to periosteum or extension into or through a suture necessitates inclusion of that area in the specimen to ensure eradication. Bony reconstruction may be necessary if associated bone is removed for access or for inclusion as pathologic specimen. Recurrence is rare after complete excision. If tearing of the cyst wall or spillage of cyst contents occurs, then postoperative review and occasional radiographs may be indicated to rule out recurrence even years later.

PILOMATRICOMA

Pilomatricoma, also known as Malherbe calcifying epithelioma, is a benign skin neoplasm arising from the outer root sheath of hair follicles.[25] Approximately 10% of cutaneous lumps in children younger than 16 years of age are pilomatricomas and are the second most common superficial tumors removed in children.[21] Over 50% of pilomatricomas occur in the head and neck area. Most common facial locations are periorbital, lateral cheek, and preauricular areas.[25,26] Pilomatricoma has a female predilection (2:1, female/male ratio) and a bimodal presentation at the first and sixth decade in life.[26] It usually presents as a single lesion. However, multiple lesions can occur and have been associated with Gardner syndrome, myotonic dystrophy, Rubinstein-Taybi syndrome, and Turner syndrome.[3]

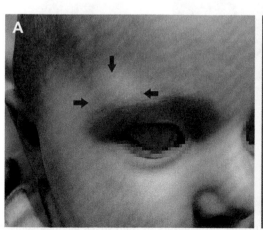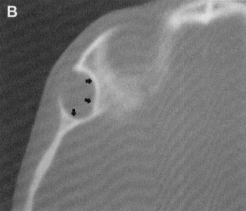

Fig. 10. (*A*) Arrows pointing to a right supraorbital dermoid cyst. (*B*) CT scan (axial) of the right orbital dermoid with arrows showing slight indentation of the underlying bone.

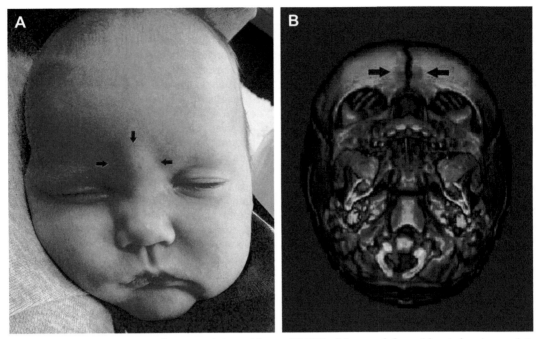

Fig. 11. (*A*) Arrows pointing to a large nasal dermoid cyst. (*B*) MRI of the nasal dermoid cyst showing no intra-cranial extension.

Clinically, pilomatricomas are asymptomatic, rock-hard masses (**Fig. 12**) slightly raised from the skin margin. Often irregularly contoured, they can have a bluish, yellowish, or reddish discoloration or ulceration (**Fig. 13**). The lesions are adherent to the dermis but mobile to the deep dermis or subcutaneous layer of the skin. Diagnosis of pilomatricoma is usually suspected after clinical examination and confirmed with histopathology. However, epidermal inclusion cyst, ossifying hematoma, giant cell tumor, dermoid cyst, chondroma, foreign body reaction, osteochondroma, trichoepithelioma, trichilemmal cyst, and basal cell epithelioma should be considered in the differential diagnosis.[26]

Surgical excision with clear margins is the definitive treatment of pilomatricoma. Adherence to the overlying skin necessitates inclusion with the specimen. Large pilomatricomas may deform or

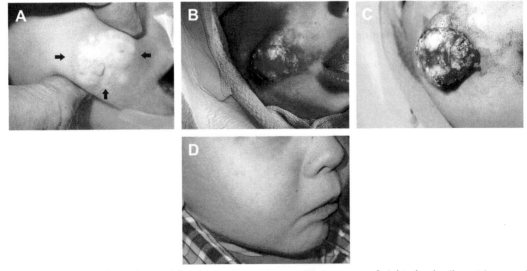

Fig. 12. (*A*) Arrows point to large right-cheek pilomatricoma. (*B*) Exposure of right-cheek pilomatricoma with inclusion of overlying skin. (*C*) Surgical excision of right-cheek pilomatricoma. (*D*) Postoperative (6 months) excision of right-cheek pilomatricoma.

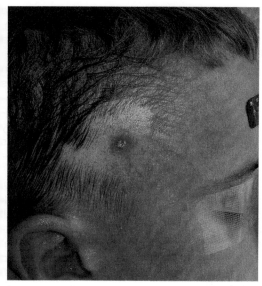

Fig. 13. Irregularly contoured, yellowish pilomatricoma of the right temporal area.

compress the surrounding skin and underlying tissues making removal tedious.[27] Recurrence does not occur if the lesion is completely excised.

MELANOTIC LESIONS
Congenital Melanocytic Nevi

Congenital melanocytic nevi (CMN) are present at birth. They are composed of nevomelanocytes and arise during early embryogenesis from melanocytic stem cells that migrate from the neural crest to the embryonic dermis and upward into the epidermis.[28,29] Although present at birth, not all CMN are apparent at birth because they lack visible pigment; these "tardive" CMN slowly develop pigment over time and become visible (**Fig. 14**).[29]

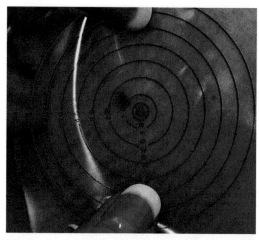

Fig. 15. Small congenital melanocytic nevus of the neck.

CMN are present in 1% to 2% of newborns[28] and usually present as round-to-oval, homogenous or heterogeneous, brown, multishaded pigmented lesions with sharply demarcated borders and thickened surface with coarse terminal hair (**Fig. 15**). Larger lesions may be multicolored with irregular topography and a nodular surface (**Fig. 16**). The color, shade, and surface of the lesion may change as the child grows but the lesion rarely regresses.[29] In general, CMN grow proportionally to the area of the body involved; however, in the craniofacial region it grows slightly faster by a factor of 1.7.[28]

Congenital melanocytic nevi are classified according to size; however, definitions of size vary. The most common definition classifies small nevi as measuring 1.5 cm or less, medium nevi as measuring from 1.5 cm to 19.9 cm, and large nevi as measuring 20 cm or greater (**Fig. 17**). Giant nevi are a subset of large nevi that measure 50 cm or greater.[28]

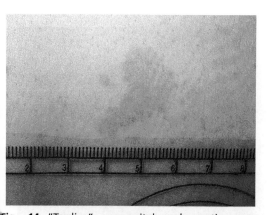

Fig. 14. "Tardive" congenital melanocytic nevus beginning to gain pigmentation.

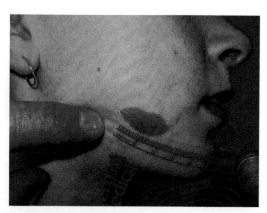

Fig. 16. Medium congenital melanocytic nevus of the face with terminal hair.

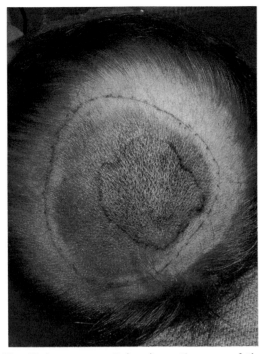

Fig. 17. Large congenital melanocytic nevus of the scalp with heterogeneous pigmentation.

There are several reasons for surgical treatment of CMN. First and foremost is the risk of dysplasia and melanoma developing in the lesion. Second, visibility of the lesion may result in psychological sequelae, especially in children. The precise prevalence rate for melanoma in CMN is not known but it seems to correlate to some degree to the size of the lesion with large CMN the greatest risk for developing melanoma.[29] The estimated lifetime risk of developing melanoma in individuals with large CMN ranges from 4.5% to 10%[29]; therefore, early surgical removal should be considered. The psychological benefit of removal of an unsightly facial CMN in early childhood should be

considered before school age if possible. Large CMN may require staged excision, reconstruction, and at times incorporate tissue expansion and local flap techniques after excision.[28]

Patients with large CMN in the axial distribution are also at risk for neurocutaneous melanocytosis (NCM). In NCM, the leptomeninges contain excessive amounts of melanocytes and melanin. Malignant degeneration of these melanocytes may result in development of primary central nervous system melanomas. Screening MRI should be considered for patients at risk for NCM.[28]

Small and medium congenital melanocytic nevi are more common than the large variety. The risk of developing melanoma associated with small and medium CMN is more controversial. Treatment choices include observation with frequent measurements and recall, laser ablation, and prophylactic excision (which is recommended) (**Fig. 18**).[29]

Spitz Nevi

Spitz nevus is an acquired nevus of childhood seen more frequently in whites. It is composed of large spindle and epithelioid melanocytes in nests or vertical fascicles.[30] Spitz nevi commonly manifest in early childhood with rapid growth with a plateau phase, which may persist for years. It is more frequently reported in white children. The head and neck and lower extremities are the most common sites for these lesions.

Clinically, Spitz nevus may be a rapidly changing red, pink, darkly pigmented brown, black or blue domed-shaped or flat lesion with smooth surface (**Fig. 19**).[31] Because of its color and its varying degree of vascularity, it may be confused with a vascular lesion. Some Spitz nevi undergo rapid growth and change in pigmentation mimicking malignancy. Histologically, Spitz nevi also share common features with melanoma, such as

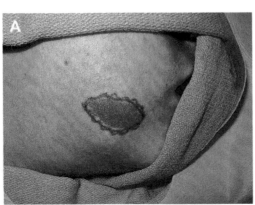
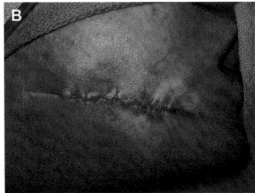

Fig. 18. (*A*) Excision of medium congenital melanocytic nevus with geometric design. (*B*) After excision.

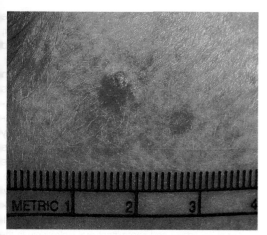

Fig. 19. Spitz nevus (*left*) and small melanocytic nevus.

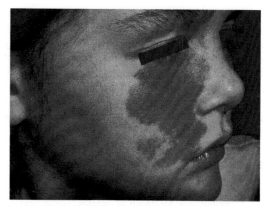

Fig. 20. PWS of the face (right maxillary distribution).

pleomorphism, large nucleoli, dropping off at the basilar level, and so forth. For these reasons, expert dermatopathological examination is required to avoid misdiagnosis.[32]

Clinical similarity between Spitz nevi and malignant melanoma dictates that Spitz nevi should be completely excised. Although these lesions may spontaneously resolve after several months, their clinical behavior pushes a family or clinician to biopsy these nevi. Dysplastic Spitz nevi have been described and should be excised with margins of 0.5 to 1.0 cm.[32]

PORT-WINE STAIN

Vascular lesions are classified either as hemangioma or vascular malformations.[33] These conditions in the pediatric population are discussed in detail in the article on vascular anomalies in children by Drs Abramowicz and Padwa elsewhere in this issue. Capillary malformations or macular stains and port-wine stain (PWS) will be briefly presented here.

Macular stains, a lighter and smaller capillary lesion, occur on the eyelids, glabella or occiput in 46% to 60% of neonates.[33] Eyelid and glabellar macular stains tend to fade over 1 to 2 years and require no treatment. Occipital lesions, termed "stork bites," are more likely to persist than those on the face or glabellar area ("angel bite"). Macular stains darken when the infant cries, reflecting their capillary features.[34]

PWS, sometimes termed nevus flammeus, are capillary malformations with normal endothelium and cellular turnover but abnormal neural and capillary architecture. This has been linked to the RASA 1 gene mutation.[35] Deficient nerve distribution at the capillary level results in persistent vascular dilation

and the intense erythema associated with PWS. This type of lesion is usually present at birth, affects approximately 3 out of 1000 people, and does not involute.[33] These lesions are generally flat and pink with a reticulated pattern that blanches on compression (**Fig. 20**).[33] As a capillary malformation, PWSs are slow flow lesions and rarely result in excessive bleeding.[34] They may ooze generously if violated but this can be controlled with pressure and topical agents. Large, nodular PWS with increased color may extend deeper, connecting to torturous venous channels, in which case ultrasound may be helpful to further delineate the extent and depth of the lesion.[34]

PWSs typically deepen in color and their surfaces become rougher or more nodular with age. Due to their prominence on the face, most children and families will elect for treatment that involves sequential pulsed dye laser (PDL) treatments over several months.[35] In most children this will require general anesthesia or deep sedation. The response is better in lighter PWS and in younger patients. Deeper PWS with varicosities may be treated with sclerotherapy to obtain some lightening of the surface epithelium, which is then treated with PDL as mentioned. This condition usually forms in later childhood or adolescence or because of inadequate or failed PDL.[36,37]

PWSs in the face, especially in the ophthalmic distribution, are associated with Sturge-Weber syndrome in which ipsilateral leptomeningeal and ocular vascular anomalies may be present.[34] These intracranial vascular anomalies may result in seizures, glaucoma, blindness, hemiplegia, and cognitive delays. CT scan or MRI is useful to confirm the extent of the intracranial involvement.

SUMMARY

Benign "lumps and bumps" are very common in children and it is prudent for the pediatric maxillofacial surgeon to be familiar with their presentation, workup (including radiographic studies), and definitive surgical management. Inflammatory and infectious lesions require prompt treatment to avoid more serious sequelae of progressive infection and scarring. For the many other less common lesions not included in this article, judicious consultation with a dermatologist is recommended.

REFERENCES

1. Rogers M, Barneston RS. Diseases of the skin. In: Campbell AG, McIntosh N, editors. Forfar and Arneil's textbook of pediatrics. 5th edition. New York: Churchill Livingstone; 1998. p. 1633–5.

2. Hawley TG. The natural history of molluscum contagiosum in Fijian children. J Hyg 1970;68:631–2.

3. Pauly CR, Artis WM, Jones HE. Atopic dermatitis, impaired cellular immunity, and molluscum contagiosum. Arch Dermatol 1978;114:3.

4. Sahl WJ, Mathewson RJ. Common facial skin lesions in children. Quintessence Int 1993;24:475–81.

5. Sidbury R. What's new in pediatric dermatology: update for the pediatrician. Curr Opin Pediatr 2004;16:410–4.

6. Lio P. Warts, molluscum and things that go bump on the skin: a practical guide. Arch Dis Child Educ Pract Ed 2007;92:ep119–24.

7. Gibbs S, Harvey I, Sterling JC, et al. Local treatments for cutaneous warts. Cochrane Database Syst Rev 2003;3:CD001781.

8. Boull C, Groth D. Update: treatment of cutaneous viral warts in children. Pediatr Dermatol 2011;28(3): 217–29.

9. Fungal and yeast infections of the skin. In: Weston WL, Lane AT, Morelli JG, editors. Textbook of pediatric dermatology. 4th edition. Philadelphia: Mosby Elsevier; 2007. p. 81–96.

10. Dagan R. Impetigo in childhood: changing epidemiology and new treatments. Pediatr Ann 1993;22: 235–40.

11. Sladden MJ, Johnston GA. Common skin infections in children. BMJ 2004;329:95–9.

12. Jansen T, Burgdorf WH, Plewig G. Pathogenesis and treatment of acne in childhood. Pediatr Dermatol 1997;14:17–21.

13. Fulton J Jr. Acne vulgaris. Emedicine. Available at: http://emedicine.medscape.com/article/1069804. Accessed January 4, 2012.

14. Paller AS, Mancini AJ, editors. Disorders of the sebaceous and sweat glands. Hurwitz clinical pediatric dermatology. 3rd edition. Philadelphia: WB Saunders; 2006. p. 195–6.

15. Antoniou C, Dessinoti C, Stratigo AJ, et al. Clinical and therapeutic approaches to childhood acne: an update. Pediatr Dermatol 2009;26:373–80.

16. Nanda S, Reddy BS, Ramji S, et al. Analytical study of pustular eruptions in neonates. Pediatr Dermatol 2002;19:210–5.

17. Yonkosky DM, Pochi PE. Acne vulgaris in childhood: pathogenesis and management. Dermatol Clin 1986;4:127–36.

18. Eady EA, Farmery MR, Ross JI, et al. Effects of benzoyl peroxide and erythromycin alone and in combination against antibiotic-sensitive and -resistant skin bacteria from acne patients. Br J Dermatol 1994;131(3):331–6.

19. Strauss JS, Krowchuk DP, Leyden JJ, et al. Guidelines of care for acne vulgaris management. J Am Acad Dermatol 2007;56(4):651–63.

20. Lee JW, Yoo KH, Park KY, et al. Effectiveness of conventional, low-dose and intermittent oral isotretinoin in the treatment of acne: a randomized, controlled comparative study. Br J Dermatol 2010;164(6):1369–75.

21. Thomson HG. Common benign pediatric cutaneous tumors: timing and treatment. Clin Plast Surg 1990; 17(1):49–64.

22. Suliman MT. Excision of epidermoid (sebaceous) cyst: description of the operative technique. Plast Reconstr Surg 2005;116(7):2042–3.

23. Pryor SG, Lewis JE, Weaver AL, et al. Pediatric dermoid cysts of the head and neck. Otolaryngol Head Neck Surg 2005;132(6):938–42.

24. Ahuja R, Azar NF. Orbital dermoids in children. Semin Ophthalmol 2006;21(3):207–11.

25. Price HN, Zaenglein AL. Diagnosis and management of benign lumps and bumps in childhood. Curr Opin Pediatr 2007;19(4):420–4.

26. Yencha MW. Head and neck pilomatricoma in the pediatric age group: a retrospective study and literature review. Int J Pediatr Otorhinolaryngol 2001; 57(2):123–8.

27. Agarwal RP, Handler SD, Matthews MR, et al. Pilomatrixoma of the head and neck in children. Otolaryngol Head Neck Surg 2001;125:510–5.

28. Bauer BS, Corcoran J. Treatment of large and giant nevi. Clin Plast Surg 2005;32:11–8.

29. Marghoob AA. Congenital melanocytic nevi: evaluation and management. Dermatol Clin 2002;20: 607–16.

30. Roth ME, Grant-Kels JM. Important melanocytic lesions in childhood and adolescence. Pediatr Clin North Am 1991;38(4):791–809.

31. Rhodes AR. Pigmented birthmarks and precursor melanocytic lesions of cutaneous melanoma identifiable in childhood. Pediatr Clin North Am 1983;30(3) 435–63.

32. Murphy ME, Boyer JD, Stashower ME, et al. The surgical management of Spitz nevi. Dermatol Surg 2002;28(11):1065–9 [discussion: 1069].

33. Higuera S, Gordley K, Metry DW, et al. Management of hemangiomas and pediatric vascular malformations. J Craniofac Surg 2006;17(4):783–9.

34. Morelli JG. Vascular disorders. In: Kliegman RM, Behrman RE, Jenson HB, et al, editors. Nelson textbook of pediatrics. 18th edition. Philadelphia: Saunders Elsevier; 2007. p. 2667–74.

35. Eerola I, Boon LM, Mulliken JB, et al. Capillary malformation-arteriovenous malformation, a new clinical and genetic disorder caused by RASA1 mutations. Am J Hum Genet 2003;73(6):1240–9.

36. Faurschou A, Olesen AB, Leonardi Bee J, et al. Lasers or light sources for treating port wine stains. Cochrane Database Syst Rev 2011;11: CD007152.

37. Minkis K, Geronemus RG, Hale EK. Port wine stain progression: a potential consequence of delayed and inadequate treatment? Lasers Surg Med 2009; 41(6):423–6.

Child Maltreatment

Bruce B. Horswell, MD, DDS, MS[a],*, Sharon Istfan, MD[b]

KEYWORDS

- Child maltreatment • Child abuse • Pattern of injury • Mandatory reporting

KEY POINTS

- Abuse of children is generally decreasing in the United States; however, negligence is increasing.
- Craniofacial fractures are uncommon in children younger than 2 years of age and are rare due to falls less than 4 feet.
- Patterns of bruising, particularly the face and ear regions, are hallmarks of physical battering in young children.
- All health professionals are held to a higher standard of surveillance and screening for abuse in children with unexplained or injuries from conflicting causes. Oral and maxillofacial surgeons are mandatory reporters by law for suspected abuse and negligence of children.

INTRODUCTION

Child maltreatment (abuse) is a disturbing component of public health domain and cost because it exerts its influence across many facets of family life, social-cultural concerns, education, and burden to the health care system. Traumatic injury is the leading cause of death in children over 1 year of age in the United States, and child abuse in all of its forms is a significant component of pediatric mortality and morbidity. Since longitudinal records were first kept by the federal government in 1979, there had been a steady increase of reported cases of child abuse until the mid 1990s when reported abuse began to plateau as recorded by medical, social service, and law enforcement officials.[1,2]

Child maltreatment includes several categories all of which overlap in relationship and intensity: physical (violence to a child by the parent or caregiver), verbal or emotional (attacks on the psychological well-being of the child), and sexual (direct and indirect harm visited on the sexual development, psyche, and body of a child).[3] Given the cultural tolerance of violence displayed on so many levels and the change of the family and domestic dynamic, it is not surprising that this has translated into the tragic outcome of abuse visited on children.

EPIDEMIOLOGY AND ECOLOGY OF CHILD MALTREATMENT

Maltreatment of children has been reported at around 1.2 million annually in the United States, of which approximately 303,000 cases are due to physical abuse.[2] The National Center on Child Abuse and Neglect estimated that 37% of abused children will develop a chronic disability or special need that will require ongoing therapy.[3] The heightened awareness of caregivers, medical personnel, and educational institutions about pediatric abuse no doubt led to increased identification and reporting of abuse.[4] Reported maltreatment occurs across all social strata and ethnicities although there are factors that have been identified as leading to increased incidence of abuse: prematurity, teenage mother, poor bonding with caregivers, special needs (learning disability, attention-deficit/hyperactivity disorder, etc), child being perceived as different or "not normal."[5]

[a] FACES, Women and Children's Hospital, CAMC, 830 Pennsylvania, Charleston, WV 25302, USA; [b] WVU Charleston, Child Advocacy Center, Children's Medicine Center, 800 Pennsylvania Avenue, Charleston, WV 25302, USA
* Corresponding author. FACES, Women and Children's Hospital, CAMC, 830 Pennsylvania, Charleston, WV 25302
E-mail address: bruce.horswell@camc.org

Oral Maxillofacial Surg Clin N Am 24 (2012) 511–517
doi:10.1016/j.coms.2012.04.002
1042-3699/12/$ – see front matter © 2012 Elsevier Inc. All rights reserved

DiScala and colleagues[6] reviewed records from the National Pediatric Trauma Registry (1988–1997) and determined that children who were physically maltreated were younger (12.8 months) than those accidentally injured (25.5 months), they were primarily injured by battering (53%), and they were more likely to have a chronic medical condition, such as delayed development or physical anomaly.

Over the last 20 years, the incidence of both physical and sexual abuse of children has steadily declined; however, the incidence of neglect and emotional abuse remains high and slightly increased over the same period (**Fig. 1**).[2,7,8] Recent evidence supports the tendency of certain observed domestic and caregiver characteristics that may contribute to this latter form of abuse and, for some children, lead to direct physical violence.[5] These characteristics include (1) caregiver's anger and uncontrolled disciplinary actions, (2) caregiver's mental illness, (3) children left with abusive baby-sitters, (4) caregiver's use of substances that disinhibit appropriate behavior, and (5) caregiver's own experience of domestic violence.

Neglect is considered an element of abuse.[8–10] It is difficult to adequately address child neglect in all of its forces and spectrum. The complex interactions of child health, caregiver knowledge and skill, socioeconomic status, and domestic and community or cultural environment combine to provide a child's welfare or lack of it.[11] The price everyone pays for the magnitude of child neglect is tragically great and indeterminable.

Negligent care is difficult to define but we recognize it when we see it as health professionals. Neglect ranges from poor parenting to obvious criminal behavior and negligence. Child neglect is basically defined as, "when a child's basic needs are not met, regardless of the circumstances leading to the inadequacy of care."[11] Negligence can be observed in the acute care setting and

outpatient visit in several forms, including obvious unhygienic dress and personal care, exposure of children to an environment of domestic violence and stress, poor living conditions, frequent missed medical appointments, and putting children at obvious risk with activities of great danger. Evidence of chronic dermatologic ailments[12] (open sores, bites or infected bites), rampant dental decay and gum disease,[13] and not using safety devices or precautions during sport or recreation[14] are indications of neglect of a child's well being.

For the maxillofacial surgeon this may present variably as signs of poor oral health, nutritional deficiencies as manifested by poor tissue healing or open skin-mucosal sores, delays in seeking treatment for obvious orofacial pathologic conditions, and so forth. Avoiding prescribed medical care is a frustrating element of some families that have a child with a craniofacial anomaly, cleft lip or palate, severe deformational plagiocephaly with accompanying occipital sores, or a chronic pathologic condition. Often times the child will have missed many appointments that are directed at optimal care during a particular developmental period, compromising the ultimate result of function, aesthetics, and a sense of well being and health for that child. Poverty, high medical costs, transportation issues, low parental health IQ, and even the child's own condition can negatively affect the sequence of obtaining good care.[11] This, sadly, is negligence and must be addressed—first as an expression of support and concern on behalf of the child and later, if clearly there is no affirmative parental or caregiver response, with child protective services and welfare agencies. The first order of business when facing noncompliance with medical treatment is to come alongside the family to inform and clarify treatment goals, inquire as to caregiver resources to comply, and voice support to the parent. These steps in providing care are necessary elements for the well-being of many children who come under the care of the pediatric maxillofacial surgeon.

Although many maxillofacial surgeons may feel that time is a limiting factor in pursuing these signs of neglect and endangerment, the law is clear that certain health practitioners (physicians and dentists are mandated reporters) are held to a higher standard in the care of patients at risk.[13,15,16]

PRESENTATION AND WORKUP

Identifying the injured child is always a highly emotional event for all involved. This is increased if battering is suspected (**Fig. 2**). As in any traumatic event, the ABCs of initial evaluation and treatment are undertaken. When the injured child

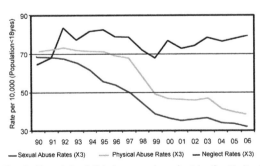

Fig. 1. Trends in child abuse and neglect in the United States, 1990 to 2006. (*Data from* US Department of Health and Human Services. National Center of Child Abuse and Neglect.)

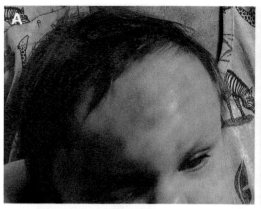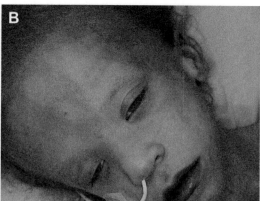

Fig. 2. Children with (*A*) battered heads and (*B*) multiple bruises.

is stable, the diagnostic sieve focuses on the plausibility, type, and pattern of injury. This is when questions addressed by medical personnel (triage nurse, emergency room [ER] physician, consultants) are helpful in corroboration of the details of the mechanism of injury, events, and time and place—all of which need to be carefully recorded. A series of routine questions are helpful in this regard and all involved treating parties should be well practiced in making these inquiries[5,7]:

- How did this injury occur?
- What was the date and time of injury?
- If an there was an inordinate amount of time between injury and care, why was there a delay in seeking treatment?
- Where did it happen?
- Who was with the child and who witnessed the injury?
- What did the child do after injury?
- What did the caregiver do after the injury?
- Has this happened before?
- If the child is verbal (about age 3 years), ask the child directly, "What happened?"

These inquiries in the ER or urgent care setting can be quickly addressed and recorded for future reference, if needed. While these early investigations are underway, several other observations are important in determining whether there is evidence for abuse:

- What is the general appearance of the child?
  - Dirty, unkempt clothes, absence of personal hygiene, foul odor.
- Is the child very withdrawn and avoiding contact with the caregiver or attendant or are they inconsolable?
  - Both of these extremes may point to the caregiver being a perpetrator and the child resisting contact due to fear.

- Is there obvious patterned or odd-shaped bruising?

These days, ER physicians are well versed about this presentation and evaluation of the injured child. When the maxillofacial surgeon is consulted for a facial injury in a child, the diagnostic process may already include appropriate medical and social service experts. The surgeon needs to be aware of this and sensitive to the emotion-laden atmosphere in the ER. This being said, the primary focus of the management team is the well-being of the child. Proper care of injuries along with control of pain and the display of genuine concern and care are very important to the child. Focus on the child is paramount and that must be communicated to the patient as well as family members standing by.

The presentation or posture of the caregiver who is present with the child may insinuate at this point. If the caregiver is also the perpetrator, then he or she may be absent or seem not interested, may be confrontational and resistant to further investigations (skeletal surveys, lab tests), or may threaten the treating personnel.[17] Again, quietly and simply putting forth the best interest of the injured child is necessary and often will defuse intimidating posture.

At this point in the evaluation, if there is suspicion of abuse, the decision tree proceeds to further document other possible injuries. A skeletal survey is helpful in further documenting other injuries. The survey consists of plain radiographs of the extremities, hands, feet, chest, spine, and skull (2–4 views) and it is mandatory for all children with suspected abuse who are younger than 2 years of age (**Fig. 3**). Further, if there is evidence of head bruising and altered mental status, a noncontrast CT scan should be obtained.[18] Older children may have a more symptom and sign-directed radiographic survey unless mental status is prohibitory. CT scan imaging is indicated for acute hemorrhage and

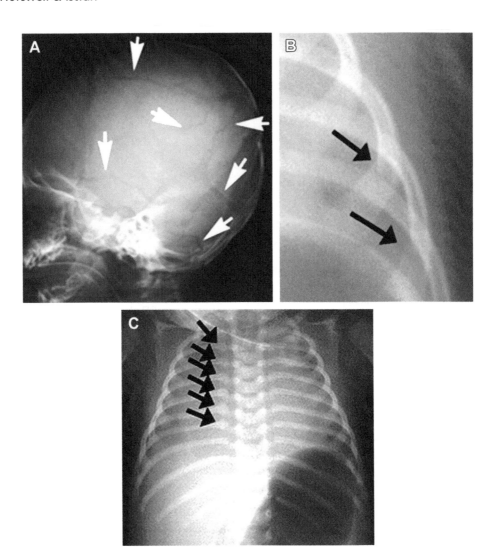

Fig. 3. Skeletal survey. (*A*) Plain skull radiograph showing multiple fractures (*arrows*). (*B*) Chest radiograph with new rib fractures (*arrows*). (*C*) Chest radiograph with old, healed posterior rib fractures (*arrows*).

fractures, whereas MRI is optimal for intraparenchymal hemorrhage, contusions, shearing injuries, and edema.[18]

If the radiographic surveys confirm a pattern of injuries suggestive of abuse, the parent is informed of the findings and the need to manage and protect the child and other children in the family who may be at risk. At this point, an institutionally-based team expert in child maltreatment generally takes over the interface and liaisons with the family while physicians manage care for the injured child.

CRANIOFACIAL INJURIES AND CHILD ABUSE

Craniofacial and neck injuries are noted in more than half of all cases of physical abuse in children.[13,16,19] Because of this, all children presenting to the ER or to the maxillofacial surgeon for care of facial injuries must be evaluated with this

in mind, unless the mechanism of injury is clearly accidental. Bruising around the head (**Fig. 4**), face, and ears in patterns (from a hand or object)

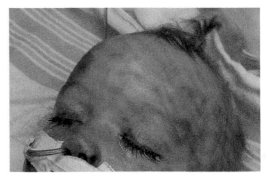

Fig. 4. Comatose infant with severe head battering resulting in traumatic brain injury.

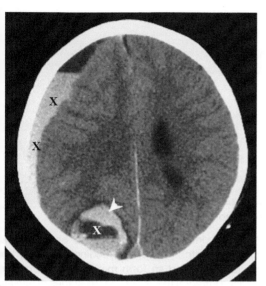

Fig. 5. CT scan demonstrating subdural and intracranial hematomas (*Xes*).

should be investigated with noncontrast CT scan imaging of the head and face.

Patterns of cranial injury in battered children often demonstrate direct blows to the head (point-counterpoint fractures or contusions) mixed with torsional and shearing-type forces (forceful shaking or throwing) evidenced by diffuse intracerebral swelling on imaging.[20,21] This combination of cranial injuries indicate severe and repeated battering and shaking. In the child with inflicted head injury, radiographic imaging will demonstrate more subdural and intraparenchymal hematomas,

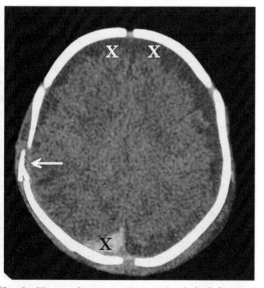

Fig. 6. CT scan demonstrating parietal skull fractures (*arrow*), subdural hematomas (*black X*), and increased extra-axial space (hygroma, *white Xes*) from resolved hematomas after battering.

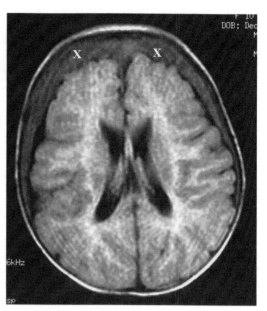

Fig. 7. MRI demonstrating large, persistent hygroma and cerebral atrophy (*Xes*).

often combined (**Fig. 5**), than seen in accidental forms of head injury.[21] Imaging may also show resolving intracerebral effacement, subdural hygroma, cerebral atrophy (**Figs. 6** and **7**), edema, or hematomas.[22] These findings, coupled with retinal hemorrhages (**Fig. 8**) and bruising, are highly associated with the battered child.

In determining the mechanism of injury, it is noteworthy that severe head injury and skull fracture generally do not result from a child "falling out of their high chair" or "falling out of bed" or being "accidentally" dropped; such injuries take greater force of impact.[23,24] In fact, Chadwick and colleagues[25] determined that it is extremely uncommon for low-height falls (<1.5 m) to result

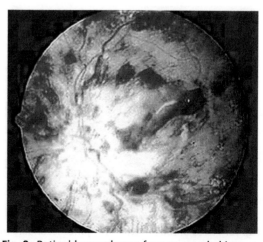

Fig. 8. Retinal hemorrhages from severe shaking.

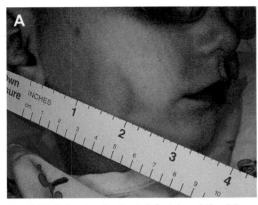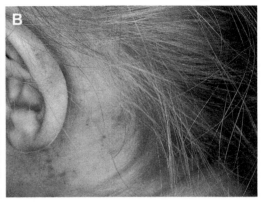

Fig. 9. Multiple bruises in the (*A*) facial and the (*B*) ear and mastoid regions.

in severe injuries in children younger than 2 years of age. This is the age when many abusive injuries that are reported as low-height falls take place. Another distinguishing feature of inflicted skull fractures is that the injury is often accompanied by intracranial extent of injury (cerebral contusion, hematoma) even though this is less common in accidental injuries.[22–25] Further inquiry should be made if this is the event relayed by the parent or caregiver.

Facial fracture patterns are not dissimilar in both inflicted and accidental mechanisms of injury; however, as in cranial fractures, the presence of old and new fractures would indicate an abusive cause. Also, facial fractures purportedly resulting from a young child running, tripping, and falling down do not fit the mechanism of injury; therefore, more inquiry must be made. Isolated facial contusions and dentoalveolar injuries are more likely accidental forms of injury.[26] Ear bruises, particularly bilateral bruises, are unusual in accidents but found more often in battering (**Fig. 9**).[26,27] Repeated abuse will generally result in injuries around the orofacial region with evidence of old and new lip injuries

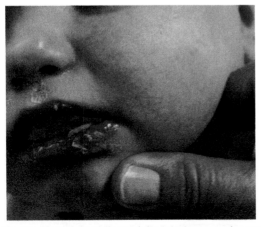

Fig. 10. Photo of toddler with lip injuries secondary to slapping.

(**Fig. 10**), intraoral lacerations and bruising, and chipped teeth.[13,16] Forced feeding, gagging, hot liquid burns, and so forth may result in torn and bruised intraoral tissues of various stages of healing and should be duly noted—particularly a torn labial frenum in a nonambulatory child.[13,16,26] If the child with suspect orofacial injuries has been seen by a dentist previously, obtaining past history, examination results, and radiographs is important in making a more clear evaluation of current status and possible cause of injury. Denial of access to records by the parent may indicate a desire to hide evidence or obstruct inquiry.[26,27]

SUMMARY

Oral and maxillofacial surgeons are in a unique position to identify and report child abuse because many children are seen for a number of dentoalveolar and orofacial conditions managed by surgeons. In the career of any practitioner, maltreated children (both physically abused and neglected) will present to the oral and maxillofacial surgeon for management of injuries and infections. Many such conditions will be ignored or missed, unfortunately, unless there is a high level of vigilance for and understanding of mechanisms of injury and skill in sorting out inflicted injuries or evidence of neglect. Because of this, the medical community, society, state law, and the legal system place oral and maxillofacial surgeons in a position of expertise and accountability in the care of children.

Contemporary OMF practice must include the ability to recognize inflicted injuries in children through an informed understanding of injury mechanism, presentation and pattern, and identify possible negligence of health and well being of a child. Proper and careful referral to protective services and to follow up on such cases is important when children are thought to be at risk of maltreated.

REFERENCES

1. Sedlak AJ. A history of the National Incidence Study of Child Abuse and Neglect. Child welfare information gateway, vol. 3. Children's Bureau, USDHHS; 2001. Available at: www.info@childwelfare.gov. Accessed January 17, 2012.

2. Fourth National Incidence Study of Child Abuse and Neglect (NIS-4; 2004-2009 Report). USDHHS 2010. Available at: http://www.acf.hhs.gov/programs/opre/abuse_neglect/nat_incid/index. Accessed February 15, 2012.

3. National Center on Child Abuse, Neglect. NCCAN data system, vol. 2. Washington, DC: Government Printing Office; 1991.

4. Prevent Child Abuse America. National child maltreatment statistics. National Center of Child Abuse Prevention Research. USDHHS, Department of Children, Youth and Families. Available at: http://member.preventchildabuse.org/site/child. Accessed January 18, 2012.

5. Giardino AP, Hudson KM, Marsh J. Providing medical evaluations for possible child maltreatment to children with special health care needs. Child Abuse Negl 2003;27(10):1179–86.

6. DiScala C, Sege R, Li G, et al. Child abuse and unintentional injuries. Pediatr Adolesc Med 2001;154:16–22.

7. Garbarino J. The human ecology of child maltreatment: a conceptual model for research. J Marriage Fam 1977;39:721–7.

8. Berger RP, Fromkin JB, Stutz H, et al. Abusive head trauma during a time of increased unemployment. Pediatrics 2011;128(4):637–43.

9. Gushurst CA. Child abuse: behavioral aspects and other associated problems. Pediatr Clin N Am 2003;50(4):919–38.

10. Helfer RE. The developmental basis of child abuse and neglect; an epidemiological approach. In: Helfer ME, Kempe RS, Krugman RD, editors. The battered child. 5th edition. Chicago: University of Chicago Press; 1997. p. 60–80.

11. Joffe MD. Child neglect and abandonment. In: Giardino AP, Giardino ER, editors. Recognition of child abuse for the mandated reporter. 3rd edition. St Louis (MO): GW Medical Publishing; 2002. p. 39–54.

12. Swerdlin A, Berkowitz C, Craft N. Cutaneous signs of child abuse. J Am Acad Derm 2007;57(3):371–92.

13. Kellogg N. Oral and dental aspects of child abuse and neglect. Pediatrics 2005;116(6):1565–8.

14. Finnoff JT, Laskowski ER, Altman KL, et al. Barriers to bicycle helmet use. Pediatrics 2001; 108(1):e24.

15. Mouden LD, Bross DC. Legal issues affecting dentistry's role in preventing child abuse and neglect. J Am Dent Assoc 1995;126:1173–80.

16. Needleman JL. Orofacial trauma in child abuse: types, prevalence, management, and the denta profession's involvement. Pediatr Dent 1986;8:71–80.

17. Perpetrators in child abuse. Child maltreatment 2010. USDHHS. Administration for children and families. Children's bureau. Available at: http://www.acf.hhs.gov/programs/cb/stats_research/index.html. Accessed February 1, 2012.

18. Sane SM, Section on Radiology, American Academy of Pediatrics. Diagnostic imaging of child abuse. Pediatrics 2000;105(6):1345–8.

19. O'Neill JA Jr, Meacham WF, Griffin JP, et al. Patterns of injury in the battered child syndrome. J Trauma 1973;13:332–9.

20. McNeese MC, Hebeler JR. The abused child: a clinical approach to identification and management. Clin Symp 1977;29(5):1–36.

21. Cox CS. Trauma from child abuse. In: Wesson DE, editor. Pediatric trauma. Pathophysiology, diagnosis and treatment. New York: Taylor and Francis; 2006. p. 73–82.

22. Reece RM, Sege R. Childhood injuries: accidental or inflicted? Arch Pediatr Adolesc Med 2000;154(1): 11–6.

23. Joffe MD, Ludwig S. Stairway injuries in children. Pediatrics 1988;82(3):457–61.

24. Lyons TJ, Oates RK. Falling out of bed: a relatively benign occurrence. Pediatrics 1993;92(1):125–7.

25. Chadwick DL, Chin S, Salerno C, et al. Deaths from falls in children: how far is fatal? J Trauma 1991;31: 1353–5.

26. Donly KJ, Nowak AJ. Maxillofacial, neck and dental lesions of child abuse. In: Reece RM, editor. Child abuse: medical diagnosis and management. Philadelphia: Lea & Febinger; 1994. p. 150–66.

27. Cairns AM, Mok JY, Welbury RR. Injuries to the head, face, mouth and neck in physically abused children in a community setting. Int J Pediatr Dent 2005;15(5):310–8.

Index

Note: Page numbers of article titles are in **boldface** type.

Oral Maxillofacial Surg Clin N Am 24 (2012) 519–524
http://dx.doi.org/10.1016/S1042-3699(12)00102-1
1042-3699/12/$ – see front matter © 2012 Elsevier Inc. All rights reserved

oralmaxsurgery.theclinics.com

Moving?

Make sure your subscription moves with you!

To notify us of your new address, find your **Clinics Account Number** (located on your mailing label above your name), and contact customer service at:

Email: journalscustomerservice-usa@elsevier.com

800-654-2452 (subscribers in the U.S. & Canada)
314-447-8871 (subscribers outside of the U.S. & Canada)

Fax number: 314-447-8029

Elsevier Health Sciences Division
Subscription Customer Service
3251 Riverport Lane
Maryland Heights, MO 63043

*To ensure uninterrupted delivery of your subscription, please notify us at least 4 weeks in advance of move.

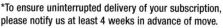

Printed and bound by CPI Group (UK) Ltd, Croydon, CR0 4YY

Printed and bound by CPI Group (UK) Ltd, Croydon, CR0 4YY

03/10/2024

01040346-0001